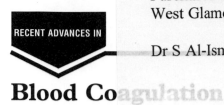

Blood Coagulation

Edited by

L. Poller DSc, MD, FRCPath
Honorary Professor, University of Manchester, UK; Project Leader, European Concerted Action on Anticoagulation

C. A. Ludlam BSc, MB, ChB, PhD, FRCP, FRCPath
Consultant Haematologist and Director, Haemophilia and Haemostasis Centre, The Royal Infirmary of Edinburgh NHS Trust, Edinburgh; Part-time Senior Lecturer, University of Edinburgh, UK

NUMBER SEVEN

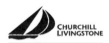

CHURCHILL LIVINGSTONE
NEW YORK EDINBURGH LONDON MADRID MELBOURNE AND TOKYO

CHURCHILL LIVINGSTONE
Medical Division of Pearson Professional Ltd

Distributed in the United States of America by Churchill
Livingstone Inc., 650 Avenue of the Americas, New York,
N.Y. 10011, and by associated companies, branches and
representatives throughout the world.

First published 1997

ISBN 0 443 05316 2

ISSN 0143-6740

British Library Cataloguing in Publication Data
A catalogue record for this book is available from the British
Library

Library of Congress Cataloging in Publication Data
is available

Note

Medical knowledge is constantly changing. As new information
becomes available, changes in treatment, procedures, equipment
and the use of drugs become necessary. The editors, contributors
and the publishers have, as far as it is possible, taken care to ensure
that the information given in this text is accurate and up to date.
However, readers are strongly advised to confirm that the information,
especially with regard to drug usage, complies with latest legislation
and standards of practice.

The
publisher's
policy is to use
paper manufactured
from sustainable forests

Produced by Longman Singapore Publishers Pte Ltd
Printed in Singapore

RECENT ADVANCES IN

Blood Coagulation

Contents

1. Regulation of coagulation by tissue factor pathway inhibitor   1
    D. Gailani, G. J. Broze

2. Developments in antiphospholipid-protein antibodies   19
    D. A. Triplett

3. The relationships of platelets to arterial thrombosis and
    atherosclerosis   33
    F. A. Ofosu

4. Inherited resistance to activated protein C as a pathogenic
    risk factor for venous thrombosis   49
    B. Zöller, B. Dahlbäck

5. Haemostatic risk factors for arterial and venous thrombosis   69
    G. D. O. Lowe

6. Thromboembolism in pregnancy and its prevention   97
    J. G. Ray, J. S. Ginsberg

7. Plasma factor VIIa   111
    J. H. Morrissey

8. Lipids and coagulation   125
    G. J. Miller

9. Changing indications for warfarin therapy   141
    C. Kearon, J. Hirsh

10. Progress in clinical fibrinolysis   161
    E. J. P. Brommer, J. J. Emeis, J. H. Verheijen, P. Brakman

11. New antithrombotic agents   183
    H. ten Cate, J. W. ten Cate

12. von Willebrand disease and its diagnosis   201
    D. J. Bowen, K. K. Hampton

13. Treatment of von Willebrand disease   221
    P. M. Mannucci, A. B. Federici

14. Treatment of haemophilia   235
   C. A. Ludlam

15. Gene therapy for haemophilia   261
   N. Salooja, E. G. D. Tuddenham

Index   277

Preface

The first edition of this series, which appeared in 1969, commented on the elaboration of investigational methods in the 15 years which had elapsed since Biggs and Macfarlane in the first edition of *Human Blood Coagulation* stated that all that was needed for blood coagulation investigations was a few glass tubes, a water bath, a supply of blood and ingenuity. The multi-disciplinary approach and the extent of the expansion of knowledge of coagulation and haemostasis is well exemplified in the present volume by the range of interests and experience of the respective contributors.

The continued success of the serial editions of this volume of Recent Advances owes much to the endeavours and enthusiasm of the contributors. We trust that the present volume will be equally useful in presenting updates of the state of the art in a selection of relevant topics. Research and development in this field has resulted in an exponential growth in recent years of the volume of published papers and reports in an ever increasing number of dedicated specialist journals. We believe that the character of *Recent Advances in Blood Coagulation* has been retained through the selection of reviews of the most important topics in the field by distinguished contributors.

The appointment of Dr Christopher Ludlam as an additional editor for this issue has proved a most welcome and opportune development. He has provided a more complete spectrum of expertise in view of the increasing diversity of haemostatic and thrombotic investigations.

Thanks are due to the publishers for their skill in typesetting and book production which has considerably lightened the task of the two editors.

Manchester   Leon Poller
Edinburgh   Christopher A Ludlam
1996

Contributors

Derek J. Bowen BSc PhD
Lecturer in Molecular Haematology, Department of Haematology,
University of Wales College of Medicine, Cardiff, UK

Pieter Brakman MD PhD
Professor of Medicine, Leiden University and Gaubius Laboratory,
TNO PG, Leiden, The Netherlands

E. J. P. Brommer MD PhD
Gaubius Laboratory, TNO PG, Division of Vascular and Connective
Tissue Research, Leiden, The Netherlands

George J. Broze Jr MD
Professor of Medicine, Haematology Research, The Jewish Hospital of
St Louis, Washington University Medical Center, St Louis, Missouri, USA

Björn Dahlbäck MD PhD
Professor of Blood Coagulation Research, Department of Clinical
Chemistry, University of Lund, University Hospital Malmö, Malmö,
Sweden

J. J. Emeis PhD
Gaubius Laboratory, TNO PG, Division of Vascular and Connective
Tissue Research, Leiden, The Netherlands

Augusto B. Federici MD
Associate Clinical Professor, A Bianchi Bonomi, Hemophilia &
Thrombosis Centre, University of Milan, Milan, Italy

David Gailani MD
Instructor in Medicine, Haematology Research, The Jewish Hospital of
St Louis, Washington University Medical Center, St Louis, Missouri,
USA

Jeffrey S. Ginsberg MD FRCPC
Director, Thromboembolism Unit, Chedoke-McMaster Hospitals,
Hamilton, Ontario, Canada

K. K. Hampton BSc MB ChB MD
Department of Haematology, University of Wales College of Medicine, Cardiff, UK

Jack Hirsh MD FRCP(C)
Director, Hamilton Civic Hospitals Research Center, Henderson General Division, Hamilton, Ontario, Canada

Clive Kearon MB MRCP(Irl) FRCP(C) PhD
Assistant Professor of Medicine, McMaster University, Henderson General Hospital, Hamilton, Ontario, Canada

Gordon D. O. Lowe
Department of Medicine, Royal Infirmary, Glasgow, UK

Christopher A. Ludlam BSc MB ChB PhD FRCP FRCPath
Consultant Haematologist and Director, Haemophilia and Haemostasis Centre, Royal Infirmary NHS Trust, Edinburgh, and Part-time Senior Lecturer, University of Edinburgh, Edinburgh, UK

Pier Mannuccio Mannucci MD
Professor of Medicine, A Bianchi Bonomi, Hemophilia & Thrombosis Centre, University of Milan, Milan, Italy

George J. Miller MD FRCP
Senior Clinical Scientist, MRC Epidemiology & Medical Care Unit, Wolfson Institute of Preventive Medicine, St Bartholomew's Hospital, London, UK

James H. Morrissey PhD
Associate Member, Cardiovascular Biology Research, Oklahoma Medical Research Foundation, Oklahoma City, Oklahoma, USA

Frederick A. Ofosu PhD
Professor of Pathology, McMaster University & Senior Scientist, Canadian Red Cross Society, Blood Services, Department of Pathology, McMaster University, Hamilton, Ontario, Canada

Leon Poller DSc MD FRCPath
Department of Pathological Sciences, the University of Manchester, Manchester, UK

Joe G. Ray
Thromboembolism Unit, Chedoke-McMaster Hospitals, Hamilton, Ontario, Canada

Nina Salooja BA MB BS MRCP DipRCPath
Clinical Scientist, Honorary Senior Registrar, Haemostasis Research Group, MRC Clinical Sciences Centre, Royal Postgraduate Medical School Hammersmith Hospital, London, UK

Hugo ten Cate MD
Internist, Centre for Haemostasis, Thrombosis, Atherosclerosis and
Inflammation Research, Academic Medical Center, Amsterdam,
The Netherlands

Jan W. ten Cate MD
Professor, Centre for Haemostasis, Thrombosis, Atherosclerosis and
Inflammation Research, Academic Medical Center, Amsterdam,
The Netherlands

Douglas A. Triplett MD FACP FCAP
Professor of Pathology and Assistant Dean, Indiana University School
of Medicine and Director of Hematology, Ball Memorial Hospital
Laboratory, Muncie, Indiana, USA

Edward G. D. Tuddenham MB BS MD FRCP FRCPath
MRC Clinical Scientific Staff, Professor of Haemostasis, Royal
Postgraduate Medical School and Honorary Consultant Haematologist,
Hammersmith Hospital, London, UK

J. H. Verheijen PhD
Gaubius Laboratory, TNO PG, Division of Vascular and Connective
Tissue Research, Leiden, The Netherlands

Bengt Zöller MD
Consultant Clinical Chemist, Department of Clinical Chemistry,
University of Lund, University Hospital Malmö, Malmö, Sweden

1. Regulation of coagulation by tissue factor pathway inhibitor

D. Gailani   G. J. Broze

The formation of a fibrin clot at a site of blood vessel injury is a critical process for the maintenance of vascular integrity. The mechanism by which soluble fibrinogen is converted to insoluble fibrin involves a series of complex and tightly regulated interactions between plasma serine proteases and their cofactors. This process results in the generation of the enzyme thrombin which converts fibrinogen to fibrin by limited proteolysis. Significant progress has been made over the last four decades in understanding the enzymatic reactions that are involved in the hemostatic process. A detailed knowledge of these events is critical as we attempt to decipher the roles of these reactions in normal coagulation and thromboembolic disease.

The classic theory of coagulation, as expounded by Schmidt and Morawitz early in this century, recognized four factors that are necessary for clot formation (Ratnoff 1991). Fibrinogen, prothrombin, and calcium ions are components of the plasma. The fourth component, tissue thromboplastin (now called tissue factor), was sequestered from the plasma in tissues. At the site of a wound, the exposure of plasma to tissue thromboplastin, which is 'extrinsic' to the blood, causes the activation of prothrombin to thrombin and subsequently the conversion of fibrinogen to fibrin. It was also recognized at this time that blood would clot when placed in a container. This process was apparently tissue thromboplastin independent, involving only factors 'intrinsic' to the blood. Early observers of intrinsic coagulation noted, however, that the nature of the container the blood was placed in affected the rate of clotting. This suggested that the container was directly participating in the coagulation process. Tissue thromboplastin (extrinsic) mediated activation of prothrombin was considered the more important mechanism for initiating coagulation for the first half of this century. The characterization of the clotting defects in plasma from patients with the severe hemorrhagic disease hemophilia (deficiency of either factor VIII or factor IX), however, made this position unsupportable. Tissue thromboplastin mediated coagulation, as measured by the prothrombin time assay, is normal in hemophiliacs, while intrinsic clotting is grossly abnormal. Based on these observations, emphasis shifted to the processes mediating intrinsic clotting as the primary mechanism for the initiation of hemostasis.

1

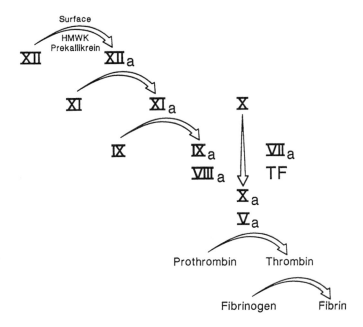

Fig. 1.1   The cascade or waterfall hypothesis of blood coagulation. The requirement for calcium and phospholipid in certain reactions is not shown. The small letter 'a' indicates the activated form of the protein. HMWK, high molecular weight kininogen; TF, tissue factor.

In 1964, Macfarlane (1964) and Davie & Ratnoff (1964) proposed the cascade and waterfall hypotheses of hemostasis (Fig. 1.1). In these schemes, coagulation proceeds through a series of sequential activations of the zymogens of plasma serine proteases culminating in the generation of thrombin which then cleaves fibrinogen to form the fibrin clot. This model separates the coagulation mechanism into an extrinsic pathway and an intrinsic pathway which converge at the activation of factor X. In the extrinsic pathway, we see the remnants of the classic theory of hemostasis. Factor VII from plasma, in the presence of its cofactor tissue factor (tissue thromboplastin) directly activates factor X. The intrinsic pathway is initiated with the activation of factor XII when blood comes into contact with a negatively charged surface, such as the wall of a glass tube. This process is referred to as contact activation. Normal contact activation requires two additional plasma components – the serine protease prekallikrein and the non-enzymatic cofactor high molecular weight kininogen. Activated factor XII activates factor XI, which in turn activates factor IX. Activated factor IX in the presence of factor VIII, then activates factor X.

   The waterfall model appears to accurately describe the major protease–substrate interactions which occur when plasma clots in vitro. Assays based on this hypothesis (the prothrombin time (PT) for the extrinsic pathway and the activated partial thromboplastin time for the intrinsic pathway) have proven enormously useful in clinical settings for diagnosing hemostatic abnormalities and for monitoring patients receiving anticoagulation therapy. It is clear, however, that the model is not an accurate representation of coagulation in vivo. Coagulation through the intrinsic pathway would appear to be important because factors VIII and IX (the proteins deficient in hemophilia A and B, respectively) are essential components of this pathway. It seems reasonable that, if the only mechanism for factor IX activation lies through the intrinsic pathway, then severe deficiencies of the proteases required for this activation (factor XII and factor XI) would result in a clinical picture similar to hemophilia. This, in fact, is not what is observed. Congenital deficiency of factor XI results in a relatively mild bleeding diathesis compared to hemophilia, while deficiencies of the contact activation factors (factor XII, prekallikrein and high molecular weight kininogen) do not predispose to bleeding. Similarly, while factor XII deficiency is not associated with excessive bleeding, a lack of factor VII (essential for extrinsic pathway initiated coagulation) may confer a hemorrhagic diathesis which is similar to hemophilia. These observations strongly indicated that coagulation is initiated predominantly through the extrinsic pathway and implied that mechanisms other than the intrinsic pathway exist for factor IX activation.

The standard PT assay is performed by adding saturating concentrations of tissue factor (concentrations in excess of the factor VII plasma concentration) to plasma to induce clotting. The tissue factor (TF) that blood would be exposed to in vivo is likely to be far more dilute. Experiments performed by Biggs & Macfarlane (1951) demonstrated that thrombin production was substantially decreased in hemophiliac plasma induced to clot with dilute tissue preparations compared to similarly treated normal plasma. This clearly showed that components of the intrinsic pathway were involved in TF mediated coagulation and implied that the intrinsic and extrinsic pathways did not function independently of each other. Osterud & Rapaport (1977) provided further support for this concept when they determined that factor VIIa–TF activated factor IX in addition to activating factor X. The new interpretation of hemostasis based solely on activation through the extrinsic pathway raised an important question. Factor VIIa–TF is a potent activator of factor X and appears to be capable of completely bypassing the intrinsic pathway to form a fibrin clot. If the factor VIIa–TF complex is the primary initiator of hemostasis, why then do hemophiliacs bleed? The recent isolation and characterization of a novel endogenous inhibitor of TF mediated coagulation offers an explanation to this conundrum (Broze et al 1988, 1990). Based on the properties of this inhibitor – tissue factor pathway inhibitor (TFPI) – a revised coagulation scheme has been proposed in which factor VII–TF initiates coagulation but factor IX and VIII are absolutely required for sustaining hemostasis.

THE FACTOR VIIa–TF PATHWAY OF COAGULATION

TF is a 45 000 Da single chain integral membrane protein which is a member of the interferon/cytokine superfamily of membrane receptors (Broze et al 1985). The protein is not normally expressed by cell types in contact with blood, such as vascular endothelial cells or peripheral blood leukocytes (Drake et al 1989, Wilcox et al 1989). Instead, TF is expressed constitutively by fibroblasts and pericytes which underlie the blood vessel endothelium (Wilcox et al 1989). These cells are normally separated from blood but are ideally located to interact with blood components if the endothelium is interrupted. TF is also found on keratinocytes in the epidermis of the skin, on fibroblasts in the capsules of organs, and on epithelial cells of the gastrointestinal and respiratory tracts. High levels of expression are seen in the brain, cardiac myocytes and renal glomeruli. Based on the observed distribution, it has been proposed that TF provides a 'hemostatic envelope' for blood vessels and organs, including the skin (Drake et al 1989). While blood vessel endothelium and monocytes, which are normally in contact with blood, do not constitutively express TF, they may be induced to express the protein by a number of stimuli such as bacterial endotoxin or interleukin-1 (Lerner et al 1971, Bevilaqua et al 1984). Monocytes have been shown to express TF in vivo in certain clinical situations such as meningococcemia and bacterial peritonitis (Osterud & Flaegstaqd 1983, Almdahl et al 1987). The foam cells found in atherosclerotic plaques, which are of monocytic origin, also express TF (Wilcox et al 1989). These findings indicate that TF may be involved in some pathological conditions associated with abnormal coagulation or thrombosis.

Factor VII is a 50 000 Da glycoprotein which circulates in plasma at a concentration of approximately 10 nM (Broze & Majerus 1982). It appears to be synthesized primarily by the liver and requires vitamin K dependent γ-carboxylation of ten glutamic acid residues at the amino-terminus for proper function. Zymogen factor VII is converted to activated factor VII (factor VIIa) by a single proteolytic cleavage between amino acids Arg152 and Ile153, resulting in a two chain disulfide linked molecule. Factors Xa, IXa, XIIa, VIIa and thrombin have all been shown to activate factor VII in vitro (Broze & Majerus 1982, Pedersen et al 1989). Coagulation is thought to be initiated when factor VII or VIIa in plasma comes into contact with TF at the site of a wound. Both the zymogen and active protein bind to TF with equal avidity in the presence of calcium ions (Ca^{2+}) (Broze 1982, Zur et al 1982). The binding of factor VII or VIIa to TF markedly alters procoagulant reactions involving these molecules. In contrast to factor VII in solution, factor VII bound to TF is rapidly activated by trace amounts of factor Xa present in plasma (Nemerson & Repke 1985, Rao & Rapaport 1989). Several hypotheses have been proposed to explain how this small amount of factor Xa is initially generated. It was suggested that zymogen factor VII has intrinsic catalytic activity (Radcliffe & Nemerson 1975). However, a recombinant factor VII in which Arg152 was changed to glutamic acid to abolish the cleavage site for factor VII activation failed to demonstrate proteolytic activity towards factor X (Wildegoose et al 1990). It seems more likely that small amounts of factor Xa are constantly being produced by factor VIIa–TF. Indeed, approximately 0.5% of plasma factor VII circulates as factor VIIa and would, therefore, be available to activate factor X (Wildegoose et al 1992).

When factor VIIa is bound to TF it hydrolyzes small synthetic substrates more rapidly (Ruf et al 1991). This effect is due mostly to an increase in the catalytic constant (k_{cat}) for the reaction and likely represents a change in factor VIIa conformation. The enzymatic activity of factor VIIa towards its plasma substrates, factors X and IX, is increased over 100-fold in the presence of TF (Bach et al 1981, Broze et al 1985). Most, but not all, investigators have found that factor X is preferred over factor IX as a substrate (Komiyama et al 1990). Most active coagulation serine proteases, when free in plasma, are rapidly inactivated by plasma serine protease inhibitors. Factor VIIa, in contrast, is quite stable with a plasma half-life almost as long as that of zymogen factor VII (Wildegoose et al 1992). Plasma inhibitors such as antithrombin III are poor inhibitors of unbound factor VIIa, even in the presence of heparin. Instead, the physiologic regulator of TF initiated coagulation, TFPI, appears to target the factor VIIa–TF complex.

HISTORY OF THE TF PATHWAY INHIBITOR

The first demonstrations of an inhibitor of tissue thromboplastin induced coagulation in plasma were reported by Thomas (1947) and Schneider (1947). These investigators noted that the lethal effect of intravenous infusions of crude tissue preparations (containing TF) into mice could be abrogated if the tissue was first incubated with serum. The inhibitory activity required Ca^{2+} and appeared to bind directly to the thromboplastin. Hjort (1954) demonstrated that the inhibitor, which he called 'anticonvertin' recognized the factor VII–Ca^{2+}–TF complex. Two decades later Marciniak & Tsukamura (1972) identified an inhibitory activity associated with low density lipoproteins (LDL) which was directed at factor Xa. Barrowcliffe et al (1982) confirmed this finding, noting that the inhibitor was present in LDL > high density lipoprotein (HDL), >> very low density lipoprotein (VLDL), and that the plasma concentration of the inhibitor appeared to increase after infusion of a heparin analog in vivo. Carson (1981) reported that plasma lipoproteins also inhibited the factor VIIa–TF complex and that the inhibitory activity was contained in the protein portion of the lipoprotein.

Following a different line of investigation, Marlar et al (1982) found that the activation of factor X in plasma induced to clot with dilute preparations of TF was greatly reduced in hemophilic plasma compared to normal plasma. This was consistent with the studies mentioned earlier, demonstrating delayed thrombin formation in hemophilic plasma under similar conditions (Biggs & Macfarlane 1951). Subsequently, Morrison & Jesty (1984) determined that the activation of factors X and IX in normal plasma induced to clot with TF was incomplete and that the apparent inhibition of factor VIIa–TF requires the presence of factor X or a brief pretreatment of the plasma with factor Xa. Studies by Sanders et al (1985) provided a link between these observations and the work documenting inhibitory activity in lipoproteins when they demonstrated that both factor X and an inhibitor in the lipoprotein fraction of plasma were required for factor VIIa–TF inhibition. Several groups confirmed these findings and subsequently demonstrated that the properties of the lipoprotein associated inhibitor were identical to those reported earlier by Hjort for anticonvertin (Hubbard & Jennings 1986, Broze & Miletich 1987a, Rao & Rapaport 1987). In 1991, a subcommittee of the International Society for Thrombosis and Haemostasis agreed to refer to the inhibitor as TFPI.

TFPI STRUCTURE

TFPI was first purified from the serum-free conditioned media of human HepG2 hepatoma cells and the amino acid sequence of the molecule was determined from cDNA sequences obtained from placental and fetal liver libraries (Fig. 1.2) (Broze & Miletich 1987b, Wun et al 1988). The mature molecule contains 276 amino acids (estimated size, 32 000 Da) and consists of an acidic amino-terminal region, three tandem Kunitz-type protease inhibitory domains, and a basic carboxy-terminal region. The identification of multiple protease inhibitory domains within TFPI is consistent with its inhibition of both factor Xa and factor VIIa–TF. Cells which produce TFPI contain TFPI mRNAs of 4.0 and 1.4 kilobases(kb) in length, which are produced through the use of alternate termination and polyadenylation signals (Girard et al 1989a).

Kunitz-type protease inhibitors are members of a superfamily of proteins with homology to bovine pancreatic trypsin inhibitor (BPTI, also referred to as aprotinin or Trasylol). The disulfide bond structure of the Kunitz inhibitory domain is highly conserved among members of the family, and the amino acid residues at the P1 positions (which define the active site cleft) are critical for the inhibitors' substrate specificity. Based on the structure of BPTI, the disulfide bonds and active site clefts for the three Kunitz domains of TFPI were determined (Fig. 1.2) (Wun et al 1988). The Kunitz-type protease inhibitors appear to work by the standard mechanism in which the inhibitor interacts with the target enzyme as a potential substrate. After binding to the enzyme, however, the cleavage between the P1 and P1' amino acids at the inhibitors' active site cleft occurs very slowly or not at all. Kunitz-type inhibitors display slow, tight-binding interactions with their targets

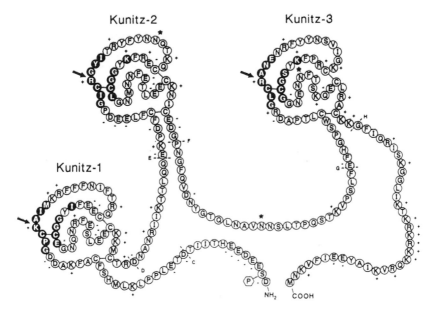

Fig. 1.2 Amino acid sequence and proposed tertiary structure for the tissue factor pathway inhibitor (TFPI). The three Kunitz-type protease inhibitory domains are labeled, and the arrows indicate their respective active site inhibitory clefts (P1 to P1′).

which are competitive and reversible. The term 'slow' indicates that inhibition is not immediate, while 'tight-binding' means that inhibitor has significant effects at concentrations near those of the target enzyme.

Site directed mutagenesis studies in which the P1 residues of the Kunitz domains of TFPI were individually changed indicate that the second Kunitz domain is involved with binding to and inhibition of factor Xa (Girard et al 1989b). The first Kunitz domain mediates the binding of the inhibitor to factor VIIa–TF; however, this inhibition also requires an intact second Kunitz domain to bind factor Xa (Girard et al 1989b). These findings are consistent with the early data indicating that inhibition of factor VIIa–TF by TFPI is dependent on factor X. An inhibitory function for the third Kunitz domain has not been identified; however, recent work by Wesselschmidt et al (1993) indicates that this region of the molecule may be involved in binding to heparin.

INHIBITORY PROPERTIES OF TFPI

TFPI directly inhibits factor Xa by binding to or near the active site serine of the enzyme (Broze et al 1988). The stoichiometry of the binding is 1:1 and does not require calcium. In fact, in recent work using a purified protein system, Ca^{2+} interfered with the interaction between factor Xa and TFPI (Huang et al 1993). While the studies mentioned above using mutant recombinant TFPI molecules indicate that the second Kunitz domain is required for factor Xa inactivation, it is now clear that other portions of the TFPI molecule are required for optimal factor Xa inhibition. A major portion of TFPI in plasma is made up of carboxyl-truncated forms which possess considerably less factor Xa inhibitory activity than full-length TFPI (Wesselschmidt et al 1992). Similarly, TFPI cleaved between the first and second Kunitz domains by leukocyte elastase shows dramatically reduced activity in a factor Xa inhibition assay (Higuchi et al 1992). These findings indicate that the positively charged carboxy-terminal region as well as portions of the molecule N-terminal to the second Kunitz domain are required for optimal interaction with factor Xa.

While factor Xa in solution is rapidly inhibited by plasma serine protease inhibitors (serpins) such as antithrombin III, it is protected from inhibition by these serpins when it is associated with the prothrombinase complex (factor Xa, phospholipid, Ca^{2+} and factor Va). In contrast, recent work indicates that, in the presence of calcium, TFPI is a more effective inhibitor of factor Xa when Xa is associated with phospholipid and factor Va (Huang et al 1993). This effect is primarily due to a decrease in the K_i for the initial factor Xa–TFPI complex, consistent with the notion that the interaction between factor Xa and TFPI involves considerably more than the second Kunitz domain. TFPI inhibition of factor Xa activity is largely responsible for the prolongation of clotting times in one-stage coagulation assays in which exogenous TFPI is added to plasma. Heparin will enhance factor Xa inhibition by TFPI at least in part by serving as a template to which factor Xa and TFPI simultaneously bind (Wesselschmidt et al 1993). The carboxy-terminal portion of TFPI is required for optimal inhibition of the prothrombinase complex as well as binding to heparin.

Inhibition of factor VIIa–TF by TFPI, at physiologic levels of the inhibitor, is factor Xa and calcium dependent and probably involves the formation of a quaternary factor Xa–TFPI–factor VIIa–TF complex (Fig. 1.3) (Broze et al 1988). Two separate mechanisms could account for the formation of such a complex. TFPI may first bind to factor Xa, via the second Kunitz domain, with subsequent binding to factor VIIa–TF. Alternatively, TFPI may bind to a tertiary complex of factor Xa–factor VIIa–TF. The quaternary complex model explains the requirement for factor Xa in TFPI mediated inhibition of factor VIIa–TF as well as the observation that active site inactivated factor Xa (which does not bind TFPI) is ineffective in mediating this inhibition (Broze & Miletich 1987a). Along similar lines, factor Xa which lacks the calcium binding amino-terminal γ-carboxyglutamic acid domain will bind to and be inhibited by TFPI, but fails to support TFPI inhibition of factor VIIa–TF (Broze et al 1988). This finding is consistent with the observation of Hjort in 1957, that the binding of 'anticonvertin' (TFPI) to factor VIIa–TF is calcium dependent.

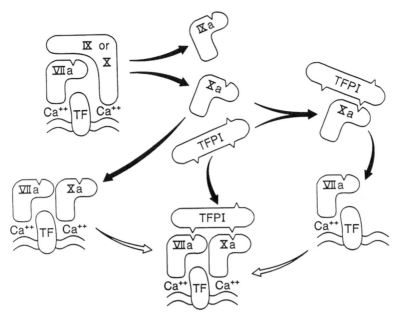

Fig. 1.3 Proposed mechanism for the formation of a quaternary complex involving membrane-bound tissue factor (TF), factor VIIa, factor Xa, and the tissue factor pathway inhibitor (TFPI). Circulating factor Xa may combine with TFPI followed by binding to the factor VIIa–TF complex. Alternatively, factor Xa may remain associated with the factor VIIa–TF complex after its activation, and be inhibited when circulating TFPI joins the complex.

TFPI PHYSIOLOGY

Three sources of TFPI have been identified in vivo: plasma (Novotny et al 1989), platelets (Novotny et al 1988), and a heparin releasable form probably from the vascular endothelium (Sandset et al 1988, Novotny et al 1991). TFPI in plasma is bound to lipoproteins: LDL (50–60% of lipoprotein associated TFPI), HDL (26–44%), and VLDL (<10%) (Hubbard & Jennings 1987, Novotny et al 1989). In addition, some unbound full-length TFPI is also present in plasma; however, it is not clear what fraction of total plasma TFPI this represents. The predominant form of TFPI associated with LDL is 34 000 Da in size, while HDL are associated with a 41 000 Da species (Novotny et al 1989, Broze et al 1990, 1994). The variation in size may be due to mixed disulfide linked complexes with apolipoprotein AII. VLDL appear to contain both the 34 kDa and 41 kDa forms. In addition, small amounts of higher molecular weight species are found, probably representing TFPI linked by disulfide bonds to other proteins. Under reducing conditions plasma TFPI is 36 kDa while recombinant TFPI is 43 kDa in size. While part of this difference may be attributed to different degrees of glycosylation, the majority of lipoprotein associated TFPI is truncated at the carboxy-terminus (Broze et al 1994). The physiologic significance of the truncation is not clear, although in vitro studies have clearly demonstrated that TFPI lacking the carboxy-terminus is a poorer inhibitor of factor Xa than is the full-length form (Wesselschmidt et al 1992).

TFPI is also carried in blood by platelets, and is released upon thrombin stimulation (Novotny et al 1988). TFPI mRNA has been detected in preparations of RNA from platelets and a megakaryocytic cell line indicating that the protein is made in megakaryocytes (Novotny et al 1988). The subcellular storage location of TFPI in platelets has not been clearly determined. Although platelets account for only 10% of TFPI in blood, the release of TFPI from aggregated platelets at the site of a wound may have a substantial effect on local TFPI concentrations. In fact, the concentration of TFPI in blood issuing from a superficial wound (template bleeding time) may reach levels 2–3 times that of peripheral blood (Novotny et al 1988). It is not clear if this increase is due exclusively to release of platelet associated TFPI or if other sources are contributing.

TFPI levels in plasma increase at least 2-fold after infusion of heparin (Sandset et al 1988, Novotny et al 1991). Since ex vivo addition of heparin to blood or plasma does not alter TFPI levels, it appears that the increase is due to release from a cellular store. Currently, it is thought that the vascular endothelium is the source of heparin releasable TFPI. The protein may be associated with heparan sulfate or other glycosaminoglycans on the cell surface. Heparin releasable TFPI is primarily the 43 kDa full-length form of the protein.

While TFPI is synthesized by a number of cultured cell lines from a variety of tissues (Broze & Miletich 1987b, Bajaj et al 1990), the cell type responsible for production of plasma TFPI in vivo is uncertain. Indeed, mRNA for TFPI may be detected on Northern blots of polyA selected RNA from most tissues (Fig. 1.4; Stanton & Broze unpublished observation). Vascular endothelial cells would seem to be a reasonable candidate for a source for TFPI. Bajaj et al (1990) have demonstrated TFPI mRNA in, and release of TFPI protein from, human umbilical endothelial cells in culture. There is conflicting data concerning hepatic production of TFPI. Several liver cell lines will express TFPI; however, polyA RNA from normal human liver and primary hepatocyte cultures has been reported not to contain detectable TFPI mRNA (Broze & Miletich 1987b, Bajaj et al 1990). In contrast, we have detected TFPI message in RNA prepared from whole liver (Fig. 1.4), although the cell type responsible for this result has not been determined. Interestingly, TFPI message is not detected in brain (Fig. 1.4). The mean plasma level of TFPI in normal adults is approximately 100 ng/ml (2.5 nmol/l) with a broad distribution from 60%–160% of the mean (Novotny et al 1991). While modest changes in TFPI levels have been reported in a number of clinical situations, it is not clear if these changes have physiologic significance. The 2-fold increase in TFPI in plasma after heparin infusion indicates that plasma TFPI is only a fraction of the total TFPI available. Endothelial cell associated TFPI, located at the interface between blood and blood vessel, may make a substantial contribution to TFPI action in vivo, but would not be measured by conventional plasma assays. Indeed, patients with hereditary abetalipoproteinemia lacking LDL have extremely low plasma levels of TFPI, but have an increase in plasma TFPI in response to heparin infusion that is similar to normal individuals (Novotny et al 1991). Furthermore, these patients do not have an increased risk of thrombosis. This finding may indicate that the TFPI normally circulating in plasma is not the most important source of this protein. Pharmacokinetic studies of recombinant TFPI infused into rabbits demonstrate a biphasic clearance of the protein, with half-lives of 2.3 and 79 min (Palmier et al 1992). The liver and kidney (primarily the outer cortex) both appear to be involved in clearance. Recently, Warshawsky et al (1994) have provided evidence that the LDL receptor related protein α_2-macroglobulin receptor (LRP) mediates the internalization and degradation of TFPI by hepatoma cells in culture. LRP is a cell membrane associated surface glycoprotein which functions as a hepatic receptor for a number of plasma proteins. LRP does not appear to be the primary binding site for TFPI, but is required for its degradation. TFPI apparently initially binds to another cell surface component which then presents the protein to LRP; however, the nature of this binding site has yet to be elucidated.

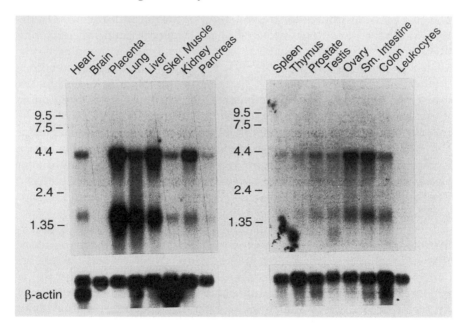

Fig. 1.4 Northern blot of mRNA from human tissues hybridized with a human TFPI cDNA probe. Northern blots of polyA enriched RNA were purchased from Clontech Laboratories (Palo Alto, CA). Hybridization with a full-length human TFPI cDNA probe was carried out as recommended by the manufacturer. A control hybridization with a β-actin probe confirms equal RNA loading in each lane. Molecular standards at the left-hand side of each blot are in kilobases.

TFPI AND THE REVISED HYPOTHESIS OF COAGULATION

The properties of TFPI indicate that it inhibits factor VIIa–TF in vivo by a novel feedback mechanism. Coagulation is probably initiated when factor VII or VIIa in blood gains access to TF at the site of a blood vessel wound. The resulting factor VIIa–TF complex would then activate some factor X to Xa and factor IX to IXa. With the initial generation of factor Xa, however, the inhibitory properties of TFPI become manifest, and inactivate factor VIIa–TF. Any additional factor Xa required for hemostasis must then be provided through the activity of factor IXa in the presence of its cofactor, factor VIII. Additional factor IXa may be produced through the activity of activated factor XI (factor XIa) as discussed below. A revised model of coagulation incorporating TFPI is shown in Figure 1.5. The revised hypothesis based on the factor Xa dependent inhibition of factor VIIa–TF by TFPI explains the need for intact extrinsic (factor VII) as well as intrinsic (factor IX and XI) pathways for proper clot formation. The aforementioned studies demonstrating decreased thrombin and factor Xa production in hemophiliac plasma induced to clot with diluted TF are consistent with this view.

The inhibitory properties of TFPI suggest an alternative interpretation of the bleeding diathesis seen in hemophilia. The waterfall model of hemostasis indicates that hemophiliacs bleed excessively because of a defect in a pathway critical for the initiation of fibrin clot formation. In the revised model, in contrast, the abnormal bleeding is due to the lack of a mechanism for sustaining coagulation, after the initiation complex, factor VIIa–TF, is inhibited by TFPI. It also predicts that the coagulation abnormalities in vitro and the excessive bleeding in vivo might be reduced if the inhibitory activity of TFPI were blocked. Recently, in assays using dilute TF, it has been demonstrated that addition of anti-TFPI IgG shortens the prolonged coagulation time of hemophiliac plasma to that of normal plasma (Nordfang et al 1991). Also, using in vivo studies involving rabbits which were made transiently deficient in factor IX by the infusion of anti-factor IX IgG, the markedly prolonged bleeding observed in a cuticle bleeding time assay was significantly shortened by the intravenous infusion of anti-TFPI antibody (Erhardtsen et al 1993).

Individuals deficient in coagulation factor XI may have a variable bleeding diathesis, indicating that this protein is required for normal hemostasis. Any revision in the coagulation scheme must, therefore, account for the contribution this molecule makes to hemostasis and explain how it would become activated in the absence of contact activation (activation mediated by factor XIIa). Observations of the bleeding tendencies of individuals deficient in factor XI have provided some information in this regard. Unlike patients with severe hemophilia A or hemophilia B, persons lacking factor XI rarely experience spontaneous hemorrhage. More commonly, bleeding follows surgery or trauma and is particularly severe when involving tissues which have high intrinsic fibrinolytic activity such as the oral cavity or urinary tract. Given these findings, factor XI appears to be required for particularly severe hemostatic challenges or in situations where processes opposing hemostasis (e.g. fibrinolysis) are active. Certainly, the bleeding pattern does not suggest that factor XI is critical for the initiation of hemostasis under most circumstances, as it would be if the classic intrinsic pathway were a major physiologic mechanism. In plasma, factor XIa is a potent activator of factor IX in the presence of Ca^{2+}. The kinetic parameters for the reaction are similar to those for factor IX activation by the factor VIIa–TF complex. During severe hemostatic challenges, therefore, the factor IX activated initially by the factor VIIa–TF complex may be insufficient for proper clot formation and supplemental factor IXa provided through the activity of factor XIa would be required. While the revised hypothesis of hemostasis is consistent with this interpretation of the clinical data, it did not initially suggest a mechanism by which factor XI would become activated in the absence of contact activation. Naito & Fujikawa (1991) and Gailani & Broze (1991) independently demonstrated that the serine protease thrombin activates factor XI in a reaction that is enhanced by the presence of negatively charged substances such as dextran sulfate, sulfatides and heparin. Furthermore, factor XI is also activated by factor XIa in the presence of these negatively charged molecules. These reactions have subsequently been shown to occur in a factor XII deficient plasma

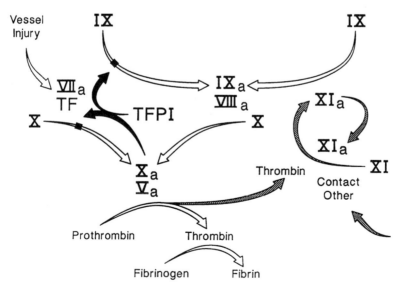

Fig. 1.5 The revised hypothesis of blood coagulation. Coagulation is initiated when factor VIIa is exposed to tissue factor (TF) at a site of blood vessel damage. Feedback inhibition of factor VIIa–TF by tissue factor pathway inhibitor (TFPI) is indicated by the black arrows and boxes. The shaded arrows indicate the proposed thrombin mediated pathway of factor XI activation. The requirement of calcium and phospholipids in certain reactions is not included.

system in which clot formation is induced withTF (Gailani & Broze 1993). The activation of factor XI by thrombin and factor XIa has been incorporated into the revised coagulation scheme (Fig. 1.5). It is important to note that the in vitro systems used to demonstrate factor XI activation by either thrombin or factor XIIa include non-physiologic negatively charged surfaces. The relevance of these reactions to in vivo hemostasis is, therefore, not clear and the physiologic conditions and cofactors required for factor XI activation and activity have yet to be determined. The revised hypothesis of coagulation differs from earlier models of hemostasis in several important respects. The cascade/waterfall hypotheses appear to accurately depict the major protease–substrate interactions which occur as blood clots in vitro. However, as we have seen, it is difficult to reconcile this model with the clinical presentation of patients deficient in various components of the intrinsic pathway. Indeed, persons lacking the proteins required for initiation of the intrinsic pathway (factor XII, prekallikrein and high molecular weight kininogen) do not have excessive bleeding. The revised model, on the other hand, incorporates only the components of the hemostatic system which appear to be important based on clinical observations. It also offers a reasonable explanation for the differences in bleeding tendencies between hemophiliacs and persons with factor XI deficiency, as well as the lack of excessive bleeding in persons missing one of the contact activation factors.

A central tenet of the revised hypothesis, in contrast to the cascade/waterfall model, is that the hemostatic process is not completed with the initial generation of factor Xa and thrombin. Instead, possibly reflecting the removal of activated coagulation factors by flowing blood, their inactivation by protease inhibitors and the competing process of fibrinolysis, the initial hemostatic response must be consolidated by the progressive generation of factor Xa and thrombin.

Available data are consistent with the concept that, in normal hemostasis, factor VIIa–TF is responsible for initial activation of factor X which provides sufficient thrombin for induction of platelet aggregation and the activation of the critical cofactors V and VIII. However, the factor Xa produced by factor VIIa–TF, dampened by TFPI, is insufficient to sustain hemostasis and must be amplified through the actions of factors IXa, VIIIa and, in certain situations, XIa, for ultimate and persistent hemostasis.

REFERENCES

Almdahl S M, Broz J H, Osterud B 1987 Mononuclear phagocyte thromboplastin and endotoxin in patients with secondary bacterial peritonitis. Scand J Gastroenterol 22: 914–918
Bach R, Nemerson Y, Konigsberg W 1981 Purification and characterization of bovine tissue factor. J Biol Chem 256: 8324–8331
Bajaj M S, Kuppuswamy M N, Saito H et al 1990 Cultured normal human hepatocytes do not synthesize lipoprotein-associated coagulation inhibitor: evidence that endothelium is the principal site of its synthesis. Proc Natl Acad Sci USA 87: 8869–8873

Barrowcliffe T W, Eggleton C A, Stocks J 1982 Studies of anti-Xa activity in human plasma II: The role of lipoproteins. Thromb Res 27: 185–195

Bevilacqua M P, Pober J S, Majean G R et al 1984 Interleukin 1 (IL-1) induces biosynthesis and cell surface expression of procoagulant activity in human vascular cells. J Exp Med 160: 618–623

Biggs R, MacFarlane R G 1951 The reaction of haemophilic plasma to thromboplastin. J Clin Pathol 4: 445–459

Broze G J Jr 1982 Binding of human factor VII and VIIa to monocytes. J Clin Invest 70: 526–535

Broze G J Jr, Majerus P W 1982 Human factor VII. Methods Enzymol 80: 228–237

Broze G J Jr, Miletich J P 1987a Characterization of the inhibition of tissue factor in serum. Blood 69: 150–155

Broze G J Jr, Miletich J P 1987b Isolation of the tissue factor inhibitor produced by HepG2 hepatoma cells. Proc Natl Acad Sci USA 84: 1886–1890

Broze G J Jr, Leykam J E, Schwartz B D et al 1985 Purification of human brain tissue factor. J Biol Chem 260: 10917–10920

Broze G J Jr, Warren L A, Novotny W F et al 1988 The lipoprotein-associated coagulation inhibitor that inhibits the factor VII-tissue factor complex also inhibits factor Xa: insight into its possible mechanism of action. Blood 71: 335–343

Broze G J, Girard T J, Novotny W F 1990 Regulation of coagulation by a multivalent Kunitz-type inhibitor. Biochemistry 29: 7539–7546

Broze G J Jr, Lange G W, Diffin K L et al 1994 Heterogeneity of plasma tissue factor pathway inhibitor. Blood Coagulat Fibrinol 5: 551–559

Carson S D 1981 Plasma high density lipoproteins inhibit the activation of coagulation factor X by factor VIIa and tissue factor. FEBS Lett 132: 37–40

Davie E W, Ratnoff O D 1964 Waterfall sequence for intrinsic blood clotting. Science 145: 1310–1312

Drake T A, Morrissey J H, Edgington T S 1989 Selective cellular expression of tissue factor in human tissues: implications for disorders of hemostasis and thrombosis. Am J Pathol 134: 1087–1097

Erhardtsen E, Madsen M T, Ezban M et al 1993 Blocking of the tissue factor pathway inhibitor (TFPI) shortens the bleeding time in rabbits with antibody induced hemophilia. Thromb Haemost 69: 556 (abstract)

Gailani D, Broze G J Jr 1991 Factor XI activation in a revised model of blood coagulation. Science 253: 909–912

Gailani D, Broze G J Jr 1993 Factor XII-independent activation of factor XI in plasma: effects of sulfatides on tissue factor-induced coagulation. Blood 82: 813–819

Girard T J, Warren L A, Novotny W F et al 1989a Identification of the 1.4 and 4.0 kb messages for the lipoprotein-associated coagulation inhibitor and expression of the encoded protein. Thromb Res 55: 37–50

Girard T J, Warren L A, Novotny W F et al 1989b Functional significance of the Kunitz-type inhibitor domains of lipoprotein-associated coagulation inhibitor. Nature 338: 518–520

Higuchi D, Wun T-C, Likert K M et al 1992 The effect of leukocyte elastase on tissue factor pathway inhibitor. Blood 79: 1712–1792

Hjort P F 1957 Intermediate reactions in the coagulation of blood with tissue thromboplastin. Scand J Clin Lab Invest 9 (suppl 27): 1–182

Huang Z-F, Wun T-C, Broze G J Jr 1993 Kinetics of factor Xa inhibition by tissue factor pathway inhibitor. J Biol Chem 268: 26950–26955

Hubbard A R, Jennings C A 1986 Inhibition of tissue thromboplastin-mediated blood coagulation. Thromb Res 42: 489–498

Hubbard A R, Jennings C A 1987 Inhibition of the tissue factor–factor VII complex: involvement of factor Xa and lipoproteins. Thromb Res 46: 527–537

Komiyama Y, Pedersen A H, Kisiel W 1990 Proteolytic activation of human factors IX and X by recombinant human factor VIIa: effects of calcium, phospholipids, and tissue factor. Biochemistry 29: 9418–9425

Lerner R G, Goldstein R, Cummings G 1971 Stimulation of human leukocyte thromboplastic activity by endotoxin. Proc Soc Exp Biol Med 138: 145–148

Macfarlane R G 1964 An enzyme cascade in the blood clotting mechanism, and its function as a biochemical amplifier. Nature 202: 498–499

Marciniak E, Tsukamura S 1972 Two progressive inhibitors of factor Xa in human blood coagulation. Br J Haematol 22: 341–351

Marlar R A, Kleiss A J, Griffin J H 1982 An alternative extrinsic pathway of human blood coagulation. Blood 60: 1353–1358

Morrison S A, Jesty J 1984 Tissue factor-dependent activation of tritium-labeled factor IX and factor X in human plasma. Blood 63: 1338–1347

Naito K, Fujikawa K 1991 Activation of human blood coagulation factor XI independent of factor XII: factor XI is activated by thrombin and factor XIa in the presence of negatively charged surfaces. J Biol Chem 266: 7353–7358

Nemerson Y, Repke D 1985 Tissue factor accelerates the activation of coagulation factor VII: the role of a bifunctional coagulation factor. Thromb Res 40: 351–358

Nordfang O, Valentin S, Bech T C, Hedner U 1991 Inhibition of extrinsic pathway inhibitor shortens the coagulation time of normal plasma and hemophilia plasma. Thromb Haemost 66: 464–467

Novotny W F, Girard T J, Miletich J P et al 1988 Platelets secrete a coagulation inhibitor functionally and antigenically similar to the lipoprotein-associated coagulation inhibitor. Blood 72: 2020–2025

Novotny W F, Girard T J, Miletich J P et al 1989 Purification and characterization of the lipoprotein-associated coagulation inhibitor from human plasma. J Biol Chem 264: 18832–18837

Novotny W F, Brown S G, Miletich J P et al 1991 Plasma antigen levels of the lipoprotein-associated coagulation inhibitor in patient samples. Blood 78: 387–393

Osterud B, Flaegstad T 1983 Increased tissue thromboplastin activity in monocytes of patients with meningococcal infection: related to unfavourable prognosis. Thromb Haemost 49: 5–7

Osterud B, Rapaport S 1977 Activation of factor IX by the reaction product of tissue factor and factor VII. Additional pathway for initiating blood coagulation. Proc Natl Acad Sci USA 74: 5260–5264

Palmier M O, Hall I J, Reisch C M et al 1992 Clearance of recombinant tissue factor pathway inhibitor (TFPI) in rabbits. Thromb Haemost 68: 33–36

Pedersen R H, Lund-Hansen T, Bisgaard-Frantzen H et al 1989 Autoactivation of human recombinant coagulation factor VII. Biochemistry 28: 9331–9336

Radcliffe R, Nemersen Y 1975 Activation and control of factor VII by activated factor X and thrombin. Isolation and characterization of a single chain form of factor VII. J Biol Chem 250: 388–395

Rao L V M, Rapaport S I 1987 Studies of a mechanism inhibiting the initiation of the extrinsic pathway of coagulation. Blood 69: 645–651

Rao L V M, Rapaport S I 1989 Activation of factor VII bound to tissue factor: a key early step in the tissue factor pathway of blood coagulation. Proc Natl Acad Sci USA 85: 6687–6691

Ratnoff O D 1991 Evolution of knowledge of hemostasis. In: Ratnoff O D, Forbes C D (eds) Disorders of hemostasis. W B Saunders, Philadelphia

Ruf W, Kalnik M W, Lund-Hansen T et al 1991 Characterization of factor VII association with tissue factor in solution. High and low affinity calcium binding sites in factor VII contribute to functionally distinct interactions. J Biol Chem 266: 15719–15725

Sanders N L, Bajaj S P, Zivelin A et al 1985 Inhibition of tissue factor/factor VIIa activity in plasma requires factor X and an additional plasma component. Blood 66: 204–212

Sandset P M, Abildgaard U, Larsen M L 1988 Heparin induces release of extrinsic coagulation pathway inhibitor (EPI). Thromb Res 50: 803–813

Schneider C L 1947 The active principle of placental toxin: thromboplastin; its inactivator in blood: antithromboplastin. Am J Physiol 149: 123–129

Thomas L 1947 Studies on the intravascular thromboplastin effect of tissue suspensions in mice: II. A factor in normal rabbit serum which inhibits the thromboplastin effect of the sedimentable tissue component. Bull Johns Hopkins Hosp 81: 26–42

Warshawsky I, Broze G J Jr, Schwartz A L 1994 The low density lipoprotein receptor-related protein mediates the cellular degradation of tissue factor pathway inhibitor. Proc Natl Acad Sci USA 91: 6664–6668

Wesselschmidt R, Likert K, Girard T et al 1992 Tissue factor pathway inhibitor: the carboxy-terminus is required for optimal inhibition of factor Xa. Blood 79: 2004–2010

Wesselschmidt R, Likert K, Huang Z et al 1993 Structural requirements for tissue factor pathway inhibitor interactions with factor Xa and heparin. Blood Coag Fibrinol 4: 661–669

Wilcox J R, Smith K M, Schwartz S M et al 1989 Localization of tissue factor in the normal vessel wall and in the atherosclerotic plaque. Proc Natl Acad Sci USA 86: 2839–2843

Wildegoose P, Berhner K, Kisiel W 1990 Synthesis, purification and characterization of an Arg^{152}-Glu^{152} site directed mutant of recombinant human blood clotting factor VII. Biochemistry 29: 3413–3420

Wildegoose R, Nemersen Y, Lyng-Hansen L et al 1992 Measurement of basal levels of factor VIIa in hemophilia A & B patients. Blood 80: 25–28

Wun T-C, Kretzmer K K, Girard T J et al 1988 Cloning and characterization of a cDNA coding for the lipoprotein-associated coagulation inhibitor shows that it consists of three tandem Kunitz-type inhibitory domains. J Biol Chem 263: 6001–6004

Zur M, Radcliffe R D, Oderdick J et al 1982 The dual role of factor VII in blood coagulation: initiation and inhibition of a proteolytic system by a zymogen. J Biol Chem 257: 5623–5631

2. Developments in antiphospholipid-protein antibodies

D. A. Triplett

Antiphospholipid-protein antibodies (APA) are a family of autoimmune and alloimmune immunoglobulins (IgG, IgM, IgA, or mixtures) that recognize phospholipid-protein complexes in in vitro laboratory test systems (Vermylen & Arnout 1992, Roubey 1994, Triplett 1995). Until recently, these antibodies were thought to have specificity for anionic or neutral phospholipids (PL). Historically, this family of antibodies has been defined by laboratory test systems using widely disparate methodologies: complement fixation assays, coagulation assays, radioimmunoassays (RIA) and enzyme-linked immunosorbent assays (ELISA). These various tests have focused on the role of PL and ignored the potential contribution of proteins present in the plasma or sera being evaluated. With the recent realization of the importance of proteins in these assays, the historical terminology presents a source of confusion to physicians and scientists who deal with the clinical complications associated with the presence of these antibodies. This review will focus on four primary areas directly related to practical clinical and laboratory advances in this field of study: definition of the antigens and antibodies, discussion of the clinical manifestations, pathophysiology, and clinical management of patients.

DEFINITION OF ANTIGENS AND ANTIBODIES

Early studies in this field were based on laboratory procedures which incorporated PL in the test systems. Reagin, the first of this family of antibodies to be described, was detected using various serologic tests for syphilis (STS) (Wassermann et al 1906). Pangborn was the first to identify acidic PL as the antigen present in alcohol extracts of bovine heart (Pangborn 1941). This extract was subsequently given the name cardiolipin. One of the most frequently used STS was the Venereal Disease Research Laboratory (VDRL) test. The VDRL reagent utilized a mixture of cardiolipin, lecithin and cholesterol. The VDRL test system was instituted for mass screening of the US population in 1938 in an effort to control syphilis. As a result of this screening program, physicians quickly became aware of many instances in which there were biological false-positive (BFP-STS) results (Arthur & Hale 1943, Davis 1944). BFP-STS were subsequently categorized as either acute or

19

chronic depending upon the transient (less than 6 months) or persistent (greater than 6 months) course of the laboratory abnormality (Moore & Mohr 1952, Moore & Lutz 1955). The STS represents the first test used to detect the presence of so-called PL antibodies. From a historical perspective, it also clearly contributed to the concept of autoimmune and alloimmune APA (Catterall 1961, Fiumara 1963). Autoimmune APA are usually persistent and often associated with clinical complications while alloimmune antibodies are usually seen in the setting of convalescence from infectious disease and are transient (Table 2.1).

Subsequently, the lupus anticoagulant (LA) was identified in patients with systemic lupus erythematosus (SLE) (Mueller et al 1951, Conley & Hartmann 1952). By definition, LA is an immunoglobulin (of varying isotypes) which interferes with one or more of the in vitro PL-dependent coagulation tests (e.g. activated partial thromboplastin time, dilute Russell viper venom time) (Exner et al 1991). LA is a misnomer since many individuals with this antibody do not have underlying SLE (Triplett 1995, Roubey 1994). Also, it is characterized by a paradoxical lack of clinical bleeding despite abnormal in vitro coagulation tests. Early studies suggested LA were specific for anionic PL (e.g. phosphatidylserine, phosphatidic acid, phosphatidylinositol) (Thiagarajan et al 1980, Pengo et al 1987).

The last member of the APA family is the anticardiolipin antibody (ACA). RIA or ELISA test systems can be used to measure ACA (Harris et al 1983). The ACA was developed to enhance sensitivity to antibodies detected in the BFP-STS.

There remains controversy regarding the antigenic target(s) for the APA family (Roubey 1994, Triplett 1995). A number of PL-binding plasma proteins have been suggested. In 1990, three groups independently described a plasma cofactor necessary for ACA testing (McNeil et al 1989, 1990,

Table 2.1   Classification of antiphospholipid-protein antibodies

I. Autoimmune
      a. Primary
             Do not fulfil criteria for systemic lupus erythematosus
      b. Secondary
             Systemic lupus erythematosus
             Other connective tissue diseases
      c. Drug-induced

II. Alloimmune
      a. Infections
             Viral
             Bacterial
             Protozoal
             Fungal
      b. Malignancies
             Hairy cell leukemia
             Lymphoproliferative
             Epithelial

Galli et al 1990, Matsuura et al 1990). This cofactor was later identified as β_2-glycoprotein I (β_2GPI) (Schultze et al 1961, Lee et al 1983). β_2GPI has a number of anticoagulant properties including the ability to inhibit the contact phase of blood coagulation, and time-dependent inhibition of the prothrombinase activity of platelets (Nimpf et al 1987, Kandiah & Krilis 1994). In the ELISA for ACA, β_2GPI is an absolute requirement for positive results in patients with autoimmune antibodies (Matsuura et al 1992, Matsuda et al 1993). In contrast, β_2GPI is inhibitory with infection-related ACA (Matsuda et al 1993). Although there is still some debate regarding the true antigen, the preponderance of evidence supports β_2GPI as the antigenic target in the ACA assay (Matsuura et al 1994). Presumably, β_2GPI binds to microtiter plate surfaces in the assay system and undergoes reconfiguration with exposure of a neotope(s) (Hunt & Krilis 1994). The genesis of ACA in vivo is presumed to be initiated by β_2GPI binding to damaged membrane surfaces with exposure of a neotope(s). Among the PL surfaces in vivo, damaged endothelial cells and activated platelets, as well as other cellular membranes, may provide surfaces to bind β_2GPI (Galli & Bevers 1994).

The second plasma protein which has been implicated as a cofactor for in vitro laboratory tests is human prothrombin (Galli & Bevers 1994). The association of LA and an acquired hypoprothrombinemic state is well established (Edson et al 1984, Simel et al 1986, Small 1988, Baudo et al 1990, Hift et al 1991). The hypoprothrombinemia is attributed to non-neutralizing antibodies which bind prothrombin in vivo leading to accelerated clearance of antigen-antibody complexes (Bajaj et al 1983, 1985). This represents one situation in which patients with LA may exhibit bleeding complications. An appreciation that LA and antiprothrombin antibodies are often the same antibodies did not occur until recent studies of Rapaport's group and work of Galli et al and Bevers et al (Fleck et al 1988, Bevers et al 1991, Galli et al 1992, Rao et al 1995). These studies suggest that LA recognizes a neotope(s) on human prothrombin bound to PL. In addition, recent studies suggest LA may recognize prothrombin in the absence of calcium ions and PL (Rao et al 1995). Also, there is some degree of species specificity with a preference for human prothrombin (Bevers et al 1991, Rao et al 1995). The observation that LA can bind to prothrombin in the absence of calcium ions and PL would seem to provide an explanation for the observed high frequency of prothrombin-LA complexes in plasma from patients with LA (Fleck et al 1988, Permpikul et al 1994). In contrast to the rare patients with hypoprothrombinemia, patients with LA-prothrombin complexes demonstrated by crossed immunoelectrophoresis commonly do not have low levels of prothrombin activity (Fleck et al 1988, Permpikul et al 1994).

There are many other candidate proteins which bind to PL. Among the proteins implicated are protein C, protein S, Annexin V, factor X, high molecular weight kininogen, factor XI and the protein core of heparan sulfate (a member of the glycosaminoglycan family) (Ruiz-Arguelles et al 1993, Oosting et al 1993, Sugi et al 1993, Matsuda et al 1994, Roubey 1994, Shibata et al 1994, Triplett & Barna 1994, Nakamura et al 1995). The diversity of potential protein-PL complexes underscores one of the most consistent observations noted clinically and in the laboratory: heterogeneity. This diversity of antigenic targets may well explain the wide spectrum of clinical findings identified in patients with APA (Triplett & Brandt 1988, Triplett 1995). With the recognition of the importance of protein components, there will be changes in nomenclature. The most appropriate designation for these antibodies will specify the protein target and laboratory test system. For example, lupus anticoagulant: prothrombin dependent or lupus anticoagulant: β_2GPI dependent. This approach will clarify the current confusing terminology. Recent studies in the ACA test system suggest β_2GPI is the antigenic target. ACA recognize β_2GPI in the absence of cardiolipin (Viard et al 1991). This group of antibodies may be designated anti-β_2GPI:ELISA.

CLINICAL MANIFESTATIONS OF APA

The association of APA and clinical complications has been well documented. The concept of an APA syndrome (APS) was first proposed in 1983 (Boey et al 1983, Harris et al 1983, Hughes 1983). These papers identified an association between thrombosis (arterial and/or venous), recurrent spontaneous abortion (RSA), thrombocytopenia and various neurologic manifestations together with positive laboratory tests for LA and/or ACA. Many of the early cases of the APS were described in the setting of SLE. However, a significant number of patients without identifiable SLE or other connective tissue diseases were observed to have the APS. These patients are now referred to as primary antiphospholipid-protein syndrome

Table 2.2   Criteria for antiphospholipid antibody (APA) syndrome

Clinical	Laboratory
Venous thrombosis	IgG anticardiolipin antibody (>10 GPL units)
Arterial thrombosis	Positive lupus anticoagulant (LA) test
Recurrent fetal loss	IgM anticardiolipin antibody (>10 MPL units) and positive LA test

Taken from Harris (1987). Patients with the APA syndrome should have at least one clinical and one laboratory finding during their disease. The APA test(s) should be positive on at least two occasions more than 8 weeks apart. The diagnosis of LA should be established using the criteria established by the SSC Subcommittee for Standardization of Lupus Anticoagulants (Exner et al 1991). GPL and MPL refer to IgG and IgM phospholipid antibodies. The units refer to the standards proposed by Harris et al at the Second International Workshop on Phospholipid Antibodies 4 April 1986 (Harris et al 1987).

(Asherson 1988, Asherson & Cervera 1994). Table 2.2 summarizes the clinical findings and laboratory results which define the necessary criteria for APS (Harris et al 1987).

The underlying pathophysiology appears to be thrombotic in the vast majority of cases. Approximately 70% of the thrombotic events are venous and 30% arterial (Triplett 1995). In the case of recurrent thrombosis, there is remarkable fidelity (i.e. arterial thrombi follow arterial thrombi, venous thrombi follow venous thrombi) (Rosove & Brewer 1992). There is a high incidence of recurrent thrombosis if the patients are not adequately anticoagulated (Rosove & Brewer 1992, Derksen et al 1993, Piette 1994, Khamashta et al 1995).

The obstetric complications associated with APA include RSA, early onset pre-eclampsia, chorea gravidarum and intrauterine fetal growth retardation (Triplett 1989). In women with a history of RSA and APA, the chance of a successful pregnancy outcome without careful monitoring and treatment is poor.

The thrombocytopenia seen in APS is thought to be immunologically mediated (Harris et al 1985, Out et al 1991). The incidence of thrombocytopenia in the APS varies from 20% to 46% of patients (Out et al 1991, Hedge 1992). There remains some question as to the role of APA in the pathogenesis of thrombocytopenia. There is direct and indirect evidence that APA may bind to platelets. Increased levels of platelet-associated immunoglobulin have been described in patients with APA (Hedge 1992). Recent studies suggested that APA do not bind to resting platelets. Binding of APA to platelets requires exposure of anionic PL and the formation of lipid-protein complexes (i.e. β_2GPI or other plasma proteins).

PATHOPHYSIOLOGIC MECHANISMS OF APA

The question of whether APA are a cause, consequence, or are coincident with clinical complications remains unresolved. However, there are emerging data which support a causative role for this group of antibodies. Indeed, one of the major areas of advances in understanding thromboembolic disease is the general concept of antibody-mediated thrombosis.

Early studies which linked APA to clinical thromboembolic events were largely retrospective (Bowie et al 1963). The concept of APS is also predicated on a history of thrombosis (Harris 1987). Thus, there is a bias based on clinical history for this group of patients. Data from recent prospective and cross-sectional studies support APA as a risk factor for thromboembolic events. Animal models and the measurement of markers of in vivo activation of coagulation (prothrombin fragment 1+2, fibrinopeptide A) also suggest APA are linked to in vivo activation of coagulation (Branch et al 1990, Smith et al 1990, Blank et al 1991, Bakiner et al 1992, Ferro et al 1993, Ginsberg et al 1993, Nakase et al 1994). Among the prospective studies, the Physicians' Health Study has provided evidence to support a causative role of APA. This randomized, double-blind study evaluated 22 071 male physicians (aged 40–84 years) in a prospective fashion. Subjects were randomized to receive either aspirin or β-carotene (Ginsberg et al 1992b). Samples that were collected at the time of entry in the study were subsequently tested for ACA. After a 5-year follow-up, individuals with a documented history of ischemic stroke, deep vein thrombosis, or pulmonary emboli were evaluated together with controls matched by age, smoking history and length of follow-up. ACA titers were higher in subjects with deep vein thrombosis and pulmonary embolus than in the matched controls. Individuals with ACA titers above the 95th percentile had a 5.3 relative risk of developing DVT or pulmonary embolism. This study suggests the relative risk for DVT in patients who are ACA+ is very similar to individuals with hereditary activated protein C (APC) resistance. Both ACA and APC resistance represent risk factors for venous thrombosis. Alone, they represent a 'weak' predisposition to venous thrombosis. It is clear that in many instances thromboembolic events are associated with 'two hits'. Thus, a patient with APC resistance who develops ACA positivity would have 'two hits' (Table 2.3).

Also, a recent study by Vaarala et al (1995) in middle-aged dyslipidemic men, who were followed over 5 years for coronary ischemic events, found that ACA levels were significantly higher in patients than in control subjects. Subjects with ACA in the highest quartile of distribution had a relative risk of myocardial infarction of 2.0 (95% confidence interval: 1.1 to 3.5) compared to the remainder of the population. This risk factor was independent of other factors such as age, smoking, systolic blood pressure, low-density lipoprotein levels (LDL) and high-density lipoprotein levels. There was also a correlation between levels of ACA and antibodies to oxidized LDL (Vaarala et al 1993). Cross-sectional studies in ACA+ SLE patients have found elevated levels of prothrombin fragment 1+2 and fibrinopeptide A (Ferro et al 1993, Ginsberg et al 1993). Ferro et al (1993) evaluated SLE patients using tests for LA and ACA. The presence of LA

Table 2.3 Risk factors predisposing to thrombosis

Stasis	Activation of coagulation	Platelet-vessel perturbation
Immobilization	Malignancies	Myeloproliferative disorders
Obesity	Pregnancy	Heparin-associated thrombocytopenia
Congestive heart failure	Nephrotic syndrome	Homocystinemia
Postoperative period	Oral contraceptives (estrogens)	APA
Air travel	APA	Atherosclerosis
	Septicemia (endotoxins)	Angioplasty
	Prosthetic valves/grafts	Thrombotic thrombocytopenic purpura

APA, antiphospholipid-protein antibodies.

was more commonly related to positive markers of in vivo activation of coagulation. In their study, patients who were LA+/ACA+ or LA+/ACA– had similarly elevated levels of fragment 1+2. Patients who were LA–/ACA+ or LA–/ACA– had similar lower levels. These results tend to confirm previous observations that LA positivity is a greater risk factor for thromboembolic events than isolated ACA positivity (Derksen et al 1988). Ginsberg et al (1992a) and Long et al (1991) have evaluated SLE patients in cross-sectional studies to correlate the role of APA in thromboembolic disease and RSA. In both studies, the presence of APA was associated with clinical complications.

These prospective studies, cross-sectional studies and analysis of markers of in vivo coagulation all support a causative role of APA in clinical thromboembolic events. Given the frequency of APA, it is likely they represent one of the more common primary or secondary 'hits' leading to clinical thrombosis. The realization of the significance of these antibodies is reflected by a marked increase in laboratory testing to identify APA (Triplett 1995). Indeed, the two tests in the coagulation laboratory which have grown exponentially over the last 2 years are analysis for APA and testing for APC-resistance (Dahlback 1995).

A variety of potential mechanisms have been proposed to explain the role of APA in thromboembolic disease, including alteration of the platelet–endothelial axis, inhibition of the heparan sulfate antithrombin III regulatory system, and abnormalities of the protein C system (Marciniak & Romond 1989, Gibson et al 1992, Derksen et al 1993, Couper & Maxwell 1994, Sorice et al 1994). Given the clinical heterogeneity (both arterial and venous thrombosis), it is reasonable to assume there are multiple pathogenic mechanisms associated with APA. On the venous side of the circulation, perturbation of the protein C system appears to account for most of the thrombotic events. On the arterial side, alteration of the platelet-endothelial axis is the most probable underlying mechanism(s).

A variety of potential sites for alteration of the protein C system have been reported. These include acquired protein S deficiency, antibodies which react to PL-bound protein C and protein S, antibodies to thrombomodulin, antibodies to factor Va and direct inhibition of APC activity based on membrane PL content (Gibson et al 1992, Couper & Maxwell 1994, Sorice et al 1994). The latter mechanism appears to be one of the more intriguing observations. Phosphatidylethanolamine enhances the expression of APC activity (Smirnov et al 1995). The phosphatidylethanolamine content of cell membranes plays a role in APC-mediated downregulation of factor Va. Also, in vitro experiments suggest that phosphatidylethanolamine enhances LA activity (Smirnov et al 1995).

Antibodies to factor Va may also predispose to thrombotic events (Lin & Zehnder 1994).

TREATMENT

APA are seen in many different clinical settings. Frequently they are alloantibodies which are transient and not associated with clinical complications (Triplett 1995). Thus, the clinical setting and persistence of APA are important criteria for interpreting potential pathogenicity of these antibodies. Treatment should be reserved for patients who have clinical evidence of APS.

Patients with persistently positive APA and a history of thrombosis are at high risk of recurrence if not treated. As noted earlier, there is remarkable consistency in terms of thrombotic recurrences (Rosove & Brewer 1992). Although there are no prospective studies, retrospective studies suggest a higher intensity of oral anticoagulation in these patients with a target INR (International Normalized Ratio) of 3.0–3.5 (Rosove & Brewer 1992, Rivier et al 1994, Khamashta et al 1995). Management of pregnancy in patients with APA and a history of RSA remains controversial. The early studies which employed high doses of prednisone or other corticosteroids together with aspirin did show improvement in the frequency of successful pregnancies (Silveira et al 1992). However, there was an unacceptable high rate of maternal morbidity (Cowchock et al 1992). Full-dose heparin together with low-dose aspirin has been used more frequently over the past several years (Rosove et al 1990, Cowchock et al 1992). The incidence of maternal morbidity with this regimen is less than with the earlier treatment employing prednisone. In particularly difficult patients, plasmapheresis or the use of intravenous immunoglobulin has been employed (Parke 1992). One of the most important aspects of management of the pregnant patient with APA is careful monitoring of the fetus.

SUMMARY

APA have emerged as one of the most important predisposing factors for clinical thromboembolic events. The relative risk of thrombosis associated with APA positivity is similar to that seen in patients with APC-resistance. Given the frequency of these two laboratory abnormalities – APA (approx. 3–5% of the population) and APC resistance (5–10% of the population) – the concordance of these two predisposing factors is not uncommon (approx. 1 in 400 individuals). However, there remains a problem in identifying which APA are pathogenic. Persistence of the antibody and perhaps IgG isotype are the only two predictive(?) criteria identified to date. With the increasing realization of multiple PL – protein target complexes, perhaps the involvement of certain proteins in these complexes will have a higher predictive value for thrombosis. Nevertheless, this remains a speculative hypothesis.

KEY POINTS FOR CLINICAL PRACTICE

* APA are a family of antibodies with varying specificity for protein–phospholipid complexes. Laboratory diagnosis requires *both* coagulation and anticardiolipin antibody (ACA) ELISA.

* APA may be classified as allo- and autoantibodies. Autoantibodies are more frequently associated with clinical complications.

* APA are associated with both venous and arterial thromboembolic events.

* APA often are a 'second hit' in patients with clinical thrombosis.

* Recurrent spontaneous abortion (RSA) has been attributed to APA.

* APA are thought to be causative in the pathogenesis of thrombosis.

* Appropriate anticoagulant therapy in APA+ patients with a history of thrombosis involves long-term oral anticoagulation (INR 3.0–3.5).

* In a pregnant women with a history of RSA, full-dose heparin (12 000 units SC b.i.d.) and low-dose aspirin (75 mg/day) are recommended.

REFERENCES

Arthur R D, Hale J M 1943 Biologic false positive tests for syphilis associated with routine army immunization. Milit Surg 92: 53–56
Asherson R A 1988 A 'primary' antiphospholipid syndrome? J Rheumatol 15: 1742–1746
Asherson R A, Cervera R 1994 Primary, secondary and other variants of the antiphospholipid syndrome. Lupus 3: 293–298
Bajaj S P, Rapaport S I, Fierer D S et al 1983 A mechanism for the hypoprothrombinemia–lupus anticoagulant syndrome. Blood 61: 684–692
Bajaj S P, Rapaport S I, Barclay S et al 1985 Acquired hypoprothrombinemia due to nonneutralizing antibodies to prothrombin: mechanisms and management. Blood 65: 1538–1543
Bakiner R, Fishman P, Blank M et al 1992 Induction of primary antiphospholipid syndrome in mice by immunization with a human monoclonal anticardiolipin antibody (H3). J Clin Invest 89: 1558–1563
Baudo F, Redaelli R, Pezzetti L et al 1990 Prothrombin-antibody consistent with lupus anticoagulant: clinical study and immunochemical characterization. Thromb Res 57: 279–287
Bevers E M, Galli M, Barbui T et al 1991 Lupus anticoagulant IgGs (LA) are not directed to phospholipids only but to a complex of lipid bound prothrombin. Thromb Haemost 66: 629–632
Blank M, Cohen J, Toder V et al 1991 Induction of antiphospholipid syndrome in native mice with mouse lupus monoclonal and human polyclonal ACA antibodies. Proc Natl Acad Sci USA 88: 3069–3073
Boey M D, Colaco C B, Gharavi A E et al 1983 Thrombosis in SLE: striking association with the presence of circulating 'lupus anticoagulant'. Br Med J 287: 1021–1023
Bowie E J W, Thompson J H, Pascuzzi C A et al 1963 Thrombosis in systemic lupus erythematosus despite circulating anticoagulants. J Lab Clin Med 62: 416–430
Branch D W, Dudley D J, Mitchell M D et al 1990 Immunoglobulin G fractions from patients with antiphospholipid antibodies cause fetal death in Balb/c mice: a model for autoimmune fetal loss. Am J Obstet Gynecol 163: 210–216
Catterall R D 1961 Collagen disease and chronic biologic false positive phenomenon. Q J Med 30: 41–55

Conley C L, Hartmann R C 1952 A hemorrhagic disorder caused by circulating anticoagulants in patients with disseminated lupus erythematosus. J Lab Clin Invest 31: 621–622

Couper R T L, Maxwell F C 1994 Anticardiolipin and acquired protein S deficiency in early childhood. J Paediatr Child Health 30: 363–365

Cowchock E S, Reece E A, Balaban D et al 1992 Repeated fetal losses associated with antiphospholipid antibodies: a collaborative randomized trial comparing prednisone with low dose heparin treatment. Am J Obstet Gynecol 166: 1318–1323

Dahlback B 1995 New molecular insights into the genetics of thrombophilia. Thromb Haemost 74: 139–148

Davis B D 1944 Biologic false positive serologic tests for syphilis. Medicine 23: 359–414

Derksen R H W M, Hasselaar P, Blokzijl L et al 1988 Coagulation screen is more specific than the anticardiolipin antibody ELISA in defining a thrombotic subset of lupus patients. Ann Rheumatol Dis 47: 364–371

Derksen R H W M, De Groot G, Kater L et al 1993 Patients with antiphospholipid antibodies and venous thrombosis should receive long term anticoagulant treatment. Ann Rheum Dis 52: 689–692

Edson J, Vogt J, Hasegawa D 1984 Abnormal prothrombin crossed immunoelectrophoresis in patients with lupus inhibitors. Blood 64: 807–816

Exner T, Triplett D A, Taberner D et al 1991 Guidelines for testing and revised criteria for lupus anticoagulants. SSC Subcommittee for Standardization of Lupus Anticoagulants. Thromb Haemost 65: 320–322

Ferro D, Quintarelli C, Valesini G et al 1993 Lupus anticoagulant and increased thrombin generation in patients with systemic lupus erythematosus. Blood 82: 304

Fiumara N J 1963 Biologic false-positive reaction to syphilis. N Engl J Med 268: 402–405

Fleck R A, Rapaport S I, Rao L V M 1988 Antiprothrombin antibodies and the lupus anticoagulant. Blood 72: 512–519

Galli M, Bevers EM 1994 Inhibition of phospholipid-dependent coagulation reactions by 'antiphospholipid antibodies': possible modes of action. Lupus 3: 223–228

Galli M, Comfurius P, Maassen C et al 1990 Anticardiolipin antibodies (ACA) directed not to cardiolipin but to a plasma cofactor. Lancet 335: 1544–1547

Galli M, Comfurius P, Barbui T et al 1992 Anticoagulant activity of β_2 glycoprotein I is potentiated by a distinct subgroup of anticardiolipin antibodies. Thromb Haemost 68: 297–300

Gibson J, Nelson M, Brown R et al 1992 Autoantibodies to thrombomodulin: development of an enzyme immunoassay and a survey of their frequency in patients with the lupus anticoagulant. Thromb Haemost 67: 507–509

Ginsburg J S, Brill-Edwards P, Johnston M et al 1992a Relationship of antiphospholipid antibodies to pregnancy loss in patients with systemic lupus erythematosus: a cross selectional study. Blood 80: 975

Ginsburg J S, Liang M H, Newcomer L et al 1992b Anticardiolipin antibodies and the risk for ischemic stroke and venous thrombosis. Ann Intern Med 117: 997–1002

Ginsburg J S, Demers C, Brill-Edwards P et al 1993 Increased thrombin generation and activity in patients with systemic lupus erythematosus and anticardiolipin antibodies: evidence for a prothrombotic state. Blood 81: 2958–2963

Harris E N 1987 Syndrome of the black swan. Br J Rheumatol 26: 324–326

Harris E N, Gharavi A E, Boey M L 1983 Anticardiolipin antibodies: detection by radioimmunoassay and association with thrombosis in systemic lupus erythematosus. Lancet ii: 1211–1214

Harris E N, Gharavi A E, Hegde U 1985 Anticardiolipin antibodies in autoimmune thrombocytopenic purpura. Br J Haematol 59: 231–234

Harris E N, Gharavi A E, Patel S P et al 1987 Evaluation of the anti-cardiolipin test: report of a standardized workshop held 4 April 1986. Clin Exp Immunol 68: 215–222

Hedge U M 1992 Platelet antibodies in immune thrombocytopenia. Blood Rev 6: 34–42

Hift R, Bird A, Sarembock B 1991 Acquired hypoprothrombinemia and lupus anticoagulant. Response to steroid therapy. Br J Haematol 30: 308–310

Hughes G R V 1983 Thrombosis, abortion, cerebral disease and the lupus anticoagulant. Br Med J 287: 1088–1089

Hunt J, Krilis S 1994 The fifth domain of β_2 glycoprotein I contains a phospholipid binding site (CYS 281–CYS 288) and a region recognized by anticardiolipin antibodies. J Immunol 152: 653–659

Kandiah D A, Krilis S A 1994 β_2 glycoprotein I. Lupus 3: 207–212

Khamashta M A, Caudrado M J, Mujic F et al 1995 The management of thrombosis in the antiphospholipid antibody syndrome. N Engl J Med 332: 993–997

Lee N S, Brewer H B, Osborne J C J 1983 β_2 glycoprotein I. Molecular properties of an unusual apolipoprotein, apolipoprotein H. J Biol Chem 258: 4765–4770

Lin R Z, Zehnder J L 1994 Acquired activated protein C resistance caused by factor Va antibody: a possible mechanism of increased thrombosis in the antiphospholipid antibody syndrome. Blood 84: 83a

Long A A, Ginsburg J S, Brill-Edwards P et al 1991 The relationship of antiphospholipid antibodies to thromboembolic disease in systemic lupus erythematosus. A cross sectional study. Thromb Haemost 66: 520

McNeil H P, Chesterman C N, Krilis S A 1989 Anticardiolipin antibodies and lupus anticoagulants comprise antibody subgroups with different phospholipid binding characteristics. Br J Haematol 73: 506–513

McNeil H P, Simpson R J, Chesterman C N et al 1990 Antiphospholipid antibodies are directed against a complex antigen that includes a lipid binding inhibitor of coagulation: β_2 glycoprotein I (apolipoprotein H). Proc Natl Acad Sci USA 87: 4120–4124

Marciniak E, Romond E H 1989 Impaired catalytic function of activated protein C: a new in vitro manifestation of lupus anticoagulant. Blood 74: 2426–2432

Matsuda J, Saitoh N, Gotchi K et al 1993 Distinguishing β_2 glycoprotein I dependent (systemic lupus erythematosus type) and independent (syphilis type) anticardiolipin antibody with tween 20. Br J Haematol 85: 799–802

Matsuda J, Saitoh N, Gohchi K et al 1994 Anti-annexin V antibody in systemic lupus erythematosus patients with lupus anticoagulant and/or anticardiolipin antibody. Am J Hematol 47: 56–58

Matsuura E, Igarashi Y, Fujimoto M et al 1990 Anticardiolipin cofactor(s) and differential diagnosis of autoimmune disease. Lancet 336: 177–178

Matsuura E, Igarashi Y, Fujimoto M et al 1992 Heterogeneity of anticardiolipin antibodies defined by the anticardiolipin cofactor. J Immunol 148: 3885–3891

Matsuura E, Igarashi Y, Yasuda T et al 1994 Anticardiolipin antibodies recognize β_2 glycoprotein I structure altered to interact with an oxygen modified solid phase surface. J Exp Med 179: 457–462

Moore J E, Mohr C F 1952 Biologically false positive serologic tests for syphilis. J Am Med Assoc 150: 467–473

Moore J E, Lutz W B 1955 The natural history of systemic lupus erythematosus: an approach to its study through chronic biologic false-positive reactions. J Chron Dis 1: 297–316

Mueller J F, Ratnoff O, Henile R W 1951 Observations on the characteristics of an unusual circulating anticoagulant. J Lab Clin Med 38: 254–261

Nakamura N, Kuragaki C, Shidara Y et al 1995 Antibody to annexin V has anti-phospholipid and lupus anticoagulant properties. Am J Hematol 49: 347–348

Nakase T, Wada H, Minamikawa K et al 1994 Increased activated protein C–protein C inhibitor complex level in patients positive for lupus anticoagulant. Blood Coagulat Fibrinol 5: 173–177

Nimpf J, Wurm H, Kostner G M 1987 β_2 glycoprotein I (apo-H) inhibits the release reaction of human platelets during ADP-induced aggregation. Atherosclerosis 63: 109–114

Oosting J D, Derksen R H W M, Bobbick I W G et al 1993 Antiphospholipid antibodies directed against a combination of phospholipids with prothrombin, protein C or protein S. An explanation for their pathogenic mechanism. Blood 81: 2618–2625

Out H J, De Groot P G, van Vliet M et al 1991 Antibodies to platelets in patients with antiphospholipid antibodies. Blood 77: 2655–2659

Pangborn M C 1941 A new serologically active phospholipid from beef heart. Proc Soc Exp Biol Med 48: 484–486

Parke A 1992 The role of IVIG in the managements of patients with antiphospholipid antibodies and recurrent pregnancy losses. In: Ballow M (ed) IVIG Therapy Today. Humana Press, Totowa, NJ, pp. 105–118

Pengo V, Thiagarajan P, Shapiro S S et al 1987 Immunological specificity and mechanism of action of IgG lupus anticoagulants. Blood 70: 69–76

Permpikul P, Rao L V M, Rapaport S I 1994 Functional and binding roles of prothrombin and β_2 glycoprotein I in the expression of lupus anticoagulant activity. Blood 83: 2878–2892

Piette J C 1994 Prevention of recurrent thrombosis in the antiphospholipid syndrome. Lupus 3: 73–74

Rao L V M, Hoang A D, Rapaport S I 1995 Differences in the interactions of lupus anticoagulant IgG with human prothrombin and bovine prothrombin. Thromb Haemost 73: 668–674

Rivier G, Herranz M T, Khamashta M A et al 1994 Thrombosis and antiphospholipid syndrome: a preliminary assessment of three antithrombotic treatments. Lupus 3: 85–90

Rosove M H, Brewer P M C 1992 Antiphospholipid thrombosis clinical course after the first thrombotic event in 70 patients. Ann Intern Med 117: 303–308

Rosove M H, Tabsh K, Wasserstrum N 1990 Heparin therapy for pregnant women with lupus anticoagulant or anticardiolipin antibodies. Obstet Gynecol 75: 630–634

Roubey R A S 1994 Autoantibodies to phospholipid-binding plasma proteins: a new view of lupus anticoagulants and other 'antiphospholipid' autoantibodies. Blood 84: 2854–2867

Ruiz-Arguelles A, Vasquez-Prado J, Deleze M et al 1993 Presence of serum antibodies to coagulation protein C in patients with systemic lupus erythematosus is not associated with antigenic or functional protein C deficiencies. Am J Hematol 44: 58–59

Schultze H E, Heide K, Haupt H 1961 Uber einbisher unbekanntes niedermole kulares β_2 globulin des human Serums. Naturwissenschaften 48: 719

Shibata S, Harpel P C, Gharavi A et al 1994 Autoantibodies to heparin from patients with antiphospholipid antibody syndrome inhibits formation of antithrombin III–thrombin complexes. Blood 83: 2537–2540

Silveira L H, Hubble C L, Jara L J et al 1992 Prevention of anticardiolipin antibody-related pregnancy losses with prednisone and aspirin. Am J Med 93: 403–411

Simel D L, St Clair E W, Adams J et al 1986 Correction of the hypoprothrombinemic by immunosuppressive treatment of the lupus anticoagulant–hypoprothrombinemia syndrome. Am J Med 83: 563–566

Small P 1988 Severe hemorrhage in a patient with circulating anticoagulant acquired hypoprothrombinemia and systemic lupus erythematosus. Arthritis Rheum 31: 1210–1211

Smirnov M D, Triplett D A, Comp P C et al 1995 Role of phosphatidyl ethanolamine in inhibition of activated protein C activity by antiphospholipid antibodies. J Clin Invest 95: 309–316

Smith H R, Hansen C L, Rose R et al 1990 Autoimmune MRL-1 pr/1 pr mice are an animal model for the secondary antiphospholipid syndrome. J Rheumatol 17: 911–915

Sorice M, Griggi T, Circella A et al 1994 Protein S antibodies in acquired protein S deficiencies. Blood 83: 2383–2384

Sugi T, Vanderpuye O A, McIntyre J A 1993 Partial purification of an anti-phosphatidylethanolamine antibody ELISA cofactor. Thromb Haemost 69: 596

Thiagarajan P, Shapiro S S, DeMano L 1980 Monoclonal immunoglobulin M lambda coagulation inhibitor with phospholipid specificity mechanism of a lupus anticoagulant. J Clin Invest 66: 397–405

Triplett D A 1989 Antiphospholipid antibodies and recurrent pregnancy loss. Am J Reprod Immunol 20: 52–67

Triplett D A 1995 Antiphospholipid-protein antibodies: laboratory detection and clinical relevance. Thromb Res 78: 1–31

Triplett D A, Barna L K 1994 Use of factor XI assay to screen for β_2GPI dependent or prothrombin dependent lupus anticoagulants. Lupus 3: 354

Triplett D A, Brandt J T 1988 Lupus anticoagulants; misnomer, paradox, riddle, epiphenomenon. Hematol Pathol 2: 121–143

Vaarala O, Alftham G, Jauhiainen M et al 1993 Cross reaction between antibodies to oxidised low-density lipoprotein and to cardiolipin in systemic lupus erythematosus. Lancet 341: 923–925

Vaarala O, Manttari M, Manninen V et al 1995 Anti-cardiolipin antibodies and risk of myocardial infarction in a prospective cohort of middle-aged men. Circulation 91: 23–27

Vermylen J, Arnout J 1992 Is the antiphospholipid syndrome caused by antibodies directed against physiologically relevant phospholipid–protein complexes? J Lab Clin Med 120: 10–12

Viard J P, Amoura Z, Bach J F 1991 Anti-β_2 glycoprotein-I antibodies in systemic lupus erythematosus — a marker of thrombosis associated with lupus anticoagulant activity. C R Acad Sci [III] 313: 607–612

Wassermann A, Neisser A, Bruck C 1906 Eine serodiagnostische Reaktion bei Syphilis. Dtsch Med Wochenschr 32: 745–746

3. The relationships of platelets to arterial thrombosis and atherosclerosis

F. A. Ofosu

Atherosclerosis is the major cause of arterial thrombosis which can precipitate a fatal myocardial infarction or stroke. A three-part review on atherosclerosis describing the intima of normal human arteries and its atherosclerosis-prone regions, initial, intermediate and advanced atherosclerotic lesions and their histological classification by the Committee on Vascular Lesions, Council on Arteriosclerosis, American Heart Association, has appeared recently (Stary et al 1992, 1994, 1995). These authors have classified six broad histologically distinct atherosclerotic lesions (types I–VI). Types I, II and III are clinically silent lesions while types IV, V and VI may be clinically silent or have significant symptoms. Type I or the initial lesion, the progression-prone type IIa lesion, and the progression-resistant type IIb lesion are early lesions evident from the first decade of life and are thus usually found at autopsy. While these initial lesions are seen in young children, they can also occur in adults. Type II lesions appear as fatty dots or streaks with the unaided eye. The macrophages (foam cells) resident in type II lesions accumulate lipoproteins intracellularly to contribute to the growth of these lesions. These foam cells express tissue factor antigen (Sueishi et al 1995) and may thus provide the initiating stimulus for the increased thrombin production seen in severe atherosclerosis. The next and clinically silent type III (intermediate or pre-atheroma) lesion is a progression from type IIa, and is characterized by small extracellular lipid pools, which are the principal means for the growth of this lesion. The lumens of the arteries with type I–III lesions usually have normal diameter and thus support blood flow normally. These early lesions are not detectable angiographically but intravascular ultrasound may detect the changes associated with these early lesions. Type IV lesions (atheromas) appear frequently from the third decade on and are characterized by a core of extracellular lipids. Type V (fibroatheroma) lesions are characterized by thickened intima, hyperplastic smooth cells and increased collagen synthesis in addition to the extracellular lipid cores of type IV lesions. Type VI (complicated) lesions have all the features of type V lesions as well as fissures, hematoma and/or thrombi. Type VI lesions may revert to type V lesions, and these late lesions appear in the fourth decade or later when their narrowed lumens frequently present clinically overt symptoms, and may be prone to sudden total occlusive events.

Associated with all stages of atherosclerosis is the abnormal growth (hyperplasia) of smooth muscle cells into the intima, primarily in response to mitogens (including platelet-derived growth factor released by activated endothelial cells, platelets and monocytes) (Katsuda et al 1990, Sumiyoshi et al 1991, Ross 1993, 1995).

This chapter will summarize mechanisms that enhance the pathogenesis of atherosclerotic lesions, the altered hemostasis seen in atherosclerosis, the evidence for increased platelet activation in atherosclerosis, and the use of antiplatelet drugs to moderate the consequences of atherosclerosis and arterial thrombosis.

PATHOGENESIS OF ATHEROSCLEROTIC LESIONS

Injury to endothelial cells stimulates the elaboration and expression by these cells of leukocyte adherence molecules, growth factors, and/or cytokines chemotactic for leukocytes and smooth muscle cells (Ross 1993, 1995). Microthrombi containing platelets and/or fibrin also form at the sites of initial endothelium injury. Many of the monocytes that are initially attracted to sites of endothelial injury also adhere to these sites from where they subsequently migrate into the intima and become converted into macrophages (foam cells) which accumulate modified (likely oxidized) lipoproteins intracellularly. Continued availability of inflammatory mediators elaborated by the injured endothelium, platelets, or macrophages enhance the intracellular accumulation of oxidized lipoproteins by the foam cells which may subsequently be seen macroscopically as fatty streaks (in type II lesions if the cause of endothelial injury persists). Tissue factor, known to be present in these foam cells (Wilcox et al 1989, Sueishi et al 1995), probably enhances thrombin production locally to increase platelet activation in situ. Focal collections of these foam cells and accumulation of extracellular lipids, migration of smooth muscle cells (in response to chemoattractants and growth factors elaborated by the macrophages, injured endothelium and activated platelets) and production of connective tissue matrix contribute to the development of, and the eventual encapsulation of, the lipid core by connective tissue, and ultimately the evolution of the fibrinolipid plaque. Some of the chemoattractants for smooth muscle cell migration elaborated by the activated macrophages (platelet-derived growth factor and insulin-like growth factor) are also potent mitogens for smooth muscle cells (Bornfeldt et al 1994). The composition of lipid, smooth muscle and collagen found in advanced (types V and VI) plaques can vary widely from being predominantly collagenous to >70% of the volume being made up of the lipid core (Hangartner et al 1986, Guyton & Klemp 1994). Microscopic study of raised plaques lacking macroscopic evidence for surface thrombus deposition demonstrates that up to 50% of advanced plaques have deep laminar deposits of fibrin associated with platelet antigens (Bini et al 1987, 1989).

When clinically significant symptoms (e.g. unstable angina, myocardial infarction or stroke) develop from advanced atherosclerotic plaques (types V and VI), they arise from two related mechanisms: namely, major thrombosis (and the associated acute arterial occlusion) and/or the natural growth of the lesions (smooth muscle cell hyperplasia, increased collagen synthesis and extracellular lipid accumulation) (Hangartner et al 1986, Davies et al 1988, 1989, Davies 1994, Ghaddar et al 1995). Obstruction of atherosclerotic vessels and the associated impaired flow of blood in these vessels result from either major thrombosis or from the consequences of minor thrombosis. Minor thrombosis arises in response to products released from activated monocytes and platelets and the actions of thrombin, all of which enhance smooth muscle proliferation (Sumiyoshi et al 1995). Minor thrombosis also arises from the recruitment of additional monocytes to sites of thrombin production and platelet activation. There are significant inflammatory events associated with plaques at risk for rupturing as evidenced by the presence of macrophages, T lymphocytes and mast cells in such lesions (Steinberg 1992).

ALTERED HEMOSTASIS IN ATHEROSCLEROSIS

When compared to sex- and age-matched controls, marked elevation in the concentrations of several of the molecular markers that reflect increased coagulation, platelet activation and endothelial cell activation in vivo are found in the plasma of patients with clinically significant atherosclerosis. In general, the severity of atherosclerosis is reflected by the elevation in the concentrations of these molecular markers of hemostasis. Elevated concentrations of plasma fibrinogen, factor VII, factor VIII, prothrombin fragment 1+2, fibrinopeptide A, von Willebrand factor, tissue plasminogen activator (tPA), D-dimer, plasminogen activator inhibitor-1 (PAI-1), platelet factor 4, β-thromboglobulin, stable metabolites of thromboxane A_2 and prostacyclin have been reported in atherosclerosis and arterial thrombosis. Elevated concentrations have been reported for plasma fibrinogen (Wilhelmsen et al 1984, Meade et al 1986, Kannel et al 1987, Yarnell et al 1991, Cortellaro et al 1992, Bini & Kudryk et al 1994, Heinrich et al 1994), factor VII (Meade et al 1986, Cortellaro et al 1993, Rugman et al 1994, Moor et al 1994, Lee et al 1995), prothrombin fragment 1+2 (Kienast et al 1993, Merlini et al 1994, Rugman et al 1994), fibrinopeptide A (Nichols et al 1982, Theroux et al 1987, Rapold et al 1989, Eisenberg et al 1990, Szczeklik et al 1992, Merlini et al 1994), and thrombin–antithrombin III (Szczeklik et al 1992, Takano et al 1992, Kienast et al 1993, Rugman et al 1994).

The high levels of fibrinogen in atherosclerosis and arterial thrombosis may reflect the chronic inflammation of atherosclerosis (Lassila 1993) since fibrinogen is an acute phase protein. The Caerphilly and Speedwell Collaborative Heart Disease Studies investigated the relationships of fibrinogen and leukocytes (among other parameters) to the incidence of ischemic heart disease in nearly 5000 middle-aged men over a period of 3–5 years, during which 251 major ischemic heart diseases occurred in this group. Age-adjusted relative odds for ischemic heart disease for the men in the top 20% of the distribution versus the bottom 20% were 4.1 for fibrinogen and 3.2 for white blood cell count. Multivariate analysis also demonstrated fibrinogen and white blood cell count to be important risk factors for ischemic heart disease (Yarnell et al 1991). The chronic inflammation of atherosclerosis likely accounts for the increased concentrations of prothrombin fragment 1+2, thrombin–antithrombin III and fibrinopeptide A in atherosclerosis and arterial thrombosis. Tissue factor is synthesized in atherosclerotic plaques (Taubman et al 1993) and functional tissue factor inhibited by anti-tissue factor antibodies is found in human atherosclerotic plaques (Wilcox et al 1989). Indeed, monocytes of patients with coronary artery disease have intrinsic tissue factor activity whereas monocytes of age-matched controls do not express tissue factor activity prior to their stimulation (Leatham et al 1995). The tissue factor of atherosclerotic plaques is predominantly located within the macrophages but tissue factor is also weakly distributed in the superficial portion of fibrous plaques and the fibrous caps over the atheroma core (Sueishi et al 1995). The resulting thrombin production in situ (reflected in elevated plasma concentrations of prothrombin fragment 1+2, thrombin–antithrombin III and fibrinopeptide A) is likely to further enhance tissue factor production by local macrophages, smooth muscle cells and fibroblast since thrombin stimulates production of the interleukins IL-1 and IL-6 by these cells (Bevilacqua et al 1984, 1985, Sower et al 1995).

Human atherosclerotic lesions have high concentrations of fibrin, and Bini et al (1989) have reported types I and II to surround vessel wall cells and macrophages in early lesions and in atherosclerotic plaques. Increased thrombin production and the subsequent fibrin production are also reflected in the elevation of plasma fibrinopeptide A and fibrin D-dimer in atherosclerosis (Lassila et al 1993, Peltonen et al 1993). Fibrinopeptides are chemoattractants for blood leukocytes, and fibrinopeptide B recruits macrophages in early lesions of atherosclerosis (Singh et al 1990). Increased fibrin formation will invariably lead to the activation of plasminogen. Plasminogen activation in atherosclerosis is catalysed by tPA and urokinase. Both enzymes are synthesized by monocytes/macrophages, and plasmin degrades the fibrin that becomes associated with these cells. These mechanisms likely explain the increased concentrations of D-dimer, tPA and PAI-1 seen in severe atherosclerosis and arterial thrombosis (Smith & Ashall 1985, Hamstein et al 1987, Takano et al 1992, Matsuda et al 1995, Thompson et al 1995). In addition to its well-known role in fibrinolysis, plasmin indirectly contributes to the degradation of the extracellular matrix, tissue remodelling and cellular differentiation. Specifically, plasmin activates procollagenases, with the collagenases in turn degrading the extracellular matrix (Saksela & Rifkin et al 1988). Enzymatic degradation of the extracellular matrix may also be catalysed by the following enzymes elaborated by activated macrophages: intestitial collagenase (which degrades types I and III collagen); a type IV collagenase which degrades basement membrane collagen; and stromelysin which degrades fibrinectin, laminin and proteoglycans (Shapiro et al 1990). Lassila (1993) reported that plasmin degrades human atherosclerotic arterial wall collagen by inducing soluble amino terminal propeptides of type III and procollagen. The actions of these proteolytic enzymes may be critical for plaque to rupture (Falk 1992). Monocyte/macrophages also produce plasminogen activator inhibitors and the protease nexin to moderate plasmin production.

Another consequence of increased thrombin production in atherosclerosis and arterial thrombosis is evident from the increased concentrations of endothelial cell metabolites made or released in response to α-thrombin. Specifically, increased synthesis of prostacyclin, nitric oxide and growth factors, and elevation in plasma concentrations of von Willebrand factor, tPA and plasminogen activator inhibitor (Jansson et al 1991a,b, Lee et al 1994, Brannstrom et al 1995, Shatos et al 1995, Margaglione et al 1994, Cortellaro et al 1993, Matsuda et al 1995, Thompson et al 1995) have been reported in atherosclerosis. Thrombin stimulates the endothelium to synthesize prostacyclin, and to release tPA, PAI-1, urokinase, von Willebrand factor, P-selectin and cytokines (Lassila 1993, Neumann et al 1995, Shatos et al 1995). P-selectin in turn stimulates tissue factor production by monocytes (Celi et al 1994), and enhances the interactions of monocytes with endothelial cells and platelets. P-selectin is also secreted by activated platelets to mediate the accumulation of leukocytes into growing experimental thrombi (Sako et al 1993).

PLATELET ACTIVATION IN ARTERIAL THROMBOSIS

Given the evidence for increased thrombin production and fibrinolysis in patients with atherosclerosis and arterial thrombosis, clear evidence for increased platelet activation in these conditions would be expected, and this has been reported in many studies. Activated platelets secrete several constituents, including β-thromboglobulin, platelet factor 4 and P-selectin, synthesize thromboxane A_2 (estimated as its stable metabolites 2,3-dinor-thromboxane B_2 and 11-dehydro-thromboxane B_2) and express the activated conformer of glycoprotein IIb/IIIa, the site on platelets to which fibrinogen binds for platelet cohesion. α-Thrombin is the most potent physiological activator of platelets, and the concentrations of thrombin (as prothrombin fragment 1+2) found in plasma of patients with significant atherosclerosis reproducibly activate platelets when added to platelet-rich plasma (Liu et al 1994). While exposure of platelets to the subendothelial matrix would also result in platelet activation (following platelet exposure to collagen and/or von Willebrand factor in this environment), the contributions of thrombin and other agonists as platelet activators during atherosclerosis remain unclear. Significant platelet activation has been reported in patients with previous myocardial infarction (Nichols et al 1982), unstable angina, or acute myocardial infarction, especially in patients with ≥50% stenosis in two or more major vessels (Van Hulsteijn et al 1984, Hamm et al 1987, Rapold et al 1989). Marked platelet activation has also been reported in ischemic stroke (Iwamoto et al 1995). Another recent study has measured plasma β-thromboglobulin and platelet factor 4 in 459 individuals with increased carotid arterial wall thickness and in 459 matched controls selected from an adhort of 15 800 men and women, aged 45–64, who participated in the Atherosclerosis Risk in Communities (ARIC) study. Plasma β-thromboglobulin was markedly elevated and this platelet product appeared to be a useful marker for early atherosclerosis in middle-aged adults. The authors also suggested that platelet activation has an independent role in the pathogenesis of atherosclerosis (Ghaddar et al 1995). Marked platelet activation has also been reported in patients with severe, angiographically confirmed, obstructive disease of the lower limb (Reilly et al 1986).

Another approach for estimating platelet activation is by measuring stable metabolites of thromboxane A_2 (synthesized by platelets) in plasma and urine. Since the concentration of the major stable metabolite of platelet thromboxane A_2 (2,3-dinor-thromboxane B_2) in urine is not subject to artefactual platelet activation, urinary concentrations of 2,3-dinor-thromboxane B_2 accurately reflect the activation state of platelets in a variety of conditions. The stable metabolite of thromboxane A_2 in plasma is 11-dehydro-thromboxane B_2. Since α-thrombin activates both platelets (to effect thromboxane synthesis) and endothelial cells (to effect prostacyclin synthesis), measurements of endothelial prostacyclin synthesis (as its stable metabolite in urine, 2,3-dinor-6-keto-prostaglandin $F_{1\alpha}$) and thromboxane A_2 synthesis (also as its stable metabolites) provide a means for estimating the balance of the interactions of thrombin with platelets and the endothelium. This balance may be especially relevant in arterial thrombosis since prostacyclin decreases the interactions of platelets with the endothelium. Jouve et al (1984) and Fitzgerald et al (1986) measured metabolites of thromboxane A_2 and prostacyclin in the urine of patients with unstable coronary disease and found marked elevation in the concentrations of 2,3-dinor-thromboxane B_2 in both unstable angina and myocardial infarction. An even higher elevation of the concentrations of 2,3-dinor-6-keto-prostaglandin $F_{1\alpha}$ was found in the urine of patients with myocardial infarction where additional vessel wall injury would also be present and, therefore, further increases in prostacyclin production would be expected. Episodic chest pain in patients with unstable angina was also associated with marked increases in the concentration of 2,3-dinor thromboxane B_2. However, less marked increases in 2,3-dinor-6-keto-prostaglandin $F_{1\alpha}$ were found, suggesting an imbalance in the synthesis of the thromboxane A_2 and prostaglandin during acute ischemic attacks.

Platelet activation in acute myocardial infarction increases further during and after pharmacological thrombolysis. Urinary 2,3-dinor-thromboxane B_2 and plasma 11-dehydro-thromboxane B_2 increased more than 20-fold and more than 10-fold, respectively, in patients with acute myocardial infarction who received streptokinase (Fitzgerald et al 1988). Similar increases were noted in patients receiving tPA (Fitzgerald & Fitzgerald 1989, Kerins et al 1989). These increases were moderated significantly (but not normalized) by co-administration of aspirin to patients receiving pharmacological thrombolysis (Fitzgerald et al 1988, Fitzgerald & Fitzgerald 1989). This suppression of platelet activation (estimated as suppression of thromboxane A_2 biosynthesis) by aspirin accords well with the established use of aspirin to prevent myocardial infarction in patients with unstable angina, and for the secondary prevention of myocardial infarction and stroke, as discussed below.

ANTIPLATELET PROPHYLAXIS AND THERAPY IN ATHEROSCLEROSIS AND ARTERIAL THROMBOSIS

The mechanism proposed for the beneficial effects of aspirin in atherosclerosis and arterial thrombosis is the ability of this drug to decrease platelet aggregation and cohesion. Platelets and products derived from or elaborated by platelets are important in acute myocardial infarction and stroke. Plaque disruption directly leads to the rapid formation of platelet deposits on the immediate areas of the disruption, followed by the formation of platelet-rich thrombi which may completely occlude the vessel. The key action of aspirin on platelet physiology is the irreversible acetylation of the active site of platelet cyclooxygenase, which is a key enzyme in the synthesis of thromboxane A_2 – a powerful platelet aggregating agent (Moncada & Vane 1979, Hennekens & Buring 1994). All platelet activators induce thromboxane A_2 synthesis by platelets (Hennekens & Eberlein 1985, Fitzgerald & Fitzgerald 1989).

In double-blind randomized trials, doses of aspirin that maximally inhibit platelet cyclooxygenase decrease myocardial infarction and cardiac death by up to 50% in patients with unstable angina (Lewis et al 1983, Cairns et al 1985, Wallentin & the RISC Group et al 1991). Numerous well-designed clinical trials carried out during the past three decades have demonstrated the effectiveness of aspirin in reducing significantly the incidence of myocardial infarction, stroke or death from unstable angina. Excellent reviews have appeared which provide details of most of the trials for which the results were available for review by 1990 (Lau et al 1992, Harker & Gent et al 1994, Hennekens & Buring 1994, Antiplatelet Trialists' Collaboration 1994a–c). Antiplatelet therapy is highly protective in preventing death, stroke or secondary myocardial infarction in high-risk patients, i.e. patients with a previous myocardial infarction, or a prior history of stroke or transient ischemic attack, or among patients with other relevant medical history (such as vascular surgery, angioplasty, unstable angina, peripheral vascular disease) (Antiplatelet Trialists' Collaboration 1994a). Doses of aspirin found to be highly effective for these indications vary from 75 mg to 325 mg. The analysis performed by the authors also suggested that the optimum duration of therapy remains undefined.

It was also concluded that there is no clear evidence on the balance of risks and benefits of antiplatelet therapy in primary prevention of non-fatal myocardial infarction since the reduction in myocardial infarction achieved with aspirin was accompanied by a non-significant increase in the risk of stroke. There is no doubt that, in the studies reviewed, the doses of aspirin used inhibited platelet thromboxane synthesis. Interestingly, Yasu et al (1993) reported that aspirin inhibited both thromboxane A_2 synthesis and thrombin–antithrombin III formation in the plasma of patients with unstable angina. These results suggest that aspirin directly or indirectly inhibits platelet-dependent prothrombinase assembly in the patients studied.

As summarized by the Antiplatelet Trialists' Collaboration (1994b), aspirin is equally effective in maintaining graft patency after coronary artery bypass grafting, and arterial patency after angioplasty, peripheral artery disease and hemodialysis. An overall event reduction of approximately 50% was observed in the above cases. Aspirin also produces a significant reduction in deep vein thrombosis and pulmonary embolism after general or orthopedic (traumatic or elective) surgery (Antiplatelet Trialists' Collaboration 1994c). The effectiveness of aspirin in preventing postoperative thrombosis highlights the potential roles of inflammation and platelets in venous thrombosis.

There are several potential reasons why inhibition of platelet activation or direct inhibition of platelet thromboxane A_2 synthesis (by aspirin) provides effective means for limiting the clinical consequences of arterial thrombosis (and possibly venous thrombosis). Thromboxane A_2 enhances the infiltration of plasma and leukocytes into arterial walls in rabbits (Numano et al 1982, 1995), and incubation of activated platelets with endothelial cells decreases endothelial cell cyclic AMP synthesis by inhibiting adenylate cyclase activity (Numano et al 1995). Activated platelets also increase intracellular Ca^{2+} concentration both by enhancing the entry of Ca^{2+} into endothelial cells (Kishi et al 1992a) and by mobilizing intracellular Ca^{2+} in these cells. Injured arterial endothelial cells in turn activate platelets to accelerate platelet adhesion to, and thrombus formation at, the injured site. In an insightful study, Kishi et al (1992b) reported concomitant increases in thromboxane B_2 and 6-keto-prostaglandin $F_{1\alpha}$ in volunteers without ischemic heart disease after treadmill exercise, demonstrating a balanced response between platelet and endothelial cell activation. In contrast to this balance, plasma thromboxane B_2 levels increased in patients with ischemic heart disease following exercise, and without any changes in the levels of 6-keto-prostaglandin $F_{1\alpha}$. These latter data suggest an impaired ability of ischemic vessels to moderate the interactions between the vessel wall and activated platelets.

The results of a large-scale, randomized, double-blind, placebo-controlled trial evaluating the effects of aspirin on evolving myocardial infarction have been reported (ISIS-2 Collaborative Group 1988). This study randomized over 17 000 patients, admitted to hospital on suspicion of evolving myocardial infarction up to 24 h earlier, to receive a single infusion of streptokinase over 1 h, or daily aspirin (162 mg) for 30 days, or both treatments, or neither drug. The authors reported that aspirin reduced non-fatal myocardial infarction or stroke by over 40%, and effected a 26% reduction in vascular death in the following 5 weeks. Aspirin (325 mg on alternate days) was also highly beneficial in reducing the risk of myocardial infarction (but not stroke) in male physicians aged 40–84 years in a study lasting over 60 months. Aspirin use did not alter the risk of angina in this study (Hennekens & Eberlein 1985).

It is worth noting that some studies have reported antithrombin drugs such as heparin to be as effective as antiplatelet therapy for treating unstable angina or acute myocardial infarction (Theroux et al 1988, 1992, 1993, Lau et al 1992). The combination of heparin and aspirin may also be more beneficial than heparin alone (Theroux et al 1992). However, doses of heparin not adjusted to prolong the activated partial thromboplastin time by approximately 2-fold may not be as effective as 75 mg of aspirin per day (The RISK Group 1990). Finally, in the context of arterial thrombosis, it may be appropriate to consider heparin as an indirect antiplatelet drug in the light of its ability to inhibit prothrombin activation and also inhibit thrombin-mediated activation of platelets.

Another antiplatelet strategy for inhibiting the adhesion of platelets to injured vessels and the subsequent recruitment of new platelets and their cohesion is the use of a monoclonal antiplatelet glycoprotein IIb/IIIa antibody. This heterodimeric glycoprotein undergoes a Ca^{2+}-dependent conformational change upon platelet activation to become a receptor for fibrinogen, which in turn bridges platelets together. A monoclonal antibody to both the native and activated conformers of glycoprotein IIb/IIIa (c7E3) abolishes platelet aggregation to all platelet agonists and prolongs bleeding (Yasuda et al 1988). The efficacy of c7E3 was evaluated in a clinical trial involving 2100 high-risk patients undergoing angioplasty or atherectomy (because of unstable angina and evolving myocardial infarction) randomized to receive either a bolus of 0.25 µg/kg c7E3 plus placebo infusion, or the same bolus of c7E3 plus an infusion of 10 µg/min for 12 h, or a bolus placebo injection followed by the infusion of placebo (The EPIC Investigators 1994). The most effective regimen for reducing non-fatal myocardial infarction, and the need for emergency PTCA (percutaneous transluminal coronary angioplasty) was the c7E3 bolus plus infusion regimen. A 6-month follow-up of the patients demonstrated a 35% reduction in major ischemic event (death, myocardial infarction, or urgent revascularization) at 30 days, and a 27% reduction at 6 months (Topol et al 1994). Thus, this antagonist of platelet GPIIb/IIIa, given for 12 h only, can markedly reduce the incidence of adverse events in arterial thrombosis.

Another receptor antagonist (ridogerel, a blocker of thromboxane A_2/prostaglandin endoperoxide receptors which also inactivates cyclooxygenase) was compared with aspirin in a study involving 907 patients with acute myocardial infarction who were all given streptokinase. A similar vessel patency (approx. 70%) was found in the two treatment arms. However, there were 32% fewer new ischemic events with ridogerel than with aspirin (The RAPT Investigators 1994). Thus, platelet receptor antagonists show reasonable promise as prophylactic and therapeutic agents in arterial thrombosis.

ANTITHROMBINS IN ARTERIAL THROMBOSIS

A few recent studies have evaluated the clinical effectiveness of hirudin and a synthetic, modified truncated hirudin (hirulog) in unstable angina (Cannon et al 1993, Topol et al 1993, GUSTO IIa Investigators 1994, Neuhaus et al 1994, Fuchs et al 1995). An unacceptably high bleeding rate with hirudin was observed in the largest planned study after approximately 25% of the patients had been randomized to receive heparin or hirudin during the initial treatment of unstable angina (GUSTO IIa Investigators 1994). The dose of hirudin used in this trial was a 0.6 mg/kg bolus followed by an infusion of 0.2 mg/kg/h[1] hirudin. In another trial comparing heparin with hirudin to prevent accumulation of thrombi in the coronary arteries of patients with unstable angina (rest ischemic pain, abnormal ECG and ≥60% stenosis of culprit vessels), the 116 patients treated with intravenous hirudin tended to show more improvement over the 3–5 days of treatment than the patients receiving intravenous heparin. The number of patients evaluated, however, was too small to justify definitive conclusions about the effectiveness of hirudin in preventing the potential consequences of unstable angina (Topol et al 1994). Another recent pilot study which compared hirudin (0.4 mg/kg body weight plus 0.15 mg/kg by infusion) with heparin (70 IU/kg body weight bolus plus 15 IU/kg/h[1]) for 48 h in 1000 patients with acute myocardial infarction was stopped after approximately 300 patients had been enrolled. Unacceptably high rates of intracranial bleeding and stroke were observed in the hirudin group (Neuhaus et al 1994). Major spontaneous hemorrhage at a non-intracranial site also occurred in a third comparative study of hirudin with heparin in myocardial infarction (Antman 1994).

Hirulog has been compared with heparin as the anticoagulant in angioplasty for unstable angina or postinfarction angina in a study involving approximately 4000 patients (Bittl et al 1995). The authors concluded that hirulog was at least as effective as heparin in preventing ischemic complications in the patients with unstable angina and with a lower bleeding risk. A total of 410 patients with unstable angina have received hirulog (up to 1 mg/kg/h[1]) for 72 h together with 325 mg of aspirin daily (Fuchs et al 1995). Non-fatal myocardial infarction was observed in 16 of 160 patients receiving 0.02 mg/kg/h[1] hirulog compared to a total of eight such events in the 250 patients who received between 0.25 and 1.0 mg/kg/h[1] hirulog during the 6 weeks of observation. Significant unsatisfactory outcomes after hospital discharge were noted in all four treatment groups (Fuchs et al 1995). Thus, both the effective dose of hirulog when used in conjunction with aspirin and the minimum duration of therapy remain to be established.

SUMMARY

The inflammatory reactions associated with clinically significant atherosclerosis and arterial thrombosis facilitate platelet activation in vivo and the participation of platelets in propagating these disease entities which are principal causes of hospitalization and death. Activated platelets synthesize thromboxane A_2 which facilitates the recruitment of other platelets and their adhesion and cohesion to atherosclerotic vessel walls and facilitates plasma and leukocyte infiltration into the arterial wall. A major inhibitor of platelet adhesion (and the subsequent cohesion) to the endothelium is prostacyclin, which is synthesized by activated endothelial cells. The chronic injury to endothelial cells compromise their ability to synthesize prostacyclin, and thus to inhibit the additional ongoing damage to the vessel wall by activated platelets and inflammatory leukocytes. Aspirin, at doses which completely inhibit platelet cyclooxygenase (and thus the synthesis of thromboxane A_2 by activated platelets), also inhibits platelet-dependent thrombin production, and thus moderates the ability of the platelets to become incorporated into occlusive platelet-dependent thrombi in arteries with narrowed lumens (as a result of severe atherosclerosis) or in arteries with ruptured atherosclerotic plaques. Several well-designed clinical trials involving tens of thousands of patients have demonstrated a significant benefit for aspirin (≥ 75 mg/day) in reducing some of the consequences of unstable angina (ischemic pain, myocardial infarction, stroke and death), and in preventing myocardial infarction in patients at risk. The adjunctive use of aspirin with thrombolytic drugs and/or heparin has also shown significant clinical benefit. Also promising are the initial results of platelet receptor (thromboxane A_2 or fibrinogen receptor) antagonists. The well-established clinical efficacy of aspirin in atherosclerosis and arterial thrombosis highlights the important role of platelets in atherosclerosis and arterial thrombosis.

REFERENCES

Antiplatelet Trialists' Collaboration 1994a Collaborative overview of randomized trials of antiplatelet therapy. I: Prevention of death, myocardial infarction, and stroke by prolonged anti-platelet therapy in various categories of patients. Br Med J 308: 81–106

Antiplatelet Trialists' Collaboration 1994b Collaborative overview of randomized trials of antiplatelet therapy. II: Maintenance of vascular graft or arterial patency by antiplatelet therapy. Br Med J 308: 159–168

Antiplatelet Trialists' Collaboration 1994c Collaborative overview of randomized trials of antiplatelet therapy. III: Reduction in venous thrombosis and pulmonary embolism by antiplatelet prophylaxis among surgical and medical patients. Br Med J 308: 235–346

Antman E M 1994 Hirudin in acute myocardial infarction. Safety report from the Thrombolysis and Thrombin Inhibition in Myocardial Infarction (TIMI) 9A trial. Circulation 90: 1624–1640

Bevilacqua M P, Pober J S, Majean G R et al 1984 Interleukin (IL-1)-induced biosynthesis and cell expression of procoagulant activity in human vascular endothelial cells. J Exp Med 160: 618–623

Bevilacqua M, Pober J S, Wheeler M E et al 1985 Interleukin-1 activation of vascular endothelium. Effects on procoagulant activity and leukocyte adhesion. Am J Pathol 121: 394–403

Bini A, Kudryk B A 1995 Fibrinogen in human atherosclerosis. Ann N Y Acad Sci 748: 461–470

Bini A, Fenoglio J J Jr, Sobel J et al 1987 Immunochemical characterization of fibrinogen, fibrin I, and fibrin II in human thrombi and atherosclerotic lesions. Blood 69: 1038–1045

Bini A, Fenoglio J, Mesa-Tejada R et al 1989 Identification and distribution of fibrinogen, fibrin and fibrin(ogen) degradation products in atherosclerosis. Use of monoclonal antibodies. Arteriosclerosis 9: 109–121

Bittl J A, Strony J, Brinker J A et al 1995 Treatment with bivalirudin (hirulog) as compared with heparin during coronary angioplasty for unstable or post infarction angina. N Engl J Med 333: 764–769

Bornfeldt K E, Raines E W, Nakano T et al 1994 IGF-1 and PDFG-BB induce directed migration of human arterial smooth muscle cells via signalling pathways that are distinct from those of proliferation. J Clin Invest 93: 1266–1274

Brannstrom M, Jansson J H, Burman K et al 1995 Endothelial haemostatic factors may be associated with mortality in patients on long-term anticoagulant treatment. Thromb Haemost 74: 612–615

Cairns J A, Gent M, Singer J et al 1985 Aspirin, sulfinpyraxone, or both in unstable angina. N Engl J Med 313: 1369–1375

Cannon C P, Maraganore J M, Loscalzo J et al 1993 Anticoagulant effects of hirulog, a novel thrombin inhibitor, in patients with coronary artery disease. Am J Cardiol 71: 778–782

Celi A, Pellegrini G, Lorenzet R et al 1994 P-Selectin induces the expression of tissue factor on monocytes. Proc Natl Acad Sci USA 91: 8767–8771

Cortellaro M, Boschetti C, Cofrancesco E et al 1992 The PLAT study: hemostatic function in relation to atherothrombotic ischemic events in vascular disease patients. Arterioscler Thromb 12: 1063–1070

Cortellaro M, Confransesco E, Boschetti C et al 1993 Increased fibrin turnover and high PAI-1 activity as predictive events in atherosclerotic patients. A case-control study. Arterioscler Thromb 13: 1412–1417

Davies M J 1994 Pathology of arterial thrombosis. Br Med Bull 50: 789–802

Davies M J, Woolf N, Rowles P M et al 1988 Morphology of the endothelium over atherosclerotic plaques in human coronary arteries. Br Heart J 60: 459–464

Davies M J, Bland M J, Hangartner W R et al 1989 Factors influencing the presence or absence of acute coronary thrombi in sudden ischemic death. Eur Heart J 10: 203–208

Eisenberg P R, Lucore C, Kaufman L et al 1990 Fibrinopeptide A levels indicative of pulmonary vascular thrombosis in patients with primary pulmonary hypertension. Circulation 82: 841–847

Falk E 1992 Why do plaques rupture? Circulation 86 (suppl III): 30–42

Fitzgerald D J, Fitzgerald G A 1989 The role of thrombin and thromboxane A_2 in vascular reocclusion following coronary thrombolysis with tissue type plasminogen activator. Proc Natl Acad Sci USA 86: 7585–7589

Fitzgerald D J, Roy L, Catella F et al 1986 Platelet activation in unstable coronary disease. N Engl J Med 315: 393–399

Fitzgerald D J, Catella F, Roy L et al 1988 Platelet activation in vivo after intravenous streptokinase. Circulation 7: 142–150

Fuchs J, Cannon C P, Cannon M D et al 1995 Hirulog in the treatment of unstable angina. Circulation 92: 727–733

Ghaddar H M, Cortes J, Salomaa V et al 1995 Correlation of specific platelet activation markers with carotid arterial wall thickness. Thromb Haemost 74: 943–948

The Global Use of Strategies to Open Occluded Coronary Arteries (GUSTO) IIa Investigators 1994 Randomized trial of intravenous heparin versus recombinant hirudin for acute coronary syndromes. Circulation 90: 1631–1637

Guyton J R, Klemp K F 1994 Development of the atherosclerotic core region. Chemical and ultrastructural analysis of microdi secreted atherosclerotic lesions from human aorta. Arterioscler Thromb 14: 1305–1314

Hamm C W, Lorenz R L, Bleifeld W et al 1987 Biochemical evidence of platelet activation in patients with persistent unstable angina. J Am Coll Cardiol 10: 998–1004

Hamstein A, DeFaire U, Walldius G et al 1987 Plasminogen activator inhibitor in plasma: risk factor for recurrent myocardial infarction. Lancet ii: 3–9

Hangartner J, Charleston A, Davies M et al 1986 Morphological characteristics of clinically significant coronary artery stenosis in stable angina. Br Heart J 56: 501–508

Harker L A, Gent M 1994 Antiplatelet agents in the management of thrombotic disorders. In: Colman R W, Hirsh J, Marder V J, Salzman E W (eds) Haemostasis and Thrombosis: Basic Principles and Clinical Practice, 3rd edn. J B Lippincott, Philadelphia, pp 1506–1513

Heinrich J, Balleisen L, Schulte H et al 1994 Fibrinogen and factor VII in the prediction of coronary risk. Results from the PROCAMA study in healthy men. Arterioscler Thromb 14: 54–59

Hennekens C H, Buring J E 1994 Aspirin in the primary prevention of cardiovascular disease. Cardiol Clin 12: 443–450

Hennekens C H, Eberlein K 1985 A randomized trial of aspirin and β-carotene among US physicians. Prev Med 14: 165–168

ISIS-2 (2nd International Study of Infarct Survival) Collaborative Group 1988 Randomized trial of intravenous streptokinase, oral aspirin, both or neither among 17,187 cases of suspected acute myocardial infarction: ISIS-2. Lancet ii: 349–360

Iwamoto T, Kubo H, Takasaki M 1995 Platelet activation in the cerebral circulation in different subtypes of ischemic stroke and Binswayer's disease. Stroke 26: 52–56

Jansson J H, Nilsson T K, Johnson O 1991a von Willebrand factor in plasma: a novel risk factor for recurrent myocardial infarction. Br Heart J 66: 351–355

Jansson J H, Nilsson T K, Olofsson B O 1991b The tissue plasminogen activator and other risk factors as predictors of cardiovascular events in patients with severe angina sectors. Br Heart J 12: 157–161

Jouve R, Rolland P H, Delboy C, Mercier C 1984 Thromboxane B$_2$, 6-keto-PGF$_{1\alpha}$, PGE$_2$, PGF$_{2\alpha}$ and PGA$_1$ plasma levels in arteriosclerosis obliterans: relationship to clinical manifestations, risk factors and arterial pathoanatomy. Am Heart J 107: 45–52

Kannel W B, Wolf P A, Castelli W P et al 1987 Fibrinogen and risk of cardiovascular disease. JAMA 258: 1183–1186

Katsuda S, Boyd H C, Flinger C et al 1990 Human atherosclerosis: immunocytochemical analysis of the cell composition of lesions of young adults. Am J Pathol 140: 907–914

Kerins D M, Roy L, FitzGerald G A et al 1989 Platelet and vascular function during coronary thrombolysis with tissue-type plasminogen activator. Circulation 80: 1718–1725

Kienast J, Thompson S G, Raskino C et al 1993 Prothrombin activation fragment 1+2 and thrombin antithrombin III complexes in patients with angina pectoris: relation to the presence and severity of coronary atherosclerosis. Thromb Haemost 70: 550–553

Kishi Y, Ashikaga T, Numano F 1992a Alteration in adenyl nucleotide metabolites in coronary smooth muscle cells by activated platelets. Thromb Res 65: 571–584

Kishi Y, Ashikaga T, Numano F 1992b Inhibition of platelet aggregation by prostacyclin is attenuated after exercise in patients with angina pectoris. Am Heart J 123: 291–297

Lassila R 1993 Inflammation in atheroma: implications for plaque rupture and platelet-collagen interaction. Eur Heart J 14: 94–97

Lassila R, Peltonen S, Lepantolo M et al 1993 Severity of peripheral atherosclerosis is associated with fibrinogen and degradation of cross-linked fibrin. Arterioscler Thromb 13: 1738–1742

Lau J, Antman E M, Jimenez-Silva J et al 1992 Cumulative meta-analysis of therapeutic trials for myocardial infarction. N Engl J Med 237: 248–254

Leatham E W, Bath P M W, Tooze J A et al 1995 Increased monocyte tissue factor expression in coronary disease. Br Heart J 73: 10–13

Lee K L, Califf R M, Simes J, van de Werf F 1994 Holding GUSTO up to the light. Ann Intern Med 120: 876–881

Lee A J, Fowkes F G R, Lowe G D O et al 1995 Fibrin D-dimer, hemostatic factors and peripheral artery disease. Thromb Haemost 74: 828–832

Lewis H D, Davis J W, Archibald D G et al 1983 Protective effects of aspirin against acute myocardial infarction and death in men with unstable angina. N Engl J Med 309: 396–403

Liu L, Freedman J, Hornstein A et al 1994 Thrombin binding to platelets and their activation in plasma. Br J Haematol 88: 592–600

Margaglione M, Di Minno G, Grandone E et al 1994 Abnormally high circulation levels of tissue plasminogen activation and plasminogen activator inhibitor-1 in patients with a history of stroke. Arterioscler Thromb 14: 1741–1745

Matsuda T, Morishita E, Jokaji H et al 1995 Plasminogen activator inhibitor in plasma and arteriosclerosis. Ann NY Acad Sci 748: 394–398

Meade T W, Mellows S, Brozovic M et al 1986 Hemostatic function and ischemic heart disease: principal results of the Northwick Park Heart Study. Lancet ii: 533–537

Merlini P A, Bauer K A, Oltrona L et al 1994 Persistent activation of coagulation mechanism in unstable angina and myocardial infarction. Circulation 90: 61–68

Moncada S, Vane J R 1979 Arachidonic acid metabolites and the interaction between platelets and blood vessel walls. N Engl J Med 300: 1142–1147

Moor E, Hamstein A, Karpe F et al 1994 Relationship of tissue factor pathway inhibitor activity to plasma lipoproteins and myocardial infarction at a young age. Thromb Haemost 71: 707–712

Neuhaus K L, von Essen R, Tebbe E et al 1994 Safety observations from the pilot phase of the randomized r-hirudin for improvement of thrombolysis (HIT-III) study. Circulation 90: 1638–1642

Neumann F J, Ott I, Gawaz M et al 1995 Cardiac release of cytokines and inflammatory responses in acute myocardial infarction. Circulation 92: 748–755

Nichols A B, Owen J, Kaplan K L et al 1982 Fibrinopeptide A platelet factor 4 and β-thromboglobulin levels in coronary heart disease. Blood 60: 650–654

Numano F, Yajima K, Nishiyama K et al 1982 Effects of thromboxane A_2 injection on the rabbit coronary artery. Atherosclerosis 76: 95–1101

Numano F, Kishi Y, Ashikaga T et al 1995 What effect does controlling platelets have on atherosclerosis. Ann N Y Acad Sci 748: 383–392

Rapold J H, Haeberl A, Kuemmerli H et al 1989 Fibrin formation and platelet activation in patients with myocardial infarction and normal coronary arteries. Eur Heart J 10: 323–333

Reilly I A G, Foran J B, Smith B et al 1986 Increased thromboxane biosynthesis in human preparation of platelet activation. Biochemical consequences of selective inhibition of thromboxane synthase. Circulation 73: 1300–1309

Ross R 1993 The pathogenesis of atherosclerosis: a perspective for the 1990s. Nature 362: 801–809

Ross R 1995 Growth regulatory mechanism and formation of the lesions of atherosclerosis. Ann NY Acad Sci 748: 1–4

Rugman F P, Jenkins J A, Duguid J K et al 1994 Prothrombin fragment F1+2: correlations with cardiovascular risk factors. Blood Coagulat Fibrinol 5: 335–340

Sako D, Chang X J, Barone K M et al 1993 Expression cloning of a functional glycoprotein ligand for P-selectin. Cell 75: 1179–1186

Saksela O, Rifkin D B 1988 Cell-associated plasminogen activator and physiological functions. Annu Rev Cell Biol 4: 93–126

Shapiro S D, Campbell E J, Kobayashi D K et al 1990 Immuno-modulation of metalloproteinase production in human macrophages. J Clin Invest 86: 1204–1210

Shatos M A, Orfeo T, Doherty J M et al 1995 α–Thrombin stimulates urokinase production and DNA synthesis in cultured cerebral microvascular endothelial cells. Arterioscler Thromb 15: 903–911

Singh T M, Kadowski M H, Glacov S et al 1990 Role of fibrinopeptide B in early atherosclerotic lesion formation. Am J Surg 160: 156–159

Smith E, Ashall C 1985 Fibrinolysis and plasminogen concentration in aortic intima and relation to death following myocardial information. Atherosclerosis 55: 171–186

Sower L E, Froelich C J, Carney D H et al 1995 Thrombin induces IL-6 production in fibroblasts and epithelial cells. Evidence for the involvement of the seven transmembrane receptor for α-thrombin. J Immunol 155: 895–901

Stary H C, Blankenhorn D H, Chandler A B et al 1992 A definition of the intima of human arteries and its atherosclerotic prone regions. Circulation 85: 391–405

Stary H C, Chandler A B, Glagov S et al 1994 A definition of initial, fatty streak, and intermediate lesions of atherosclerosis. Arterioscler Thromb 14: 840–856

Stary H C, Chandler A B, Dinsmore R E et al 1995 A definition of advanced types of atherosclerotic lesions and a histological classification of atherosclerosis. Circulation 92: 1355–1374

Steinberg D 1992 Antioxidants and atherosclerosis. A current assessment. Circulation 84: 1420–1425

Sueishi K, Ichikawa K, Nagakawa K et al 1995 Procoagulant properties of the atherosclerotic aorta. Ann N Y Acad Sci 748: 185–192

Sumiyoshi A Y, Asada Y, Tayashi K 1991 Platelets and intimal thickening. In: Tanaka T (ed) Advances in Thrombosis and Fibrinolysis. Academic Press, Tokyo, pp 169–180

Sumiyoshi A, Asada Y, Marutsuka K 1995 Platelets and intimal thickening. Ann NY Acad Sci 748: 74–85

Szczeklik A, Dropinski J, Radwan J et al 1992 Persistent generation of thrombin after acute myocardial infarction. Arterioscler Thromb 12: 548–553

Takano K, Yamaguchi T, Uchida K 1992 Markers of a hypercoagulable state following acute ischemic stroke. Stroke 23: 194–198

Taubman M B, Marmur J D, Rosenfield C-L et al 1993 Agonist-mediated tissue factor expression in cultured vascular smooth muscle cells. J Clin Invest 91: 547–552

The EPIC Investigators 1994 Use of a monoclonal antibody directed against the platelet glycoprotein IIb/IIIa receptor in high-risk coronary angioplasty. N Engl J Med 330: 956–961

The RAPT Investigators 1994 Randomized trial of ridogerel, a combined thromboxane A₂/prostaglandin endoperoxide receptor antagonist versus aspirin as adjunct to thrombolysis in patients with acute myocardial infarction. Circulation 89: 588–595

The RISK Group 1990 Risk of myocardial infarction and death during treatment with low dose aspirin and intravenous heparin in men with unstable coronary artery disease. Lancet 336: 827–830

Theroux P, Latour J G, Leger-Gauthier C et al 1987 Fibrinopeptide A and platelet factor levels in unstable angina pectoris. Circulation 75: 156–162

Theroux P, Oumet H, McCans J et al 1988 Aspirin, heparin, or both to treat acute unstable angina. N Engl J Med 319: 105–111

Theroux P, Waters D, Lam J et al 1992 Reactivation of unstable angina after the discontinuation of heparin. N Engl J Med 327: 141–145

Theroux P, Waters D, Qiu S et al 1993 Aspirin versus heparin to prevent myocardial infarction during the acute phase of unstable angina. Circulation 88: 2045–2048

Thompson S G, Kienast J, Pyke S D M et al 1995 Hemostatic factors and the risk for myocardial infarction or sudden death in patients with angina pectoris. N Engl J Med 332: 635–641

Topol E J, Bonan R, Jewitt R et al 1993 Use of a direct antithrombin, hirulog, in place of heparin during coronary angioplasty. Circulation 87: 1622–1629

Topol E J, Califf R M, Weisman H F et al 1994 Randomized trial of coronary intervention with antibody against platelet IIb/IIIa integrin for reduction of clinical restenosis: results at 6 months. Lancet 343: 881–886

Van Hulsteijn H, Kolff J, Briet E et al 1984 Fibrinopeptide A and β-thromboglobulin in patients with angina pectoris and acute myocardial infarction. Am Heart J 107: 39–45

Wallentin L C, the RISC Group 1991 Aspirin (75 mg/day) after an episode of unstable coronary artery disease: long term effects on the risk for myocardial infarction, occurrence of severe angina and the need for revascularization. J Am Coll Cardiol 18: 1587–1593

Wilcox J N, Smith K M, Schwartz S M et al 1989 Localization of tissue factor in the normal vessel wall and in the atherosclerotic plaque. Proc Natl Acad Sci USA 86: 2839–2843

Wilhelmsen L, Svardsudd K, Korsan-Bengtsen K et al 1984 Fibrinogen as a risk factor for stroke and myocardial infarction. N Engl J Med 311: 501–505

Yarnell J W G, Baker I, Sweetman P M et al 1991 Fibrinogen viscosity and white blood cell count are major risk factors for ischemic heart disease. Circulation 83: 836–844

Yasu T, Oshima S, Imanishi M et al 1993 Effects of aspirin DL-lysine on thrombin generation in unstable angina pectoris. Am J Cardiol 71: 1164–1168

Yasuda T, Gold H K, Fallon J T et al 1988 Monoclonal antibody against the platelet glycoprotein (GP) IIb/IIIa receptor prevents coronary artery reocclusion after reperfusion with recombinant tissue-type plasminogen activator in dogs. J Clin Invest 81: 1284–1291

4. Inherited resistance to activated protein C as a pathogenic risk factor for venous thrombosis

B. Zöller   B. Dahlbäck

Venous thromboembolism is an important health problem, annually affecting 1 per 1000 individuals (Kirkegaard et al 1980), as well as being the most common cause of death associated with major orthopedic surgery (Bertina 1988). Although acquired risk factors, such as surgery, pregnancy and oral contraceptives, often precipitate thrombosis (Malm et al 1992), a positive family history can be found in 24–40% of thrombosis patients (Heijboer et al 1990, Malm et al 1992). This suggests that venous thrombosis is a multifactorial disease affecting genetically predisposed individuals when exposed to circumstantial risk factors. Until recently, the major known genetic risk factors were deficiencies of protein C, protein S, and antithrombin III, which together only accounted for 5–10% of those with thrombosis (Gladson et al 1988, Ben-Tal et al 1989, Heijboer et al 1990, Tabernero et al 1991, Malm et al 1992). Progress has been made with the recent discovery of inherited resistance to activated protein C (APC resistance) as a pathogenic risk factor for thrombosis (Dahlbäck et al 1993). APC resistance is caused by a single point mutation in the factor V gene, which predicts replacement of $Arg(R)^{506}$ in one of the APC cleavage sites with a Gln(Q) (Bertina et al 1994, Greengard et al 1994, Voorberg et al 1994, Zöller & Dahlbäck 1994, Zöller et al 1994). Mutated activated factor V ($FVa:Q^{506}$) is less efficiently degraded by APC than normal factor Va (factor $Va:R^{506}$), which leads to increased thrombin generation and a hypercoagulable state (Bertina et al 1994, Majerus 1994, Sun et al 1994, Kalafatis et al 1995). APC resistance is now known to be a major risk factor for venous thrombosis (Griffin et al 1993, Koster et al 1993, Svensson & Dahlbäck et al 1994). Unlike other genetic risk factors for thrombosis, APC resistance is highly prevalent in the general population. The recent observation of APC resistance in a high proportion of thrombosis-prone families with inherited protein C or protein S deficiency suggests that thrombophilia may be the result of multiple genetic defects (Koeleman et al 1994, Zöller et al 1995a). APC resistance and other genetic defects of the protein C anticoagulant system associated with inherited thrombophilia will be reviewed. For a description of antithrombin III deficiency the reader is referred to a recent review (Lane et al 1992).

THE PROTEIN C ANTICOAGULANT PATHWAY

The cascade of proteolytic events that leads to explosive thrombin generation is controlled by several physiologically important mechanisms, one of which is the protein C anticoagulant system (Fig. 4.1) (reviewed in Esmon 1989, Dahlbäck and Stenflo 1994, Dahlbäck 1995). Thrombin generated at sites of vascular injury has procoagulant effects as it activates factors V and VIII (to Va and VIIIa, in a positive feedback reaction), activates platelets and converts fibrinogen to insoluble fibrin. In contrast, thrombin generated at sites of intact vasculature attains anticoagulant properties as a result of its binding to the endothelial membrane protein thrombomodulin (TM). Binding of thrombin to TM is associated with modulation of the proteolytic specificity of thrombin; procoagulant properties are lost and the ability to activate protein C is gained. APC inhibits blood coagulation by proteolytic inactivation of factor Va and factor VIIIa. These reactions are stimulated by two cofactors: protein S and the unactivated form of factor V (Shen & Dahlbäck 1994, Dahlbäck et al 1995). The major physiological importance of the protein C anticoagulant system is illustrated by the severe thromboembolic disorder which affects individuals with homozygous protein C deficiency already in the neonatal period (Marlar et al 1988).

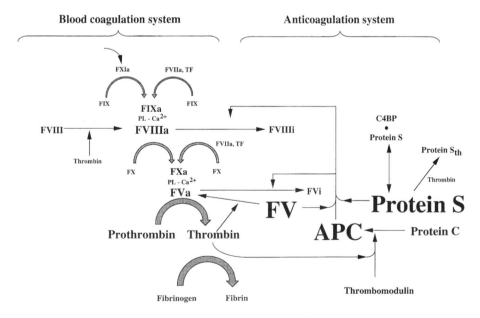

Fig. 4.1 Schematic representation of reactions involved in blood coagulation and the protein C anticoagulant system. Activated protein C (APC), together with its two cofactors protein S and intant factor V, degrades the activated forms of factors V and VIII. The APC cofactor function of factor V is lost upon thrombin cleavage. Thrombin cleavage of protein S also results in the loss of APC cofactor activity. TF denotes tissue factor which triggers the reactions involving factor VII. (Modified from Dahlbäck & Stenflo 1994 with permission.)

PROTEIN C DEFICIENCY

Heterozygous protein C deficiency is found in 2–5% of patients with deep venous thrombosis (Heijboer et al 1990, Tabernero et al 1991, Malm et al 1992). In thrombosis-prone families with protein C deficiency, approximately 50% of the affected members have suffered a thrombotic episode before the age of 30–45 years, which suggests an autosomal dominant mode of inheritance and protein C deficiency as a strong risk factor for thrombosis (Broekmans & Conard 1988, Bovill et al 1989, Reitsma et al 1991, Allaart et al 1993). This idea was challenged by the identification of protein C deficiency in 0.3% of healthy blood donors, the families of whom did not have a high incidence of thrombosis (Miletich et al 1987). In these families, only individuals with homozygous or compound heterozygous protein C deficiency had severe thrombotic disease, suggesting a recessive mode of inheritance (Seligsohn et al 1984). The molecular basis for the difference between dominant and recessive protein C deficiency has been enigmatic and it was particularly puzzling when the same mutation was identified in both types of families (Reitsma et al 1991). It has been proposed that thrombosis-prone families with protein C deficiency may suffer from additional genetic risk factors of thrombosis (Miletich et al 1993). This concept gained support by the recent demonstration of APC resistance as an additional genetic risk factor in 19% of Dutch thrombosis-prone protein C deficient families (nine out of 48 families) (Koeleman et al 1994). In six families, two-locus linkage analysis supported the assumption that the factor V and protein C genes were the two loci responsible for the thrombophilia.

Two types of protein C deficiency have been described: both protein C antigen and functional activity are reduced in type I deficiency, whereas only the functional activity is reduced in type II deficiency. The genetic defects have been identified in many cases and a mutation database is available (Reitsma et al 1993). Of a total of 67 different single base-pair substitutions, 29(43%) occur in CpG dinucleotides – compatible with a model of methylation-mediated deamination.

During the initiating phase of oral anticoagulant therapy, individuals with protein C deficiency are at risk of developing skin necrosis (Broekmans & Conard 1988). This is believed to be due to a temporary imbalance between pro- and anticoagulant forces which is the result of the shorter half-life of protein C ($t_{1/2} \approx 8$ h) compared to those of factors IX, X and prothrombin. High initial doses of coumarin should therefore be avoided (Broekmans & Conard 1988).

PROTEIN S DEFICIENCY

Protein S deficiency, which is now a well-established cause of familial thrombophilia (Comp & Esmon 1984, Comp et al 1984, Schwarz et al 1984, Engesser et al 1987, Briet et al 1988, Zöller et al 1995a,b), is found in 1.5–7% of patients with thromboembolic disease (Broekmans et al 1986,

Heijboer et al 1990, Tabernero et al 1991, Malm et al 1992). The prevalence of protein S deficiency in the general population is not known. As in the case of protein C deficiency, APC resistance has been found to be an additional genetic risk factor in several thrombosis-prone families with protein S deficiency (Zöller et al 1995b).

In plasma, 60–70% of protein S is bound to C4b-binding protein (C4BP) – a regulatory protein of the classical complement pathway (reviewed in Dahlbäck & Stenflo 1994). Only the free form of protein S is active as cofactor to APC. Some protein S deficient patients have low plasma levels of free protein S, whereas their total protein S levels are normal (Comp et al 1984, Chafa et al 1989, Iijima et al 1989, Lauer et al 1990, Malm et al 1992); this is referred to as type III deficiency (nomenclature proposed by Bertina at the ISTH Subcommittee Meeting 1991). Other patients present with decreased plasma levels of both free and complexed protein S (Comp & Esmon 1984, Bertina 1985, Briet et al 1988) – referred to as type I. Type II is characterized by a functional defect in individuals having normal protein S antigen levels (Mannucci et al 1989, Maccaferri et al 1991). Recently, it has been shown that most individuals previously classified as having type II deficiency do no have a defect in their protein S gene, but that they instead suffer from APC resistance (Faioni et al 1993, 1994, Cooper et al 1994). The reason for this misclassification is that $FV:Q^{506}$, which is present in APC-resistant plasma, affects coagulation-based functional assays for protein S.

The molecular difference between type I and type III protein S deficiencies has until recently remained elusive. In the course of characterizing thrombosis-prone families with protein S deficiency, we found coexistence of type I and type III deficiency in 14 out of 18 families (Zöller et al 1995b) (Fig. 4.2). This suggested that the two types of protein S deficiency are phenotypic variants of the same genetic disease. There was a perfect autosomal dominant pattern of inheritance of free protein S deficiency, whereas the penetrance of total protein S deficiency was incomplete. Thus, it can be concluded that measurements of free protein S is a sine qua non in the characterization of protein S deficiency. In these families, protein S deficiency was associated with an increased risk of thrombosis, 50% of protein S deficient relatives having had one or more thrombotic events before the age of 45 years; the corresponding number among normal relatives was 12%. There was no significant difference in thrombosis-free survival between type I and type III deficient relatives.

To understand the molecular mechanisms involved in the expression of the two phenotypes of protein S deficiency types I and III, a detailed knowledge of the C4BP subunit structure and of the physiological regulation of the plasma levels of the C4BP isoforms and protein S is required. In plasma, C4BP is composed of six or seven α-chains and one or no β-chain; only the latter contains the protein S binding site (Dahlbäck 1991, Härdig et al 1993). Thus, of the different C4BP isoforms that are present in plasma,

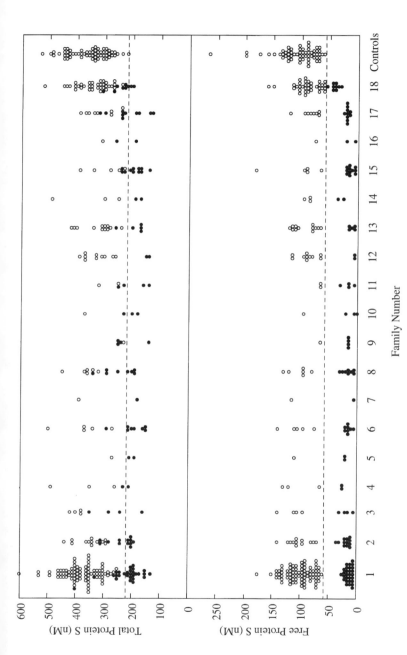

Fig. 4.2 Type I and type III protein S deficiencies are phenotypic variants of the same genetic disease. Plasma levels of free and total protein S in 307 non-anticoagulated members from 18 unrelated families with protein S deficiency. The lower normal reference levels for free and total protein S are indicated by dashed lines (56 nM and 219 nM, respectively). Individuals with free protein S below 56 nM are considered to be protein S deficient (●). In all families, the difference between protein S deficient and normal relatives was most evident from results of measurements of free protein S. The overlap in total protein S levels between normal and protein S deficient cases illustrates the coexistence of type I and type III deficiencies in 14 of the families. (From Zöller et al 1995b with permission.)

only those containing the β-chain (C4BPβ+) bind protein S (Hillarp & Dahlbäck 1988, Hillarp et al 1989). Under physiological conditions, the protein S–C4BP interaction is of high affinity and the equilibrium is shifted towards complex formation (Dahlbäck 1991). The concentration of free protein S in plasma is equal to the molar excess of protein S over C4BPβ+ (Griffin et al 1992, Garcia de Frutos et al 1994). Thus, the concentrations of protein S and C4BPβ+ are the only parameters which determine the level of free protein S. During acute phase reactions, the relative proportion of C4BP isoforms lacking the β-chain increases, which ensures stable levels of free protein S despite the high plasma levels of total C4BP (Garcia de Frutos et al 1994).

In protein S deficiency, the low free protein S concentration (16 ± 10 nmol/l) is the result of equimolar concentrations of total protein S (215 ± 50 nmol/l) and C4BPβ+ (228 ± 51 nmol/l) in combination with a high-affinity interaction between the two proteins (Zöller et al 1995b). In protein S deficient cases, as well as in normal individuals, there is a high correlation between the plasma concentrations of protein S and C4BPβ+, suggesting the plasma concentrations of these two proteins are regulated by similar mechanisms. The two types of protein S deficiency differ in that individuals with type III deficiency have higher plasma concentrations of both total protein S and C4BPβ+ than those with type I deficiency. This may partly be an age-dependent phenomenon because individuals with type III deficiency tended to be older than those with deficiency of type I (Zöller et al 1995b).

Genetic studies of protein S deficiency have been complicated by the existence of two homologous genes for protein S on chromosome 3. The nucleotide sequences of the active PSα gene and the inactive PSβ pseudogene are 97% and 95.4% identical in coding and non-coding parts, respectively (reviewed in Dahlbäck & Stenflo 1994). Only two large deletions of the PSα gene have been shown to be associated with protein S deficiency (Ploos van Amstel et al 1989, Schmidel et al 1991). Recently, several point mutations in the protein S gene were described (Hayashi et al 1994, Reitsma et al 1994, Gandrille et al 1995, Gómez et al 1995). Using denaturing gradient gel electrophoresis in screening of exons II, IV, V, VIII, X and XV of the PSα gene from 100 protein S deficient patients, Gandrille et al (1995) found 15 novel point mutations and three polymorphisms. Three of the mutations were associated with true type II phenotypes (Arg-2 to Leu, Arg-1 to His and Thr-103 to Asn). In a study of eight Dutch protein S deficient patients, mutations were only found in five cases even though all exons of the PSα gene were sequenced (Reitsma et al 1994).

THROMBOMODULIN DEFECTS

So far, no cases with TM deficiency or functionally defective TM molecules have been described. As TM is an endothelial cell membrane protein there are obvious difficulties in measuring TM activity. In an effort to elucidate whether genetic defects of the TM gene are involved as pathogenic risk factors for thrombosis, the TM gene has been screened for mutations. A dimorphism, Ala[455] to Val, was found, but was shown not to be associated with thrombosis (Van der Welden et al 1991). Recently, a point mutation in the TM gene, which predicts replacement of Asp[468] with a Tyr, was identified in a 45-year-old man with thromboembolic disease (Öhlin & Marlar 1995). Whether this mutation affects the TM function or the level of protein expression and whether it is a risk factor for thrombosis remains to be elucidated.

RESISTANCE TO ACTIVATED PROTEIN C AS A PATHOGENIC RISK FACTOR FOR THROMBOPHILIA

Based on an hypothesis of thrombosis being due to a poor anticoagulant response to APC, the APC resistance test was devised, which measures the anticoagulant effect of exogenous APC in individual patient plasmas (Dahlbäck et al 1993). In normal plasma, the clotting time is prolonged because APC cleaves and inactivates factors VIIIa and Va. However, resistance to APC was observed in a middle-aged man with recurrent venous thrombosis. Similar APC resistance was found in several of his relatives, suggesting a new genetic cause of familial thrombophilia.

The APC resistance test was used to elucidate the prevalence of APC resistance in patients with venous thrombosis (Svensson & Dahlbäck 1994). In a consecutive series of 104 patients with venous thrombosis, 40% were found to manifest APC resistance, whereas the corresponding number in a control population was only 7% (Svensson & Dahlbäck 1994). The results indicate that, not only is APC resistance very frequent in thrombosis patients, but also that it is highly prevalent in the general population. Investigation of relatives of APC resistant probands confirmed the inherited nature of the phenotype and demonstrated an association between APC resistance and an increased risk of thrombosis (Svensson & Dahlbäck 1994). In the same cohort of thrombosis patients, deficiencies of protein S, protein C and antithrombin III were together found in only 5%, suggesting APC resistance is at last ten times more prevalent than any of the other known genetic defects. The conclusion that APC resistance is by far the most prevalent cause of venous thrombosis has been confirmed by studies from several laboratories (Griffin et al 1993, Faioni et al 1993, Koster et al 1993, Halbmayer et al 1994). Among 301 unselected patients with deep venous thrombosis, APC resistance was found in 21% of cases, with a corresponding frequency in matched controls of only 3%; the matched odds ratio was calculated to be 6.6 (Koster et al 1993). These results suggest that APC resistance is associated with a 5–10-fold increased risk of thrombosis.

A number of possible molecular mechanisms for the APC resistance were initially investigated (Dahlbäck et al 1993). It was observed that a protein fraction of normal plasma when mixed with APC resistant plasma corrected the APC resistance phenotype, whereas a corresponding fraction of APC resistant plasma was without effect. The protein was purified and demonstrated to be the intact form of factor V (Dahlbäck & Hildebrand 1994), which suggested that APC resistance is caused by a molecular defect of factor V. This concept gained further support from a close linkage between a neutral polymorphism in the factor V gene and the APC resistance phenotype found in a large Swedish family (Zöller & Dahlbäck 1994). Other researchers also came to the conclusion that APC resistance is caused by a defect in the factor V molecule (Bertina et al 1994, Sun et al 1994). In plasma-mixing experiments, they found APC resistance to be corrected by all coagulation factor deficiency plasmas except that deficient in factor V. The Dutch group demonstrated a linkage between APC resistance and a polymorphism located close to the factor V gene and were the first to report an association between APC resistance and a point mutation in the factor V gene, a substitution of G with an A at nucleotide position 1691 predicting replacement of $Arg(R)^{506}$ with a Gln(Q) (Bertina et al 1994). The same mutation was subsequently found in a Swedish family (Zöller & Dahlbäck 1994). Almost at the same time, two other laboratories reported an association between $FVa:Q^{506}$ and APC resistance (Greengard et al 1994, Voorberg et al 1994). R^{506} is located in one of three APC cleavage sites in the heavy chain of factor Va. $FVa:Q^{506}$ is not cleaved at position 506, but is slowly degraded by APC mediated cleavages at R^{306} and R^{679} (Kalafatis et al 1995). The rate of inactivation of $FVa:Q^{506}$ by APC is 10–20-fold lower compared to the rate of degradation of $FVa:R^{506}$ (Aparicio & Dahlbäck 1996).

In several countries, the allele frequency of $FV:Q^{506}$ is reported to be around 2%, in The Netherlands 2% (Bertina et al 1994), in the UK 1.7% (Beuchamp et al 1994), in Australia 2% (Van Bockxmeer et al 1995), in Germany 2% (März et al 1995) and in the USA 3% (Ridker et al 1995). A multicentre study found allele frequencies of 2.8% in Belfast, 0.3% in Lille, 1.4% in Toulouse and 4.7% in Strasbourg (Emmerich et al 1995). Even higher allele frequencies have been found in southern Sweden: 5.9% in Malmö and 7.9% in Kristianstad (unpublished data). Linkage disequilibrium of the $FV:Q^{506}$ mutation with the common *Hinf1* allele of factor V (nucleotide 2298) polymorphism suggested a founder effect to be involved in the spread of this allele in the population (Bertina et al 1994). The high prevalence of the $FV:Q^{506}$ allele in the population suggests that it has conferred a survival advantage during evolution, possibly due to a hypercoagulable state and lower bleeding tendency. So far, APC resistance has not been reported in African, Japanese or Asian populations. It is tempting to speculate that the lower incidence of venous thromboembolism in Asia (Woo et al 1988) and Africa (Thomas et al 1960), compared to that found in Western communities (Goldhaber 1994), is related to a lower prevalence of APC resistance in these populations.

In more than 90% of cases, the APC resistance phenotype is associated with the FV:Q^{506} allele (Zöller et al 1994). The molecular defects of the remaining 10% are as yet unknown. In a study of 50 thrombosis-prone families with inherited APC resistance, the FV:Q^{506} allele was identified in 47 families. The sensitivity of the APC resistance test for the FV:Q^{506} mutation was 87% and the specificity 85% (Fig. 4.3). The Dutch group,

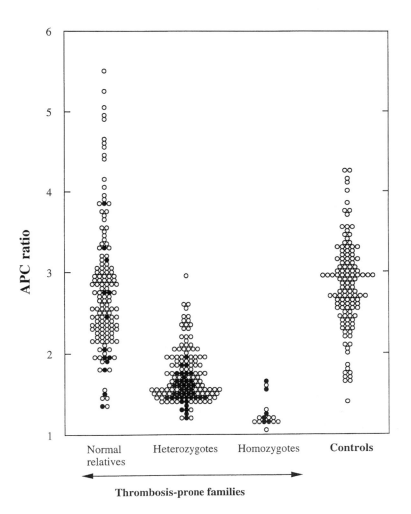

Fig. 4.3 Relationships between the FV:Q^{506} mutation and APC ratios in families with APC resistance. •, family members with a history of thrombosis. Differences in APC ratios (number, mean ± SD) between normals (n = 143, 2.8 ± 0.8), heterozygotes (n = 142, 1.7 ± 0.3) and homozygotes (n = 16, 1.3 ± 0.2) were highly significant ($P > 0.001$). (Modified from Zöller et al 1994 with permission.)

Families with APC resistance and FV mutation

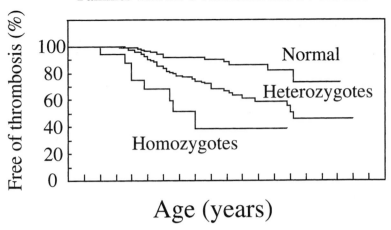

Fig. 4.4   Relationship between the factor V genotype and thrombosis-free survival curves. The probability to be free from thrombotic events at a certain age for 146 normals, 144 heterozygotes and 18 homozygotes is presented in the Kaplan–Meier analysis. Differences between normals and heterozygotes and between heterozygotes and homozygotes were highly significant ($P > 0.001$ and $P = 0.01$, respectively). (Modified from Zöller et al 1994 with permission.)

using another APTT (activated partial thromboplastin test) reagent, have reported even higher specificity and sensitivity for the FV:Q[506] mutation (Bertina et al 1994, De Ronde & Bertina 1994), which may be related to the choice of APTT reagent. A modified APC resistance test, in which the patient plasma is diluted in factor V deficient plasma, appears to yield higher sensitivity and specificity for the FV:Q[506] mutation; this modified assay is also useful for patients on oral anticoagulation (Jorquera et al 1994, Trossaërt et al 1994). However, the original unmodified APC resistance test is still very useful because APC resistance that is not caused by the FV:Q[506] mutation has also been found to be associated with an increased risk for thrombosis (Zöller et al 1994). Moreover, it is noteworthy that thrombosis-prone heterozygotes have significantly lower APC ratios than heterozygotes who have never experienced thrombosis. This may be a post-thrombotic phenomenon or may possibly be caused by other genetic risk factors for thrombosis which segregate in these families and which also contribute to the severity of the APC resistance.

Clinical manifestations of APC Resistance

Heterozygosity and homozygosity for FV:Q[506] are associated with a 5–10 and a 50–100-fold increased risk of thrombosis, respectively (Bertina et al 1994, Majerus 1994). This demonstrates that it is of clinical importance to determine whether an APC-resistant patient is heterozygous or homozygous for the FV:Q[506] mutation. In 50 families with APC resistance, eight of 18

(44%) homozygotes, 43 of 144 (30%) heterozygotes, and 14 of 146 (10%) individuals without the FV:Q^{506} mutation had experienced one or more venous thrombotic events (Zöller et al 1994), and there were significant differences in thrombosis-free survival curves between heterozygous, homozygous and normal individuals (Fig. 4.4). The mean age at the first thrombotic episode was 36 years (range 18–71 years) for heterozygotes compared to 25 years (range 10–40 years) for homozygotes. By 33 years of age, 8% of those not carrying the mutation, 20% of heterozygotes and 40% of homozygotes had had at least one venous thromboembolic episode (Zöller et al 1994). This is higher than expected from population data taken together with an estimated 5–10-fold increased thrombosis risk of heterozygous APC resistance and suggests that thrombosis-prone families with APC resistance are affected by more than one genetic defect.

In APC-resistant families, deep venous thrombosis was the most common manifestation, but pulmonary embolism and superficial thrombophlebitis also occurred (Table 4.1) (Zöller et al 1994). Other rare thrombotic events, such as Budd–Chiari syndrome, which have been reported in association with APC resistance (Denninger et al 1995, Mahmoud et al 1995), were not observed in these families. The multifactorial etiology of thrombosis was illustrated by the observation that the first thrombotic episode was associated with a circumstantial risk factor in eight of 14 normals, in 25 of 43 heterozygotes, and in seven out of eight homozygotes. The most common risk factors were pregnancy, surgery, trauma and oral contraceptives (Zöller et al 1994). That APC resistance is a risk factor for thrombosis in association with pregnancy is further reflected by an observed 60% prevalence of APC resistance among women who have had thrombosis during pregnancy (Hellgren et al 1995). Oral contraception in combination with APC resistance due to heterozygosity for FV:Q^{506} is associated

Table 4.1 Clinical manifestations in symptomatic family members with APC resistance and FV:Q^{506}

	Normals No. (%)	Heterozygotes No. (%)	Homozygotes No. (%)
History of thrombosis	14 (100)	43 (100)	8 (100)
Patients with a thrombotic symptom[a]			
DVT	8[c] (57)	36[b] (84)	8 (100)
PE	3 (21)	8 (19)	4 (50)
STP	5 (36)	8 (19)	1 (12)
Recurrence	7 (50)	17 (40)	4 (50)

Modified from Zöller et al (1994).
[a]Since a patient may have suffered from several different thrombotic events, the numbers do not add up to 100%.
[b]One heterozygous individual had had central retinal venous thrombosis.
[c]One patient had a superior sagittal sinus thrombosis as first episode. He was APC resistant but lacked the FV:Q^{506} mutation.
DVT, deep venous thrombosis; PE, pulmonary embolism; STP, superficial thrombophlebitis.

with a 35-fold increased risk of thrombosis compared to an 8-fold increased risk in heterozygous carriers not using oral contraceptives (Vandenbroucke et al 1994).

A large prospective study of apparently healthy men has confirmed the conclusion that APC resistance due to heterozygosity for $FV:Q^{506}$ is a risk factor for venous thromboembolism (Ridker et al 1995). The overall relative risk of venous thrombosis among the heterozygous men was 2.7 (95% CI (confidence interval), 1.3 to 5.6). In heterozygous men over the age of 60 years, the relative risk for primary venous thrombosis was even higher (relative risk, 7.0; 95% CI, 2.6 to 19.1). From a clinical point of view, these data pose important questions, such as whether it is worthwhile to screen older individuals before surgery. It is not yet known whether patients with the $FV:Q^{506}$ mutation should be treated with prolonged anticoagulant therapy after a thromboembolic episode and whether they benefit from aggressive prophylactic treatment in high-risk clinical situations.

It is at present not clear whether APC resistance is associated with an increased risk of arterial thrombosis. Only one of several case-control studies has found an association between myocardial infarction and an increased prevalence of APC resistance (Samani et al 1994, Emmerich et al 1995, März et al 1995, Van Bockxmeer et al 1995). In the large cohort study of apparently healthy men, no association between myocardial infarction or stroke and heterozygosity for $FV:Q^{506}$ was observed (Ridker et al 1995). So far, no study has excluded the possibility that homozygosity for $FV:Q^{506}$ is a risk factor for premature arterial thrombosis and, indeed, homozygous APC resistance has been found in a few cases with arterial thrombosis (Holm et al 1994, Lindblad et al 1994).

FAMILIAL THROMBOPHILIA IS THE RESULT OF MULTIPLE GENETIC DEFECTS

It is noteworthy that more than one genetic defect was segregated in the two families that were used to link the APC resistance phenotype to the factor V gene (Zöller & Dahlbäck 1994, Bertina et al 1994). The Swedish family had protein S deficiency, whereas the Dutch family carried a protein C deficiency in addition to APC resistance. These reports were the first clear demonstrations of familial thrombophilia being caused by multiple genetic defects. More recently, this concept has gained further support by the identification of APC resistance in six out of 32 (19%) thrombosis-prone protein C deficient families (Koeleman et al 1994). In these families, 73% of individuals with combined defects had had venous thrombosis; the corresponding numbers in individuals with isolated protein C deficiency or APC resistance were 31% and 13%, respectively. A similar situation has been demonstrated in families with protein S deficiency (Zöller et al 1995a). The $FV:Q^{506}$ allele was found in seven out of 18 (39%) Swedish protein S deficient families, and significant differences in thrombosis-free survival

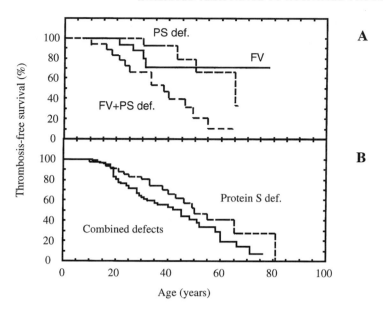

Fig. 4.5 Thrombosis-free survival curves in protein S deficiency. **A** In seven out of 18 families with protein S deficiency, APC resistance was also found. Thrombosis-free survival curves in 21 family members with only APC resistance (FV:Q^{506}), 21 with only protein S deficiency and 18 with both defects. The difference between those having only the factor V gene mutation or protein S deficiency and those with combined defects was significant ($P = 0.0084$ and $P = 0.0019$, respectively). There was no significant difference between those with only the factor V gene mutation and those with isolated protein S deficiency ($P = 0.47$). **B** Thrombosis-free survival curve of all patients with isolated protein S deficiency from 18 families compared with that of 18 patients with combined protein S deficiency and APC resistance. There was no significant difference between the curves ($P = 0.09$), suggesting unknown risk factors to be present in the 11 families who did not have APC resistance. (Modified from Zöller et al 1995c with permission.)

curves between individuals with combined defects and those with isolated defects were noted (Fig. 4.5A). The youngest protein S deficient patient to suffer from thrombosis, at the age of 10 years, had a combination of protein S deficiency and APC resistance due to homozygosity for FV:Q^{506} (Zöller et al 1995c). In the thrombosis-prone protein S families lacking APC resistance, other as yet unknown genetic risk factors may segregate. This is suggested by the observation that when all 18 families were compared there was no significant difference in thrombosis-free survival curves between individuals with combined defects (protein S deficiency plus APC resistance) and those with only protein S deficiency (Fig. 4.5B). Similarly, in the six Dutch families carrying both protein C deficiency and APC resistance, not all thrombosis cases could be explained by the combination of the two defects, and the presence of a third genetic risk factor segregating in these families was suggested (Koeleman et al 1994).

To accept a genetic defect as a pathogenic risk factor for thrombosis, the defect must be demonstrated to cosegregate with the clinical manifestations (i.e. thrombosis) in a pedigree. This has been demonstrated in a large number of families with deficiencies of antithrombin III (Lane et al 1992), protein C (Broekmans & Conard 1988, Allaart et al 1993), protein S (Engesser et al 1987, Briet et al 1988, Zöller et al 1995a) and APC resistance (Svensson & Dahlbäck 1994, Zöller et al 1994). The observation that familial thrombosis is often the result of at least two genetic defects (Koeleman et al 1994, Zöller et al 1995a) suggests that two-locus linkage analysis and methods such as allelic association, using polymorphic markers close to candidate genes, should be used in studies aimed at the identification of other unknown genetic risk factors for thrombosis.

LABORATORY INVESTIGATION OF THROMBOPHILIC PATIENTS AND TREATMENT OF PATIENTS WITH INHERITED THROMBOPHILIA

Based on our present knowledge, we suggest that the laboratory investigation of patients should at least include determination of free protein S antigen, protein C activity, antithrombin III activity, APC resistance test, $FV:Q^{506}$ mutation analysis (if positive APC resistance test) and screening tests for lupus anticoagulant. Following identification of an inherited defect in a patient should a family investigation be initiated? We believe the answer to this is 'yes' because identification in a healthy individual of a genetic risk factor for thrombosis may allow appropriate preventive measures to be taken in association with circumstantial risk situations. The justification of this being that circumstantial risk factors often provoke first thrombotic events in a large proportion of patients with genetic risk factors. When asymptomatic, but biochemically affected, relatives to patients with protein S, protein C or antithrombin III deficiency are given prophylaxis in risk situations such as surgery, trauma and pregnancy, and if oral contraceptives are avoided, the incidence of thrombosis has been found to decrease (De Stefano et al 1994a,b). Guidelines for treatment of asymptomatic and symptomatic patients with protein C, protein S and antithrombin III deficiencies are available (Broekmans & Conard 1988, Briet et al 1988, Marlar et al 1988, Lane et al 1994). There are no internationally accepted guidelines available for the management of symptomatic and asymtomatic individuals with APC resistance. Based on several years of experience in our laboratory, we have adopted the following practical guidelines:

1. The APC resistance test is used as a screening assay and a PCR (polymerase chain reaction) based analysis for the $FV:Q^{506}$ allele is performed when the APC resistance test is positive (Zöller et al 1994).

2. Individuals with heterozygosity for the $FV:Q^{506}$ allele who have no other anticoagulant defects and no personal or family history of thrombosis are given prophylactic treatment only in thrombosis-predisposing situations such as major surgery.

3. Patients with APC resistance having a history of thrombosis are treated like thrombosis patients with deficiencies of protein C, protein S or antithrombin III; i.e. preventive anticoagulation therapy is given in high-risk situations and long-term therapy is considered if thrombosis is recurrent, spontaneous or life-threatening.

4. Homozygous cases, and heterozygous patients with a second congenital prothrombotic disorder, are given therapy in all-risk situations and extended or lifelong therapy is considered even after a single thrombotic episode.

An important challenge for future research is to elucidate how individuals with inherited APC resistance should be managed and to investigate whether APC resistance should be screened for before surgery, pregnancy, oral contraception and hospitalization. Indeed, the results of a recent prospective study of apparently healthy men suggest that it may be useful to screen for APC resistance, particularly in elderly people because the risk for venous thromboembolism in APC resistant individuals increases with age (Ridker et al 1995).

KEY POINTS FOR CLINICAL PRACTICE

- Activated protein C resistance (APCR) is found in up to 60% of patients with venous thrombosis.

- In most patients APCR is due to a single base change in the gene for factor V leading to a replacement at 506 arginine (FVaR 506) with glutamine (FVaQ 506) at the site of cleavage by activated protein C. With a result the rate of inactivation of FVaQ506 is 10–20 fold slower than FVaR506.

- Individuals with APCR but with the normal allele (FVaR506) also have an increased risk of thrombosis.

- Heterozygosity for FVaQ506 confers a 5–10 fold risk of venous thrombosis whilst homozygosity is associated with a 50–100 fold risk.

- Those who are heterzygous for FVaQ506 and on the combined oral contraceptive pill have a 30 fold risk of thrombosis compared to non pill takers who are negative for this allele.

- Possession of protein C, S or ATIII deficiency, as well as FVaQ506, also markedly increases the risk of thrombosis.

- The data reviewed in this Chapter confirms the multifactional aetiology of venous thrombembolic disease.

REFERENCES

Allaart C F, Poort S R, Rosendaal F R et al 1993 Increased risk of venous thrombosis in carriers of hereditary protein C deficiency defect. Lancet 341: 134–138

Aparicio C, Dahlbäck B 1996 Molecular mechanisms of activated protein C resistance. Properties of factor V isolated from an individual with homozygosity for the Arg^{506} to Gln mutation in the factor V gene. Biochem J 313: 467–472

Ben-Tal O, Zivelin A, Seligsohn U 1989 The relative frequency of hereditary thrombotic disorders among 107 patients with thrombophilia in Israel. Thromb Haemost 61: 50–54

Bertina R M 1985 Hereditary protein S deficiency. Haemostasis 15: 241–246

Bertina R M 1988 Molecular basis of thrombosis. In: Bertina R M (ed) Protein C and related proteins. Churchill Livingstone, Edinburgh, p 1

Bertina R M, Koeleman B P C, Koster T et al 1994 Mutation in blood coagulation factor V associated with resistance to activated protein C. Nature 369: 64–67

Beuchamp N J, Daly M, Hampton K K et al 1994 High prevalence of mutation in the factor V gene within the UK population; relationship to activated protein C resistance and familial thrombosis. Br J Haematol 88: 219–222

Bovill E G, Bauer K A, Dickermann J D et al 1989 The clinical spectrum of heterozygous protein C deficiency in a large New England kindred. Blood 73: 712–717

Briet E, Broekmans A W, Engesser L 1988 Hereditary protein S defiency. In: Bertina R M (ed) Protein C and related proteins. Churchill Livingstone, Edinburgh, p 203

Broekmans A W, Conard J 1988 Hereditary protein C deficiency. In: Bertina R M (ed) Protein C and related proteins. Churchill Livingstone, Edinburgh, p 160

Broekmans A W, van der Linden I K, Jansen-Koeter Y et al 1986 Prevalence of protein C (PC) and protein S (PS) deficiency in patients with thromboembolic disease. Thromb Res Suppl 6: 135a

Chafa O, Fischer A M, Meriane F et al 1989 A new case of 'type II' inherited protein S deficiency. Br J Haematol 73: 501–505

Comp P C, Esmon C T 1984 Recurrent thromboembolism in patients with a partial deficiency of protein S. N Engl J Med 311: 1525–1528

Comp P C, Nixon R R, Cooper M R et al 1984 Familial protein S deficiency is associated with recurrent thrombosis. J Clin Invest 74: 2082–2088

Cooper P C, Hampton K K, Makris M et al 1994 Further evidence that activated protein C resistance can be misdiagnosed as inherited functional protein S deficiency. Br J Haematol 88: 201–203

Dahlbäck B 1991 Protein S and C4b-binding protein: components involved in the regulation of the protein C anticoagulant system. Thromb Haemost 66: 49–61

Dahlbäck B 1995 The protein C anticoagulant system: inherited defects as basis for venous thrombosis. Thromb Res 77: 1–43

Dahlbäck B, Hildebrand B 1994 Inherited resistance to activated protein C is corrected by anticoagulant cofactor activity found to be a property of factor V. Proc Natl Acad Sci USA 81: 1396–1400

Dahlbäck B, Stenflo J 1994 The protein C anticoagulant system. In: Stamatoyannopoulos G, Nienhuis A W, Majerus P W, Varmus H (eds) The molecular basis of blood diseases. WB Saunders, Philadelphia, p 599

Dahlbäck B, Carlsson M, Svensson P J 1993 Familial thrombophilia due to a previously unrecognized mechanism characterized by poor anticoagulant response to activated protein C: prediction of a cofactor to activated protein C. Proc Natl Acad Sci USA 90: 1004–1008

Denninger M H, Beldjord K, Durand F et al 1995 Budd–Chiari syndrome and factor V Leiden mutation. Lancet 345: 525–526

De Ronde H, Bertina R M 1994 Laboratory diagnosis of APC resistance: a critical evaluation of the test and the development of diagnostic criteria. Thromb Haemost 72: 880–886

De Stefano V, Leone G, Mastrangelo S et al 1994a Thrombosis during pregnancy and surgery in patients with congenital deficiency of antithrombin III, protein C, protein S. Thromb Haemost 71: 799–800

De Stefano V, Leone G, Mastrangelo S et al 1994b Clinical manifestations and management of inherited thrombophilia: retrospective analysis and follow-up after diagnosis of

238 patients with congenital deficiency of antithrombin III, protein C, protein S. Thromb Haemost 72: 352–358

Emmerich J, Poirier O, Evans A et al 1995 Myocardial infarction, Arg[506] to Gln factor V mutation, and activated protein C resistance. Lancet 345: 321

Engesser L, Broekmans A W, Briët E et al 1987 Hereditary protein S deficiency: clinical manifestations. Ann Intern Med 106: 677–682

Esmon C T 1989 The roles of protein C and thrombomodulin in the regulation of blood coagulation. J Biol Chem 264: 4743–4746

Faioni E M, Franchi F, Asti D et al 1993 Resistance to activated protein C in nine thrombophilic families: interference in a protein S functional assay. Thromb Haemost 70: 1067–1071

Faioni E M, Boyer-Neumann C, Wolf M et al 1994 Another protein S functional assay is sensitive to resistance to activated protein C. Thromb Haemost 72: 648

Gandrille S, Borgel D, Eschwege-Gufflet V et al 1995 Identification of 15 different candidate causal point mutations and three polymorphisms in 19 patients with protein S deficiency using scanning method for analysis of the protein S active gene. Blood 85: 130–138

Garcia de Frutos P, Alim R I M, Härdig Y et al 1994 Differential regulation of α and β chains of C4b-binding protein during acute-phase response resulting in stable plasma levels of free anticoagulant protein S. Blood 84: 815–822

Gladson C L, Scharrer I, Hach V et al 1988 The frequency of type I heterozygous protein S and protein C deficiency in 141 unrelated young patients with venous thrombosis. Thromb Haemost 59: 18–22

Goldhaber S Z 1994 Epidemiology of pulmonary embolism and deep vein thrombosis. In: Bloom A L, Forbes C D, Thomas D P, Tuddenham E G D (eds) Haemostasis and thrombosis. Churchill Livingstone, Edinburgh, p 1327

Gómez E, Ledford M R, Pegelow C H et al 1995 Homozygous protein S deficiency due to a one base pair deletion that leads to a stop codon in exon III of the protein S gene. Thromb Haemost 71: 723–726

Greengard J S, Sun X, Xu X et al 1994 Activated protein C resistance caused by Arg[506]Gln mutation in factor Va. Lancet 343: 1362–1363

Griffin J H, Gruber A, Fernández J A 1992 Reevaluation of total, free and bound protein S and C4b-binding protein levels in plasma anticoagulated with citrate or hirudin. Blood 79: 3203–3211

Griffin J H, Evatt B L, Wideman C et al 1993 Anticoagulant protein C pathway defective in a majority of thrombophilic patients. Blood 82: 1989–1993

Halbmayer W M, Haushofer A, Schön R et al 1994 The prevalence of poor anticoagulant response to activated protein C (APC resistance) among patients suffering from stroke or venous thrombosis and among healthy subjects. Blood Coagulat Fibrinol 5: 51–57

Hayashi T, Nishioka J, Shigekiyo T et al 1994 Protein S Tokushima: abnormal molecule with a substitution of Glu for Lys-155 in the second epidermal growth factor-like domain of protein S. Blood 83: 683–690

Heijboer H, Brandjes D, Büller H R et al 1990 Deficiencies of coagulation-inhibiting and fibrinolytic proteins in outpatients with deep-vein thrombosis. N Engl J Med 323: 1512–1516

Hellgren M, Svensson P J, Dahlbäck B 1995 Resistance to activated protein C as a basis for venous thromboembolism associated with pregnancy and oral contraceptives. Am J Obstet Gynecol 173: 210–213

Hillarp A, Dahlbäck B 1988 Novel subunit in C4b-binding protein required for protein S binding. J Biol Chem 263: 12759–12764

Hillarp A, Hessing M, Dahlbäck B 1989 Protein S binding in relation to the subunit composition of human C4b-binding protein. FEBS Lett 259: 53–56

Holm J, Zöller B, Svensson P J et al 1994 Myocardial infarction associated with homozygous resistance to activated protein C. Lancet 344: 952–953

Härdig Y, Rezaie A R, Dahlbäck B 1993 High affinity binding of human vitamin K-dependent protein S to a truncated recombinant β-chain of C4b-binding protein expressed in *Escherichia coli*. J Biol Chem 268: 3033–3036

Iijima K, Inoue N, Nakamura K et al 1989 Inherited deficiency of functional and free form protein S. Acta Haematol Jpn 52: 126–133

Jorquera J I, Montoro J M, Fernández M A et al 1994 Modified test for activated protein

C resistance. Lancet 344: 1162–1163

Kalafatis M, Bertina R M, Rand M D et al 1995 Characterization of the molecular defect in factor VR506Q. J Biol Chem 270: 4053–4057

Kirkegaard A 1980 Incidence of acute deep venous thrombosis in two districts: a phlebographic study. Acta Chir Scand 146: 267–269

Koeleman B P C, Reitsma P H, Allaart C F et al 1994 Activated protein C resistance as an additional risk factor for thrombosis in protein C-deficient families. Blood 84: 1031–1035

Koster T, Rosendaal F R, de Ronde F et al 1993 Venous thrombosis due to poor response to activated protein C: Leiden thrombophilia study. Lancet 342: 1503–1506

Lane D A, Olds R R, Thein S L 1992 Antithrombin and its deficiency states. Blood Coagulat Fibrinol 3: 315–341

Lane D A, Olds R J, Thein S L 1994 Antithrombin and its deficiency. In: Bloom A L, Forbes C D, Thomas D P, Tuddenham E G D (eds) Haemostasis and thrombosis. Churchill Livingstone, Edinburgh, p 655

Lauer C G, Reid T J, Wideman C S et al 1990 Free protein S deficiency in a family with venous thrombosis. J Vasc Surg 12: 541–544

Lindblad B, Svensson P J, Dahlbäck B 1994 Arterial and venous thromboembolism with fatal outcome in a young man with inherited resistance to activated protein C. Lancet 343: 917

Maccaferri M, Legnani C, Preda L et al 1991 Protein S activity in patients with heredofamilial protein S deficiency and in patients with juvenile venous thrombosis. Results of a functional method. Thromb Res 64: 647–658

Mahmoud A E A, Wilde J T, Elias E 1995 Budd–Chiari syndrome and factor V Leiden mutation. Lancet 345: 526

Majerus P W 1994 Bad blood by mutation. Nature 369: 14–15

Malm J, Laurell M, Nilsson I M et al 1992 Thromboembolic disease – critical evaluation of laboratory investigation. Thromb Haemost 68: 7–13

Mannucci P M, Valsecchi C, Krashmalnicoff A et al 1989 Familial dysfunction of protein S. Thromb Haemost 62: 763–766

Marlar R A, Montgomery R R, Madden R M 1988 Homozygous protein C deficiency. In: Bertina R M (ed) Protein C and related proteins. Churchill Livingstone, Edinburgh, p 182

März W, Seydewitz H, Winkelmann B et al 1995 Mutation in coagulation factor V associated with resistance to activated protein C in patients with coronary artery disease. Lancet 345: 526–527

Miletich J P, Sherman L, Broze G J Jr 1987 Absence of thrombosis in subjects with heterozygous protein C deficiency. N Engl J Med 317: 991–996

Miletich J P, Prescott S M, White R et al 1993 Inherited predisposition to thrombosis. Cell 72: 477–480

Öhlin A K, Marlar R A 1995 The first mutation identified in the thrombomodulin gene in a 45-year-old man presenting with thromboembolic disease. Blood 85: 330–336

Ploos van Amstel H K, Huisman M V, Reitsma P H et al 1989 Partial protein S gene deletion in a family with hereditary thrombophilia. Blood 73: 479–483

Reitsma P H, Poort S R, Allaart C F et al 1991 The spectrum of genetic defects in a panel of 40 Dutch families with symptomatic protein C deficiency type I: heterogeneity and founder effects. Blood 78: 890–894

Reitsma P H, Poort S R, Bernardi F et al 1993 Protein C deficiency: a database of mutations. Thromb Haemost 69: 77–84

Reitsma P H, Ploos van Amstel H K, Bertina R M 1994 Three novel mutations in five unrelated subjects with hereditary protein S deficiency type I. J Clin Invest 93: 486–492

Ridker P M, Hennekens C H, Lindpaintner K et al 1995 Mutation in the gene coding for coagulation factor V and the risk of myocardial infarction, stroke, and venous thrombosis in apparently healthy men. N Engl J Med 332: 912–917

Samani N, Lodwick D, Martin D et al 1994 Resistance to activated protein C and risk of premature myocardial infarction. Lancet 344: 1709–1710

Schmidel D K, Nelson R M, Broxson E H et al 1991 A 5.3-kb deletion including exon XIII of the protein S a gene occurs in two protein S-deficient families. Blood 77: 551–559

Schwarz H P, Fischer M, Hopmeier P et al 1984 Plasma protein S deficiency in familial thrombotic disease. Blood 64: 1297–1300

Seligsohn U, Berger A, Abend A et al 1984 Homozygous protein C deficiency manifested by massive thrombosis in the newborn. N Engl J Med 310: 559–562

Shen L, Dahlbäck B 1994 Factor V and protein S as synergistic cofactors to activated protein C in degradation of factor VIIIa. J Biol Chem 269: 18735–18738

Sun X, Evatt B L, Griffin J H 1994 Blood coagulation factor Va abnormality associated with resistance to activated protein C in venous thrombophilia. Blood 83: 3120–3125

Svensson P J, Dahlbäck B 1994 Resistance to activated protein C as a basis for venous thrombosis. N Engl J Med 330: 517–521

Tabernero M D, Tomas J F, Alberca I et al 1991 Incidence and clinical characteristics of hereditary disorders associated with venous thrombosis. Am J Hematol 36: 249–254

Thomas W A, Davies J N P, O'Neal R M et al 1960 Incidence of myocardial infarction correlated with venous and pulmonary thrombosis and embolism. A geographic study based on autopsies in Uganda, East Africa and St Louis, USA. Am J Cardiol 5: 41–47

Trossaërt M, Conard J, Horellou M H et al 1994 Modified APC resistance assay for patients on oral anticoagulants. Lancet 344: 1709

Van Bockxmeer F M, Baker R I, Taylor R R 1995 Premature ischaemic heart disease and the gene for coagulation factor V. Nature Med 1: 185

Vandenbroucke J P, Koster T, Briët E et al 1994 Increased risk of venous thrombosis in oral-contraceptive users who are carriers of factor V Leiden mutation. Lancet 344: 1453–1457

Van der Welden P A, Krommenhoek-Van Es T, Allaart C F et al 1991 A frequent thrombomodulin amino acid dimorphism is not associated with thrombophilia. Thromb Haemost 65: 511–513

Voorberg J, Roelse J, Koopman R et al 1994 Association of idiopathic thromboembolism with single point mutation at Arg^{506} of factor V. Lancet 343: 1535–1536

Woo K S, Tse L K K, Tse C Y et al 1988 The prevalence and pattern of pulmonary thromboembolism in the Chinese in Hong Kong. Int J Cardiol 20: 373–380

Zöller B, Dahlbäck B 1994 Linkage between inherited resistance to activated protein C and factor V gene mutation in venous thrombosis. Lancet 343: 1536–1538

Zöller B, Svensson P J, He X et al 1994 Identification of the same factor V gene mutation in 47 out of 50 thrombosis-prone families with inherited resistance to activated protein C. J Clin Invest 94: 2521–2524

Zöller B, Berntsdotter A, Garcia de Frutos P, Dahlbäck B 1995a Resistance to activated protein C as an additional genetic risk factor in hereditary deficiency of protein S. Blood 85: 3518–3523

Zöller B, Garcia de Frutos P, Dahlbäck B 1995b Evaluation of the relationship between protein S and C4b-binding protein isoforms in hereditary protein S deficiency demonstrating type I and type III deficiencies to be phenotypic variants of the same genetic disease. Blood 85: 3524–3531

Zöller B, He X, Dahlbäck B 1995c Resistance to activated protein C due to homozygous factor V gene mutation combined with protein S deficiency in a young boy with severe thrombotic disease. Thromb Haemost 73: 743–745

5. Haemostatic risk factors for arterial and venous thrombosis

G. D. O. Lowe

Epidemiological studies increasingly show that there is a range of variables relevant to haematology which are predictive of thrombosis, arterial or venous (Table 5.1). Some of these variables are primary risk predictors: that is, they predict thrombotic events in persons with no history of thrombotic or vascular disease. Some are secondary risk predictors: that is, they predict thrombotic events in persons with a previous thrombotic event or pre-existing vascular disease. These haematological variables include rheological variables which affect blood flow, and haemostatic variables related to the platelet, endothelial, coagulation and fibrinolytic systems (Table 5.1).

RISK PREDICTION OF DISEASE: STATISTICAL ISSUES

Establishing that a haematological (or any other) variable is a predictor of thrombotic risk is initially a statistical exercise. The 'statistical significance' of a biological variable as a risk predictor depends not only on the strength of the association, but also on the power (size) of the study, the biological variability of the measure, and the variability in its measurement (Table 5.2). Since the introduction of the concept of risk factors for cardiovascular disease was first introduced by the prospective Framingham Study (Kannel et al 1961), it has been shown that the strength of association for

Table 5.1 Haematological predictors of thrombotic risk (modified from Lowe 1993a)

Rheology	Haematocrit, white cell count, erythrocyte sedimentation rate, plasma viscosity (fibrinogen)
Platelets	Platelet count, volume, aggregation, release
Endothelium	von Willebrand factor (tPA, PAI), thrombomodulin, tissue factor, tissue factor pathway inhibitor
Coagulation	Fibrinogen, factor VII:C, factor VIII:C
	Antithrombin, protein C, protein S
	Activated protein C resistance (factor V Leiden)
	Lupus anticoagulants (antiphospholipid antibodies)
	Fibrin(ogen) degradation products
Fibrinolysis	Clot lysis times, PAI activity, tPA antigen
	(Fibrin(ogen) degradation products)

tPA, tissue plasminogen activator; PAI, plasminogen activator inhibitor.

each of the three major risk factors – cigarette-smoking (Doll et al 1994, Parish et al 1995), serum cholesterol (Law et al 1994) and blood pressure (MacMahon et al 1990) – has been underestimated statistically due to failure to correct for the variability of these measures, and hence for the imprecision of a single estimation. Haematological variables are at least as variable (biologically and methodologically) as these 'classical' risk factors (Vickers & Thompson 1985, Thompson et al 1987); hence epidemiological studies are even more likely to underestimate their true predictive value. This predictive value will, of course, increase with the number of measurements. For example, accurate (over 90%) classification of persons undergoing cardiovascular risk stratification may require four measurements of plasma fibrinogen over a period of several weeks – in a similar fashion to the accepted clinical practice of repeated measurement of serum cholesterol or arterial blood pressure over several weeks before classifying individuals as 'hypercholesterolaemic' or 'hypertensive' prior to the institution of lifestyle advice or risk factor lowering medication (Rosenson et al 1994).

Table 5.2   Some statistical, biological and utilitarian considerations in assessment of the predictive value of haemostatic variables for thrombotic events

- Statistical: risk predictor, or not?
  Strength of association
  Power (size) of study
  Biological variability
  Measurement variability
  – Preanalytical
  – Analytical

- Biological: causal risk factor, or not?
  Strength of association
  – Relative risk
  – Dose–response effect
  Consistency
  – In different populations, studied by different observers, at different times, by different methods
  Presence of factor predates onset of disease
  – Primary prediction (or statistical adjustment for presence of baseline prevalent disease)
  – Genetic studies
  Biological plausibility
  Reduction in factor results in reduction in disease

- Clinical utility: practical applications?
  Stratification of thrombotic risk
  – General population
  – Hypertensives
  – Hyperlipidaemics
  – Diabetics
  – Arterial disease
  – Preoperative patients
  – (Outpatient clinic users/pregnancy)
  Definition of groups who may benefit from antithrombotic prophylaxis.

RISK FACTORS CAUSING DISEASE: BIOLOGICAL ISSUES

When does a statistical risk predictor become established as a biologically significant risk factor, which is defined as a biological variable which plays a truly causal role in the development of cardiovascular disease, including thrombosis (Shaper 1988)? Table 5.2 shows some criteria for establishing causal relationships, including the strength of the association, its consistency, the presence of the factor prior to the onset of disease, the biological plausibility that the potential risk factor might promote disease, and finally the demonstration that reduction in risk factor exposure results in reduction of disease (Bradford Hill 1965; Shaper 1988).

It should be recognized that 'the presence of the factor prior to the onset of disease' refers to clinically detectable disease. Necropsy studies of young adults after sudden traumatic death show an appreciable prevalence both of small thrombi in leg veins (Rössle 1937) and of atherosclerotic lesions and mural thrombi in the aorta and coronary arteries (Chandler 1974, Wissler et al 1993); hence to some extent thrombosis and atherosclerosis are part of normal adult life.

In the past, there has been a regrettable tendency to confuse the 'statistical independence' of risk predictors with their biological significance. Throwing a number of biological variables into a multivariate analysis, finding that some remain 'independent predictors' while others do not, then concluding that the former are 'biologically significant' while the latter are not, is silly. Multivariate analysis tends to reject measures that are more biologically variable and hence, paradoxically, possibly of greater pathophysiological significance since they are (according to chaos theory) more likely to disturb homeostasis and result in a biological catastrophe such as thrombosis. All risk factors for cardiovascular disease tend to be related; hence 'declaring statistical independence' is dangerous (Davey-Smith & Phillips 1990). Few clinicians doubt the importance of obesity in hypertension and in hyperlipidaemia (weight reduction is first-line treatment); however, obesity tends to show less 'independent' prediction of ischaemic heart disease than do blood pressure or serum cholesterol, probably because its adverse effects are partly mediated by these two variables. The inter-relationships of obesity, blood pressure, serum triglyceride, glucose intolerance and serum insulin in the 'insulin resistance syndrome' make it difficult to define their relative biological significance (Godsland & Stevenson 1995); this also applies to their relationships with the haemostatic variables coagulation factor VII, plasminogen activator inhibitor type 1 (PAI-1) and tissue plasminogen activator (tPA) antigen (see below).

Another example of interpreting the results of multivariate analyses is the relationship between cigarette-smoking, fibrinogen and ischaemic heart disease (IHD). Three prospective studies have now observed that, when smoking and fibrinogen are compared as predictors of IHD events, smoking is no longer an 'independent risk factor', whereas fibrinogen is (Kannel et al 1987, Meade et al 1987, Cremer et al 1994). The likely interpretation is that increased fibrinogen is an important biological mechanism through which smoking increases IHD risk. It would be wrong to conclude that smoking is no longer a causal risk factor for IHD because epidemiological studies have also started to measure one of its associated mechanisms.

Haematological variables are certainly plausible candidates as biologically significant risk factors for both venous and arterial thrombosis. Both haemostasis and thrombosis involve the interaction of blood platelets and coagulation factors with the endothelium and subendothelium, regulated by inhibitors of platelets and activated coagulation factors, and by the fibrinolytic system. If thrombosis is 'haemostasis in the wrong place' (Macfarlane 1977), then these haemostatic variables are also potentially thrombotic variables. Both haemostasis and thrombosis involve localization of vascular plugs in areas of disturbed blood flow; hence rheological variables (including blood viscosity and blood cell deformability) are also plausible candidates for risk factor status (Lowe 1994a).

Furthermore, epidemiologists recognize that established major risk factors such as smoking, hypertension and high serum cholesterol 'explain' only a minority of arterial thrombotic events; in one study such 'high-risk' persons accounted for only 32% of subsequent myocardial infarctions (Heller et al 1984). Even if the predictive value of such established risk factors has been underestimated (as discussed above), there is clearly scope for improving the prediction of arterial thrombosis by including haematological variables. There is even greater scope for assessing their predictive value for venous thromboembolism, which was not predicted by smoking, hypertension or hyperlipidaemia in the Framingham Study; only obesity in women predicted pulmonary embolism (Goldhaber et al 1983).

CLINICAL UTILITY OF RISK PREDICTION: PRACTICAL ISSUES

Having reviewed the statistical aspects of haematological tests as risk predictors, and their biological significance as causal risk factors, one can also investigate their potential utility in clinical practice (Lowe 1993a; Table 5.2). As noted above, major risk predictors currently used to identify persons at high risk of thrombosis in the general population are inefficient; hence the addition of haematological variables to current risk screening (measurement of smoking habit, blood pressure, body weight, serum cholesterol) may improve risk stratification, to select referral of 'high-risk' persons to prevention clinics. Within 'high-risk' persons who attend such 'risk-factor clinics' for hypertension, hyperlipidaemia, or diabetes, further risk stratification is again desirable, so that the costs and risks of lifestyle modifications and medications to lower blood pressure or blood lipids can be focused on high-risk persons who are most likely to benefit (Davey-Smith et al 1993); again, haematological variables merit assessment in such persons.

While persons with evidence of established arterial disease have a much higher risk of further arterial thrombotic events than similar persons without such evidence, haematological variables again can predict a high-risk group for thrombotic events. For example, two studies have shown that plasma fibrinogen level was the strongest predictor of death in persons with intermittent claudication (Banerjee et al 1992, Fowkes et al 1993), while another study found that von Willebrand factor (vWF) levels added to clinical prediction of graft occlusion or death when measured prior to infrainguinal bypass graft surgery (Woodburn et al 1994). Fibrinogen, vWF and tPA levels also predicted cardiovascular events in the European Concerted Action against Thrombosis (ECAT) Angina Pectoris Study (Thompson et al 1995).

There is now a general consensus that patients admitted to hospital for major surgery or medical illness should be prescribed prophylaxis for venous thromboembolism (at least during the period of immobilization), when their risk is significant as assessed on clinical grounds (Thromboembolic Risk Factor Consensus (THRIFT) Group 1992). Again preoperative measurement of haematological variables may increase the predictability of postoperative deep venous thrombosis (DVT) in gynaecological (Crandon et al 1980), general (Sue-Ling et al 1986) and elective orthopaedic surgery (Paramo et al 1985); however, the effects of preoperative illness on preoperative blood tests should also be considered (Lowe et al 1982). A wide range of preoperative haemostatic tests has been performed in 400 patients undergoing elective hip replacement in the ECAT DVT Study, and their predictive values for postoperative DVT (detected by routine venography) will be of interest.

Venous thromboembolism continues to be an increased risk in users of the combined oestrogen–progesterone contraceptive pill. The recent finding (Vandenbroucke et al 1994) that this risk is greatly increased in the 3–6% of the population who have a prothrombotic mutation in coagulation factor V ($Arg^{506}Gln$, factor V Leiden), which confers resistance to its inactivation by activated protein C, raises the future possibility of screening for this condition when advising on contraceptive measures. If this gene polymorphism also confers an increased risk of venous thromboembolism during pregnancy, screening may also be a future consideration to identify women for thrombotic surveillance and/or prophylaxis.

If haematological variables are used in clinical medicine as predictors of thrombotic risk, consideration has to be given to the practicalities of measurement, as well as their power to discriminate persons who develop thrombosis from those who do not. Ideally, haematological predictors should be already widely available, standardized (so that uniform criteria to define increased risk can be recommended), reproducible, cheap, user-friendly, and should have well-defined effects of age, gender, etc. (Lowe 1993a). User-friendliness is obviously greater for variables which do not require careful standardization of preanalytical variables (e.g. fasting, time of day, resting, careful venepuncture, special tubes, rapid transport of samples to the laboratory for processing).

Apart from merely being predictors of thrombotic risk, haematological variables might also identify persons who merit specific types of antithrombotic prophylaxis. Antithrombotic prophylaxis has been remarkably successful, despite the lack of routine tests to predict a prothrombotic state (in contrast to hypotensive, hypolipidaemic and antidiabetic agents; Lowe 1993a). It is, however, possible that the balance of benefit over risk with antithrombotic prophylaxis may be higher in persons found to have markers of a prothrombotic state. Stratification with such markers might in future identify those at low risk (for no antithrombotic prophylaxis), moderate risk (for low-risk prophylaxis; e.g. aspirin, or low-dose heparin for short-term prophylaxis of venous thromboembolism), or high-risk (for high-risk prophylaxis; e.g. oral anticoagulants).

A topical example of such risk stratification is non-rheumatic atrial fibrillation (AF) which carries increased thromboembolic (especially cardioembolic) risk. Several recently reported randomized controlled trials have shown that warfarin prophylaxis is highly effective (Albers 1994); however, there is concern about the balance of antithrombotic benefits and bleeding risk, as well as the practical implications and costs of long-term anticoagulation of large numbers of elderly people (Sudlow et al 1995). Aspirin is less effective, but safer, and low-risk groups of persons with AF have been defined in whom no antithrombotic prophylaxis appears appropriate. Patients with AF should therefore be stratified on clinical grounds into high-, moderate- and low-risk groups in whom, respectively, warfarin, aspirin or no prophylaxis may be appropriate (Albers 1994). Recent studies (Lip et al 1995) have shown that persons with AF have elevated plasma levels of fibrinogen, vWF, and D-dimer (a marker of cross-linked fibrin turnover), each of which has now been shown to predict thrombosis in the general population (Lowe et al 1995a,b). These haemostatic variables therefore merit prospective evaluation of their prediction of thrombotic risk in persons with AF, and possibly thereafter evaluation of their value in risk stratification and choice of thromboprophylactic regimen (Lip et al 1995). Warfarin prophylaxis variably reduces the elevated plasma D-dimer levels in persons with AF (Lip et al 1995), and this test also merits evaluation in indicating, and in monitoring the efficacy of, oral anticoagulation.

If elevated plasma fibrinogen levels are a causal risk factor for thrombosis, then controlled trials of plasma fibrinogen reduction in prevention of thrombosis are indicated. Likewise, increased platelet activity might indicate prophylaxis with antiplatelet agents; elevated vWF levels might indicate trials of particular antiplatelet agents which reduce the binding of vWF to platelets and/or subendothelium; elevated fibrinogen levels might indicate trials of agents which reduce the binding of fibrinogen to platelets; and elevated PAI levels might indicate trials of agents which reduce such levels and increase fibrinolytic potential, such as anabolic steroids (Lowe & Small 1988).

PREDICTIVE VALUE OF INDIVIDUAL HAEMOSTATIC FACTORS

Rheological variables

'Routine' haematological tests including haematocrit (or the closely related haemoglobin concentration), white cell count, erythrocyte sedimentation rate and plasma viscosity are consistent primary predictors of IHD events and of total mortality in the general population (for reviews see Lowe 1993a, 1994a). Figure 5.1 illustrates the strong predictive value of plasma viscosity, fibrinogen (which is one determinant of plasma viscosity) and white cell count in the Caerphilly and Speedwell Studies (Yarnell et al 1991). They also have strong predictive value in secondary prediction of recurrent IHD events and mortality following recovery from a first myocardial infarction (Martin et al 1991).

These four haematological tests may reasonably be termed 'rheological' because they all affect the flow properties of blood. An increase in each of these four variables is likely to affect blood flow behaviour in the microcirculation and/or macrocirculation, and hence to increase the risks of thrombosis and/or ischaemia following arterial occlusion (Lowe 1993a, 1994a). While not generally considered 'haemostatic' variables, it should be noted that haematocrit is an important determinant of platelet adhesion and aggregation in whole blood, that the interactions of leucocytes with the endothelium, platelets, coagulation and fibrinolysis are of increasing interest to workers in haemostasis and thrombosis, and that plasma viscosity influences platelet adhesion, as well as representing one biological mechanism through which increased plasma fibrinogen may promote IHD events (Lowe 1993a, 1994a).

The predictive value of rheological tests for venous thromboembolism is uncertain, with the exception that the high haematocrit in primary proliferative polycythaemia is related to increased thrombotic risk (Lowe 1984).

These haemorheological tests have potential practical advantages over haemostatic tests in the clinical prediction of thrombosis, being widely available, standardized, reproducible, cheap and robust (except the erythrocyte sedimentation rate, ESR), and having well-defined population distributions and effects of age, gender and smoking (Lowe 1993a). Plasma viscosity has several advantages over the ESR (Lowe 1994b); it may be a stronger predictor of IHD events than fibrinogen, perhaps because it is also a measure of other acute-phase proteins and lipoproteins (Fig. 5.1), and unlike fibrinogen has standardized methodology and units (Lowe 1994b).

No large randomized trials of reduction in haematocrit, white cell count or plasma viscosity in prevention of arterial thrombosis have been reported; however, trials of haemodilution with dextran, or defibrinogenation and plasma viscosity reduction with ancrod, have reported efficacy in prophylaxis of venous thrombosis following hip surgery (Lowe 1994a).

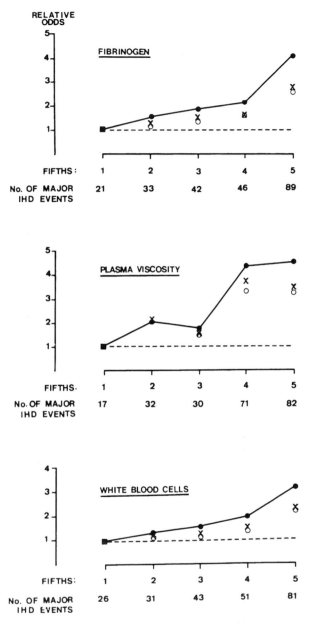

Fig. 5.1   Risk (relative odds) of major IHD events by fifths (quintiles) of plasma fibrinogen, plasma viscosity, and white blood cell count in 4641 men in the Caerphilly and Speedwell Collaborative Heart Disease Studies. Data linked by solid lines are adjusted for age and area; crosses show data adjusted also for smoking habit and pre-existent IHD; open circles show data adjusted also for diastolic blood pressure, body mass index and total serum cholesterol. (Reproduced, with permission, from Yarnell et al 1991.)

Platelets

There are few reported studies of the predictive value of platelet count, mean platelet volume (MPV) or measures of platelet reactivity for arterial thrombotic events (Wilhelmsen 1991, Lowe 1993a). In the only large reported study of primary prediction, the relative risk of IHD mortality in the quartile (25%) with the highest platelet counts was 2.5 compared to the quartile with the lowest platelet counts (Thaulow et al 1991). In contrast, platelet count was not a secondary predictor of recurrent IHD events or mortality in a larger study of infarct survivors, although MPV was (Martin et al 1991). The increasing routine availability of platelet counts and MPV as part of the 'full blood count' in modern cell counters may facilitate performance of further studies, although there are important methodological issues in MPV measurement.

Measurements of platelet reactivity (in vivo or in vitro) also have methodological problems, as well as large biological variability (Vickers & Thompson 1985), including the effects of aspirin, other non-steroidal anti-inflammatory drugs (NSAIDs) and alcohol. Nevertheless, some recent epidemiological studies have suggested that platelet aggregability in vitro may predict arterial thrombosis. In a random subsample of the Norwegian prospective study (Thaulow et al 1991), ADP-induced platelet aggregation was predictive of fatal myocardial infarction. This observation is consistent with the cross-sectional data from the Caerphilly Study, in which ADP-induced platelet aggregation in 1811 fasting men with no history of recent aspirin or NSAID drug use was associated with a past history of myocardial infarction (Elwood et al 1991). On the other hand, a larger, 10-year follow-up of men in the Northwick Park Heart Study was recently reported to show no association of either ADP- or adrenaline-induced platelet aggregation with IHD events (Meade 1995). Two studies have reported that platelet aggregability was a secondary predictor of arterial thrombotic events. Breddin et al (1986) observed that platelet aggregation was predictive of cardiovascular events in diabetics, while Trip et al (1990) reported that spontaneous platelet aggregation was predictive of recurrent myocardial infarction. With the increasing use of prophylactic aspirin (or alcohol!) in persons with arterial disease, it may be difficult to perform such prospective studies in the future.

Despite the paucity of prospective studies of platelet-related variables, the biological importance of platelets in arterial thrombosis is in little doubt, as shown by both morphological studies (necropsy and angioscopy) and by meta-analyses of platelet-inhibitor drugs, notably aspirin (Antiplatelet Trialists' Collaboration 1994a,b). As noted above, the widespread use of aspirin limits the potential utility of platelet activity tests. However, the recently described resistance to the antiplatelet effects of aspirin in some persons with cerebrovascular disease may indicate a potential role for such tests in monitoring the antiplatelet effects of antiplatelet drugs during prophylaxis.

Interest in the role of platelets in venous thrombogenesis has recently been re-awakened by the results of the Antiplatelet Trialists' Collaboration (1994c) meta-analysis, which showed a greater reduction in pulmonary embolism than had been anticipated as a complication of deep venous thrombi, which are largely composed of fibrin. Nevertheless, platelet-rich thrombi can be present at the onset of venous thrombogenesis, and plasma levels of the platelet-release marker β-thromboglobulin were predictive of postoperative DVT when measured on the day after surgery, although not preoperatively (Douglas et al 1985).

Endothelium

The vascular endothelium has several haemostatic, antithrombotic and prothrombotic activities which may play important roles in both haemostasis and thrombosis. These include synthesis of prostacyclin, nitric oxide, platelet-activating factor, ectonucleotidases, vWF, thrombomodulin, tissue factor and tissue factor pathway inhibitor (TFPI), tPA and PAI-1 (Pearson 1994). The latter two variables are considered below under the heading of fibrinolysis. Measurement in plasma of soluble thrombomodulin, tissue factor and TFPI may in the future elucidate the roles of these endothelial products in arterial and venous thrombosis. However, at present plasma vWF is the most commonly measured marker of endothelial disturbance.

Two recent studies have observed that plasma von Willebrand factor antigen (vWF:Ag) was a primary predictor of IHD events. In the Northwick Park Heart Study, Meade et al (1994a) found that vWF:Ag was not significantly associated with IHD events (84 events among 1020 men aged 46–70 years over 10 years) on univariate analysis; however, after adjustment for the effect of blood group on vWF levels, an increase by one approximate standard deviation (38.6% of standard) was associated with an increase in incidence of fatal IHD events of 1.34 ($P = 0.05$), although there was no association with non-fatal events. Because of the strong association of plasma vWF with coagulation factor VIII activity (VIII:C, as expected from the carrier function of vWF for factor VIII:C in the circulation), it was not possible to distinguish the predictive values of vWF and factor VIII:C, although the latter showed a stronger association with fatal IHD events. While this study confirmed the findings of several previous studies that ABO blood groups other than group O were associated with increased risk of IHD, the associations between IHD and factor VIII:C–vWF, and between IHD and blood group, appeared to be independent (Meade et al 1994a).

In the Caerphilly Study, the risk of all IHD events (129 fatal and non-fatal events) in 2086 men aged 50–64 years, followed for 5 years, increased progressively by quintile (20%) of plasma vWF:Ag; the relative risk was 1.8 in the highest compared to the lowest quintile (Lowe et al 1995b). Multivariate analysis showed very little effect of the standard risk factors on this association, which was statistically significant ($P = 0.05$).

Four secondary prediction studies support the findings of these two primary prediction studies, that plasma vWF levels predict arterial thrombotic events. Breddin et al (1986) observed that vWF levels predicted vascular complications in diabetics, while Jansson et al (1991a) reported that vWF levels predicted recurrent myocardial infarction. In the ECAT multicentre study of 3043 patients with angina pectoris who underwent coronary angiography and were followed for 2 years, during which time 106 had definite coronary events, the risk of coronary events increased progressively with quintiles of vWF:Ag; after adjustment for all confounding variables the relative risk was 1.85 in the highest compared to the lowest quintile (Thompson et al 1995). These findings are very similar to those of the Caerphilly Study (Lowe et al 1995b). In the ECAT Study, factor VIII:C levels were not predictive of coronary events (Thompson et al 1995). In a study of 160 patients undergoing infrainguinal bypass grafting for peripheral arterial disease, plasma vWF level was the only haematological variable which added significantly to the predictive value of clinical variables for graft occlusion or death in the first postoperative year, and was used to derive a potentially useful predictive index (Woodburn et al 1994).

The association of plasma vWF:Ag level with venous thrombosis was recently investigated in the Leiden Thrombophilia Study: a population-based case-control study of 301 unselected consecutive patients, aged under 70 years, with a first, objectively confirmed episode of DVT and without underlying malignant disease (Koster et al 1995). The risk of previous DVT increased progressively with increasing vWF levels, the relative risk being 3.0 in subjects with vWF levels greater than 1.50 IU/dl, compared to subjects with vWF levels less than 1.0 IU/dl. The association of DVT with factor VIII activity was stronger, and there was also an association with blood group non-O. After adjustment for factor VIII:C levels and blood group, the association of DVT with vWF levels was not statistically significant, and the authors concluded that these two variables 'mediated' the association of DVT with vWF levels (Koster et al 1995). Preoperative plasma vWF levels have also been reported to predict postoperative DVT (Nilsson et al 1986).

The elevation of vWF levels in AF (Lip et al 1995) has already been noted.

Plasma vWF:Ag levels therefore merit further study in prediction of arterial and venous thrombotic risk, particularly as assays are relatively robust. As noted previously, these associations may suggest a role for endothelial disturbance in arterial and venous thrombogenesis; elevated vWF levels may promote thrombogenesis via platelet adhesion and aggregation, and might in theory suggest a prophylactic role for antiplatelet agents which reduce the interaction of vWF with its platelet and vessel wall receptors. However, the confounding effects of factor VIII and blood group should be considered in interpreting the associations of vWF levels and thrombosis.

Fibrinogen

Of all haemostatic variables, plasma fibrinogen is the best established predictor of arterial thrombotic events. The evidence that fibrinogen is a cardiovascular risk factor has been extensively reviewed in the published proceedings of two international symposia in 1992 (Ernst et al 1992) and 1994 (Lowe et al 1995a); only a brief review is given here. At the time of writing, it appears that such biennial international symposia will continue until the millennium, indicating the continued interest of epidemiologists, laboratory scientists, clinicians and pharmaceutical companies in this field.

Since the pioneering report in 1980 from the Northwick Park Heart Study that plasma fibrinogen (as well as coagulation factors VII and VIII) were predictive of cardiovascular death (Meade et al 1980), at least 20 prospective studies have reported that fibrinogen is a strong, consistent, primary or secondary predictor of arterial thrombotic events (IHD and stroke). The results of two meta-analyses of the early published reports of the seven primary predictive studies (Ernst & Resch 1993, Resch & Ernst 1995) are illustrated in Fig. 5.2. At the time of the second meta-analysis, these seven studies collectively included 15 700 individuals followed for a mean observation time of 6.4 years (102 168 patient-years) during which 838 major cardiovascular events occurred. Figure 5.2 shows that the results of these studies were highly consistent, in that there was a clinically significant increase in cardiovascular risk in the upper tertile (third, 33%) of the study population. These consistent results occurred despite wide differences between studies in country, selection of subjects, mean age of subjects, absolute cardiovascular risk (Fig. 5.2), or method of fibrinogen assay. The latest meta-analysis found that persons in the upper tertile of the population distribution of fibrinogen had a relative risk of cardiovascular events of 2.45 (95% confidence intervals (CI) 2.05–2.93) (Resch & Ernst 1995). More recent reports from four of these studies (Meade et al 1993, Cremer et al 1994, Heinrich et al 1994, Sweetnam et al 1994) do not appear to change these estimates appreciably (see also Fig. 5.1).

Confirmation and extension of the results of these seven studies comes from the Scottish Heart Health Study, in which men and women aged 40–59 years were chosen by random sampling of general practice registers across 50% of districts in Scotland; 74% (10 359) attended and 8824 had plasma fibrinogen assays performed by the automated Clauss method (Lee et al 1990, 1993a,b). A provisional analysis was performed after an 8-year follow-up, during which 438 coronary events (Tunstall-Pedoe et al 1994) and 412 deaths (Woodward et al 1994) had occurred – a total of 850 events. As shown in Figure 5.3, both IHD events and total mortality increased progressively with quartiles of plasma fibrinogen, in both men and women (Lowe 1995). It is therefore apparent, from these eight studies with almost 2000 events in 25 000 persons, that fibrinogen is as strong and consistent a primary predictor of IHD events and death as any other potentially modi-

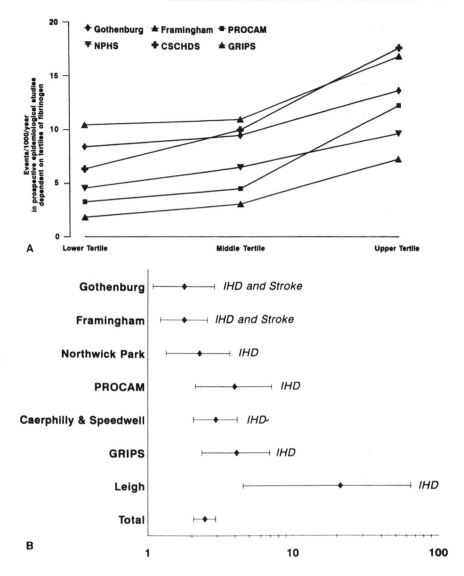

Fig. 5.2 A Cardiovascular events by thirds (tertiles) of plasma fibrinogen in six of seven primary prospective studies. **B** Odds ratios and 95% confidence intervals for risk of IHD and stroke (upper tertile relative to lower tertile) in these seven studies. (Reproduced, with permission, from Resch & Ernst 1995.)

fiable risk factor. Fibrinogen levels have also been reported to predict peripheral arterial disease (Bainton et al 1994).

As previously discussed, three of these studies have suggested that a major part of the increased risk of IHD events in smokers is mediated through increased fibrinogen levels (Kannel et al 1987, Meade et al 1987, Cremer

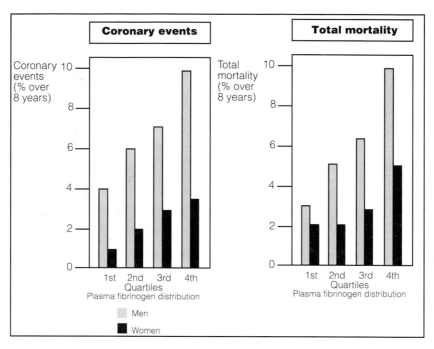

Fig. 5.3 Association of plasma fibrinogen with IHD and total mortality in men and women in the Scottish Heart Health Study. Data from Tunstall-Pedoe et al (1994) and Woodward et al (1994). (Reproduced, with permission, from Lowe 1995.)

et al 1994). A fall in fibrinogen levels after smoking cessation parallels a fall in IHD risk (Lowe 1993b). Furthermore, fibrinogen and cholesterol may have additive effects on IHD risk (Stone & Thorp 1983, Heinrich et al 1994, Thompson et al 1995), fibrinogen and systolic blood pressure may have additive effects on stroke risk (Wilhelmsen et al 1983), and fibrinogen and diabetes have additive effects on cardiovascular risk (Breddin et al 1986, Kannel et al 1990). The addition of plasma fibrinogen measurement to the standard cardiovascular risk assessment is therefore likely to improve risk stratification (Heinrich et al 1994).

However, several practical issues must be addressed before fibrinogen assays are used routinely to assess cardiovascular risk in the general population. The need to perform several assays to obtain an accurate (over 90%) assessment of an individual's mean plasma fibrinogen level (as with other major risk factors) has already been discussed (Rosenson et al 1994). Standardization of fibrinogen assays is required, so that uniform criteria to define increased risk (e.g. upper tertiles; Fig. 5.2) can be agreed. An international standard for the commonly used Clauss assay of thrombin-clottable fibrinogen has been developed (Gaffney & Wong 1992); using such a standardized assay, one study (Lowe et al 1994) suggested that a plasma fibrinogen level of about 3.0 g/l defines the upper tertile in middle-aged men, who have a 2–3-fold increase in risk of IHD events and mortality (Fig. 5.2) – a potentially simple 'rule of threes'.

On the other hand, clotting assays in citrated plasma, although used routinely in haematology laboratories to detect low fibrinogen levels and predict risk of bleeding, may be inferior to other types of assay, such as nephelometry, for prediction of arterial thrombotic events (Yarnell et al 1991, Sweetnam et al 1994). Nephelometric fibrinogen assays can be performed in the same dipotassium edetate anticoagulated sample tubes that are used for routine full blood counts and for blood lipid and lipoprotein analyses, and which are more robust during sample transport and processing (unpublished observations). Hence they would be relatively simple to incorporate into existing primary cardiovascular risk screening in general practice and in hospital 'risk-factor' clinics, in which such samples are already sent for lipid and lipoprotein analyses to biochemistry laboratories (and could be also sent to haematology laboratories for measurement of haematological predictors such as haematocrit, white cell count, plasma viscosity or ESR, and possibly platelet count and mean platelet volume; see above). Whether nephelometric assays of fibrinogen should be performed by biochemical laboratories or by haematological laboratories will be an interesting future issue!

The plasma fibrinogen level is not only a strong and consistent primary risk factor for arterial events, it is also an equally strong and consistent secondary risk factor for arterial events in persons with established arterial disease. Examples include persons with peripheral arterial disease (Banerjee et al 1992, Fowkes et al 1993, Woodburn et al 1994), angina (Thompson et al 1995), previous myocardial infarction (Cooper & Douglas 1991, Martin et al 1991, Benderly 1994), or previous stroke (Ernst et al 1991).

The case that fibrinogen is a causal risk factor for arterial thrombosis, rather than simply a risk predictor, can be examined according to the classical criteria of Bradford Hill (1965) (Table 5.2). There is now little doubt that fibrinogen is a strong, dose-dependent and consistent risk predictor (Figs 5.1–5.3). It is equally strong as a primary and a secondary risk predictor, suggesting that hyperfibrinogenaemia predates the onset of thrombosis. Cross-sectional studies have shown that fibrinogen is related to the extent of arterial disease (Lowe 1993b, Lowe et al 1993) and to increasing evidence of IHD (Lee et al 1993a). That high fibrinogen levels precede the onset of disease is supported by the findings of two epidemiological studies that a genetic polymorphism for the Bβ chain of fibrinogen (synthesis of which is the rate-limiting step in fibrinogen synthesis; Green & Humphries 1994), which is associated with increased fibrinogen levels, is associated with peripheral arterial disease (Fowkes et al 1992) and with the angiographic extent of coronary artery disease (Evans et al 1995). These findings are consistent with the observations of two other studies that a family history of premature IHD is associated with higher fibrinogen levels in asymptomatic persons (Hoffman et al 1993, Lee et al 1993a).

The association of fibrinogen with arterial thrombotic events is also biologically plausible (Lowe 1993b, Lowe et al 1995a). Increased plasma fibrinogen levels may promote atherosclerosis by infiltration of the arterial wall and by incorporation of mural thrombi; they may promote arterial thrombosis not only by promoting formation of arterial plaques, but also by increasing platelet aggregation and the volume and rigidity of fibrin thrombi, as well as decreasing the lysability of thrombi; and finally they may promote ischaemia by increasing plasma and blood viscosity. The evidence for these processes has been reviewed recently (Lowe 1993b, Lowe et al 1995a).

The final proof of whether or not elevated plasma fibrinogen levels promote thrombosis will come from large, randomized trials of drugs which lower fibrinogen concentration. These agents include fibrates, ticlopidine and hormone replacement therapy (HRT).

Certain fibrates (bezafibrate, ciprofibrate, clofibrate and fenofibrate, but not gemfibrozil) lower plasma fibrinogen levels by about 25% (Meade 1995) which from epidemiological studies is associated with a potentially substantial reduction in cardiovascular risk. Clofibrate reduced the risk of myocardial infarction in one primary prevention study, although mortality was increased; however, its effects on lowering fibrinogen were most marked in high-risk subjects such as smokers, in whom it appeared to prevent the smoking-induced increase in fibrinogen (Green et al 1989).

Two studies of secondary prevention by bezafibrate, for which there is most evidence for fibrinogen reduction, are in progress: one in survivors of myocardial infarction (Benderly 1994), the other in persons with peripheral arterial disease (Meade 1995).

The antiplatelet agent ticlopidine also lowers plasma fibrinogen levels, by about 10% (Drouet et al 1994), which may be relevant to its possibly greater prophylactic effect against arterial thrombosis than aspirin (Antiplatelet Trialists' Collaboration 1994a).

Cross-sectional studies have suggested that HRT appears to attenuate the postmenopausal rise in fibrinogen, which accompanies increased cardiovascular risk (Meilahn et al 1992, Lee et al 1993b, Nabulsi et al 1993). A recently reported randomized trial of HRT has confirmed that it reduces plasma fibrinogen levels (PEPI Trial 1995). Together with the effects of HRT on blood lipids, this effect may partly explain the apparent protective effects of HRT against risk of IHD and stroke.

It will be appreciated that currently available agents which lower plasma fibrinogen levels also reduce blood lipids (fibrates, HRT) or have antiplatelet effects (ticlopidine). Hence large trials will be required to differentiate the effects of fibrinogen reduction from the other biological effects of these agents.

Fibrinogen levels (and high-fibrinogen genotypes) have also been associated with risk of venous thrombosis (Crandon et al 1980, Lowe 1984, Balendra 1990, Koster et al 1994a). Defibrinogenation with ancrod reduced the risk of DVT after surgery for hip fracture (Lowe 1984).

Factor VII

Factor VII activity (VII:C) has been shown to predict IHD events in the Northwick Park Heart Study (Meade et al 1980, 1986, 1993) and in the PROCAM Study (Heinrich et al 1994). The stronger predictive value of factor VII:C in the Northwick Park Heart Study may reflect the use in that study of an assay more sensitive to the active, two-chain form of factor VII (VIIa) whose circulating concentration is much lower than that of inactive, single chain factor VII (Miller et al 1994). This possibility could be tested in prospective studies of recently developed specific assays of factor VIIa. Factor VII:C may be more predictive of fatal IHD events than of non-fatal events, possibly by promoting large coronary thrombi (Ruddock & Meade 1994). Combined activity of factors II, VII and X did not predict IHD or stroke events in the Göteborg study (Wilhelmsen et al 1983).

Factor VII activity is related to dietary fat intake, blood lipids, obesity and glucose intolerance; hence it is one potential link between these risk factors and thrombosis (Meade 1995). The causal role of factor VII activity in IHD events is currently being tested in a primary prevention trial of low-dose warfarin (which lowers high factor VII:C levels) in high-risk men, defined by high levels of factor VII:C and fibrinogen as well as conventional risk factors (Meade et al 1988).

Neither factor VII activity nor factor VII genotype were related to venous thrombosis in the Leiden case-control study (Koster et al 1994a).

Factor VIII

Factor VIII activity (VIII:C) was not predictive of IHD or stroke in the Göteborg Study (Wilhelmsen et al 1983) but, as noted above, was predictive of IHD events, after adjustment for the effect of blood group, in the Northwick Park Heart Study (Meade et al 1994a). As with factor VII:C, factor VIII:C appeared more predictive of fatal events than of non-fatal events. As noted above, very large studies will be required to differentiate the predictive effects of factor VIII:C from vWF because of their strong correlation (Meade et al 1994a). Nevertheless, an independent direct effect of factor VIII:C on arterial thrombosis is suggested by other evidence:

1. The protective effect of low factor VIII:C levels (in the presence of normal vWF levels) in haemophilia A, which carries a relative risk of IHD mortality of 0.2 (Rosendaal et al 1989) and in which myocardial infarction is rare (Small et al 1983).
2. Increased in vivo thrombin generation after low–normal factor VIII levels are elevated to high–normal factor VIII levels by desmopressin

infusion (Ibbotson et al 1992), which is occasionally followed by myocardial infarction.
3. The independent association of factor VIII:C levels with venous thrombosis, in both prospective (Crandon et al 1980) and case-control studies (Balendra 1990, Koster et al 1995). Factor VIII:C levels over 150 IU/dl showed a strong association with DVT in case-control studies (Balendra 1990, Koster et al 1995), although it is possible that some of this elevation might result from previous venous thrombosis. Koster (1995) calculated that high factor VIII:C levels accounted for 16% of the population-attributable risks of DVT.

Factor XII deficiency

Factor XII is involved in the initiation of both the intrinsic coagulation pathway and in fibrinolysis. However, deficiency is rarely associated with either a bleeding tendency or a thrombotic tendency (Koster et al 1994b).

Antithrombin, protein C and protein S deficiencies

Congenital heterozygous deficiencies of the natural coagulation inhibitors, antithrombin (antithrombin III), protein C and protein S, are well-established risk factors for venous thrombosis. What is less clear is the prevalence of such deficiencies in the general population, the relative risk of venous thrombosis associated with each type of deficiency, and to what extent these deficiencies contribute to the population-attributable risks of DVT. In the Leiden thrombophilia case-control study, Koster and colleagues identified from the initial measurement antithrombin deficiency in 4.2% of patients and 1.9% of controls (odds ratio 2.2, 95% CI 1.0–4.7), protein C deficiency in 4.6% versus 1.5% (odds ratio 3.1, 1.7–7.0), total protein S deficiency in 1.7% versus 2.3% (odds ratio 0.7, 0.3–1.8), and free protein S deficiency in 3.1% versus 2.1% (1.6, 0.6–4.0) (Koster 1995). Repeated measurements of these variables reduced the apparent frequency of these deficiencies in both cases and controls, presumably due to the effect of 'regression to the mean'. Nevertheless, antithrombin and protein C deficiencies (but not protein S deficiencies) were significant potential predictors of thrombotic risk, although in combination these deficiencies accounted for only 5% of the population-attributable risks of DVT. Hence, while important for individual patients and their families, identification and management of these deficiencies will have only a small impact on DVT prevention in the community.

In the smaller case-control study of Balendra (1990), no cases of antithrombin or protein C deficiency were encountered, again suggesting their limited contribution to DVT in the population. In contrast, a significant independent relationship of lower mean total protein S to DVT was observed, suggesting that analysis of the total distributions of coagulation deficiencies to thrombosis is of interest, rather than the relative frequencies of arbitrarily defined 'deficiencies' (Balendra 1990).

The association of coagulation inhibitors with arterial thrombosis is unclear. While two prospective studies have associated low antithrombin levels with risk of IHD (Cortellaro 1991, Meade et al 1991), Meade et al (1991) also associated high antithrombin levels with risk of IHD, possibly as a 'compensatory' rise associated with high fibrinogen levels.

Activated protein C resistance (factor V Leiden)

The recent discovery by Dahlbäck and colleagues that activated protein C (APC) resistance is associated with venous thrombosis, and is highly correlated with a prothrombotic mutation in coagulation factor V identified by Bertina et al (Arg^{506}Gln, factor V Leiden), is a major advance in the discovery of genetic mutations promoting risk of venous thrombosis (Bertina et al 1995, Dahlbäck 1995). In the Leiden Thrombophilia Study, APC resistance was associated with an odds ratio for DVT risk of 6.6 (95% CI 3.6–12.0) (Koster et al 1993), and accounted for 17% of the population-attributable risk of DVT (Koster 1995). In a nested case-control study using stored DNA from the US Physicians' Health Study, Ridker et al (1995) observed a somewhat lower relative risk (Fig. 5.4). As previously noted, Vandenbroucke et al (1994) observed that factor V Leiden is associated

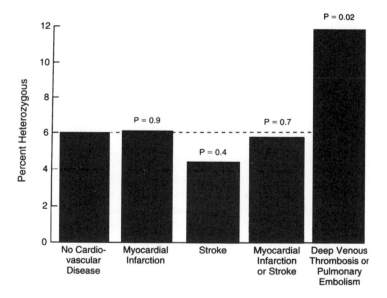

Fig. 5.4   Prevalence of factor V Leiden genotype in nested case-control study of myocardial infarction, stroke and venous thromboembolism in the US Physicians' Health Study. (Reproduced, with permission, from Ridker et al 1995.)

with increased risk of venous thromboembolism associated with the contraceptive pill, raising the possibility of screening for the mutation to detect increased risk in persons exposed to acquired thrombotic risk factors (e.g. pill use, pregnancy).

Two epidemiological studies have suggested that factor V Leiden is not associated with risk of arterial thrombosis (Emmerich et al 1995, Ridker et al 1995; Fig. 5.4).

Antiphospholipid antibodies/lupus anticoagulants

Antiphospholipid antibodies, especially if present in persistently high titres, associated with the lupus anticoagulant phenomenon, or associated with systemic lupus erythematosus (SLE) in which this phenomenon was first described, are associated with increased risk of both venous and arterial (especially cerebrovascular) thrombosis (Muir 1995). Their associations with premature and recurrent thrombosis in non-SLE patients have been proposed as a causal 'primary antiphospholipid syndrome' (Harris et al 1987). In a recent critical review, Muir (1995) has queried the causal role of these antibodies, and emphasized the selection bias in many studies. There is a need for further epidemiological studies to determine the primary and secondary predictive value of antiphospholipid antibodies, such as a nested case-control study using stored sera from the US Physicians' Health Study, which found anticardiolipin titres to be predictive of subsequent development of DVT, but not of ischaemic stroke (Ginsburg et al 1992).

Fibrin(ogen) degradation products

Fibrin(ogen) degradation products reflect degradation of fibrin(ogen), usually by plasmin, and often as a secondary fibrino(geno)lytic response to primary activation of the coagulation system. Very high levels are seen in disseminated intravascular coagulation (DIC), therapeutic fibrinolysis (e.g. with streptokinase), and occasionally in primary pathological fibrinolysis (e.g. tumours releasing tPA or urokinase). Moderately high levels are observed in venous thromboembolism. Currently, commercially available specific antibodies against D-dimer (present in cross-linked fibrin degradation products), fibrinogen degradation products, or other fibrin degradation products are frequently used in diagnosis of these conditions, using plasma samples instead of the traditional approach of measuring serum fibrinogen-related antigen (Nieuwenhuizen 1991).

For several years, we have studied plasma levels of D-dimer in epidemiological studies and cohort studies of healthy persons and persons with arterial or cardiac disease, on the premise (1) that plasma D-dimer is quantifiable in all adults, and (2) that in the absence of DIC, venous thrombosis, or diseases in which there is appreciable generation of extravascular cross-linked fibrin causing elevation of D-dimer (e.g. tissue damage due to trauma, surgery, infections, cancer or sterile inflammatory conditions such as rheumatoid arthritis) plasma D-dimer level may quantify ongoing activation of blood coagulation, thrombin formation and function of cross-linked intravascular fibrin which is most likely intra-arterial or intracardiac in origin. This hypothesis has been supported by our findings, in population-controlled studies, of 'dose-dependent' elevations of plasma D-dimer in arterial disease (Reid 1991, Al-Zahrani et al 1992, Smith et al 1993, Rumley et al 1994, Lee et al 1995) and atrial fibrillation (Lip et al 1995). Prospective cohort studies have shown that plasma D-dimer is a strong, independent risk predictor of IHD events in patients with peripheral arterial disease (Fowkes et al 1993), and in the Caerphilly Study (Lowe et al 1995b). Similar results were reported in the PLAT Study of atherosclerotic patients (Cortellaro et al 1993), and the US Physicians' Health Study (Ridker et al 1994).

The consistency and strength of these associations, as well as the weak correlations between plasma D-dimer and classical risk factors for IHD (Lee et al 1995), suggest that plasma D-dimer may be a useful addition to the cardiovascular risk profile (Lip & Lowe 1995). In addition, it may identify persons with high intravascular fibrin turnover who may benefit from prophylactic full-dose anticoagulant therapy, which normalizes elevated D-dimer levels (Lip et al 1995). Neither aspirin nor minidose (1 mg/day) warfarin lower raised D-dimer levels in patients with arterial disease (Reid 1991). The elevation of D-dimer levels in AF, and the possibility that they might be used to monitor efficacy of oral anticoagulant therapy, have been previously noted (Lip et al 1995). Plasma D-dimer levels also predict progression of atherosclerosis (Fowkes et al 1993), consistent with the Rokitansky–Duguid hypothesis which suggests that arterial fibrin formation contributes to atherogenesis. Both serum fibrin(ogen) degradation products (Crandon et al 1980) and plasma D-dimer (Rowbotham et al 1992) have been shown to predict postoperative DVT, when measured preoperatively.

Fibrinolytic variables

While levels of fibrin(ogen) degradation products are a measure of ongoing fibrin turnover (fibrin formation and fibrinolysis), traditional 'fibrinolytic tests' such as clot lysis times, PAI activity, or tPA activity or antigen are a measure of fibrinolytic potential. Many cross-sectional studies have associated these variables with arterial disease or venous thrombosis (Lowe & Small 1988), but few prospective studies have been reported.

In the long-term follow-up of men in the Northwick Park Heart Study, Meade et al (1993) found that global fibrinolytic activity (measured by the dilute whole blood clot lysis time) was predictive of IHD events in men aged 40–54 years, but not in men aged 55–64 years. The latter finding is consistent with the results of the Göteborg Study of men aged 54 years and over, that the euglobulin clot lysis time was not predictive of IHD or stroke (Wilhelmsen et al 1984). The former finding is consistent with the findings of Hamsten et al (1987) that PAI activity predicted recurrence in 109 young (age under 45 years) survivors of myocardial infarction; high PAI activity is a major determinant of long clot lysis times (Meade et al 1994b). However, the study of Hamsten et al (1987) was a secondary prediction study (recurrent infarction) in a highly selected group of infarct survivors (those aged under 45 years). Furthermore, PAI activity did not predict events at the 6-year follow-up (Wiman & Hamsten 1990). PAI activity also predicted events in atherosclerotic patients in the PLAT Study (Cortellaro et al 1993), but not in the study of Janssen et al (1993). Neither PAI activity nor PAI antigen predicted IHD events in the ECAT Angina Pectoris Study (Thompson et al 1995). Two other studies (Ridker et al 1992a, Lowe et al 1995b) have found that PAI activity was not a significant primary predictor of IHD events in healthy men, regardless of age. Any association of PAI activity with IHD in these studies was accounted for by their mutual associations with hyperlipidaemia and other associations of insulin resistance, as were the associations of PAI activity with prevalent peripheral arterial disease in the Edinburgh Artery Study (Smith et al 1995). While increased PAI activity (decreasing thrombolysis) might be one mechanism by which insulin resistance might promote atherothrombosis (Juhan-Vague & Alessi 1993), at present it does not appear a useful predictor of IHD events, possibly due to its high biological variability.

Plasma tPA antigen may also be a marker of impaired fibrinolytic activity, because much tPA circulates as inactive complexes, formed as a result of excess PAI-1 (Meade et al 1994b). While predictive of IHD events in a nested case-control study from the US Physicians' Health Study (Ridker et al 1993) and in the Caerphilly Study (Lowe et al 1995b), this was largely explained by its associations with hyperlipidaemia, as was its association with prevalent arterial disease in the Edinburgh Artery Study (Smith et al 1995). The ECAT Angina Pectoris Study, however, found an independent secondary predictive value of tPA antigen for IHD events in patients with angina (Thompson et al 1995), confirming the previous reports of Jansson et al (1991b, 1993). Furthermore, a case-control study from the US Physicians' Health Study showed that tPA antigen was an independent predictor of stroke risk (Ridker et al 1994a).

With regard to venous thrombosis, preoperative prolonged euglobulin clot lysis times were predictive of postoperative DVT in some studies (e.g. Crandon et al 1980, Sue-Ling et al 1986), as were preoperative PAI and tPA assays (Paramo et al 1985). However, a critical review emphasized the lack of epidemiological studies (Prins & Hirsh 1991), and neither case-control studies (Balendra 1990, Levi et al 1991) nor the prospective US Physicians' Heart Study (Ridker et al 1992b) observed significant associations of fibrinolytic activity, PAI activity or tPA antigen; the associations in the study of Balendra (1990) appeared once again to be due to hyperlipidaemia.

KEY POINTS FOR CLINICAL PRACTICE

- Present evidence suggests that certain haemorheological tests (haematocrit, white cell count and possibly plasma viscosity and ESR) and haemostatic tests (fibrinogen, vWF, D-dimer and possibly tPA antigen, factor VII:C and factor VIII:C) are predictive of arterial thrombosis, and may add to the cardiovascular risk profile.

- Potential predictors of venous thrombosis include APC resistance/factor V Leiden, fibrinogen, factor VIII:C, and deficiencies of antithrombin or proteins C or S.

- Ongoing studies should clarify the predictive value, biological significance and clinical utility of haematological variables in relation to thrombotic risk.

REFERENCES

Albers G 1994 Atrial fibrillation and stroke. Arch Intern Med 154: 1143–1148
Al Zahrani H, Lowe G D O, Douglas J T et al 1992 Increased fibrin turnover in peripheral arterial disease: comparison with a population study. Clin Hemorheol 12: 867–872
Antiplatelet Trialists' Collaboration 1994a Collaborative overview of randomised trials of anti-platelet therapy – I. Prevention of death, myocardial infarction, and stroke by prolonged antiplatelet therapy in various categories of patients. Br Med J 308: 81–106
Antiplatelet Trialists' Collaboration 1994b Collaborative overview of randomised trials of antiplatelet therapy – II. Maintenance of vascular graft or arterial patency by antiplatelet therapy. Br Med J 308: 159–168
Antiplatelet Trialists' Collaboration 1994c Collaborative overview of randomised trials of antiplatelet therapy – III. Reduction of venous thrombosis and pulmonary embolism by antiplatelet prophylaxis among surgical and medical patients. Br Med J 308: 235–246
Bainton D, Sweetnam P, Baker I, Elwood P 1994 Peripheral vascular disease: consequence for survival and association with risk factors in the Speedwell prospective heart disease study. Br Heart J 72: 128–132
Balendra P R 1990 Deep vein thrombosis of the leg: natural history and haemostatic variables. M D Thesis, University of Belfast
Banerjee A K, Pearson J, Gilliland E L et al 1992 A six year prospective study of fibrinogen and other risk factors associated with mortality in stable claudicants. Thromb Haemost 68: 261–263
Benderly M 1994 Fibrinogen as predictor of mortality in coronary heart disease patients. Blood Coagulat Fibrinol 5 (suppl 2): 16
Bertina R M, Reitsma P H, Rosendaal F R, Vandenbroucke J P 1995 Resistance to activated protein C and factor V Leiden as risk factors for venous thrombosis. Thromb Haemost 74: 449–453
Bradford Hill A 1965 The environment and disease: association or causation? Proc R Soc Med 58: 295–300
Breddin H K, Krzywanek H J, Atthof P et al 1986 Spontaneous platelet aggregation, von Willebrand factor antigen and fibrinogen as risk factors for new vascular occlusions in type I and II diabetics. Thromb Res 6 (suppl): 154
Chandler A B 1974 Mechanisms and frequency of thrombosis in the coronary circulation. Thromb Res 4: 3–23
Cooper J, Douglas A S 1991 Fibrinogen level as a predictor of mortality in survivors of myocardial infarction. Fibrinolysis 5: 105–108
Cortellaro M 1991 Antithrombin III and arterial disease. Lancet 338: 1525–1526
Cortellaro M, Confrancesco E, Boschetti C et al 1993 Increased fibrin turnover and high

PAI-1 activity as predictors of ischaemic events in atherosclerotic patients: a case-control study. Arterioscler Thromb 13: 1412–1417

Crandon A J, Peel K R, Anderson J A et al 1980 Post-operative deep vein thrombosis: identifying high-risk patients. Br Med J 2: 343–344

Cremer P, Nagel D, Labrot B et al 1994 Lipoprotein Lp(a) as predictor of myocardial infarction in comparison to fibrinogen, LDL cholesterol and other risk factors: results from the prospective Göttingen Risk Incidence and Prevalence Study (GRIPS). Eur J Clin Invest 24: 444–453

Dahlbäck B 1995 New molecular insights into the genetics of thrombophilia. Thromb Haemost 74: 139–148

Davey-Smith G, Phillips A 1990 Declaring independence: why we should be cautious. J Epidemiol Community Health 44: 257–258

Davey-Smith G, Song F, Sheldon T A 1993 Cholesterol lowering and mortality: the importance of considering initial level of risk. Br Med J 306: 1367–1373

Doll R, Peto R, Wheatley K et al 1994 Mortality in relation to smoking: 40 years' observations on male British doctors. Br Med J 309: 901–911

Douglas J T, Blamey S L, Lowe G D O et al 1985 Plasma beta-thromboglobulin, fibrinopeptide A and Bβ 15–42 antigen in relation to postoperative DVT, malignancy and stanozolol treatment. Thromb Haemost 53: 235–238

Drouet L, Mazoyen E, Ripoll L et al 1994 Does the fall in plasma fibrinogen during ticlopidine treatment depend on the initial level? Blood Coagulat Fibrinol 5 (suppl 2): 18

Elwood P C, Renaud S, Sharp D S et al 1991 Ischaemic heart disease and platelet aggregation: the Caerphilly Collaborative Heart Disease Study. Circulation 83: 38–44

Emmerich J, Poirier O, Evans A et al 1995 Myocardial infarction, Arg 506 to Gln factor V mutation, and activated protein C resistance. Lancet 345: 321

Ernst E, Resch K L 1993 Fibrinogen as a cardiovascular risk factor: a meta-analysis and review of the literature. Ann Intern Med 118: 956–963

Ernst E, Resch K L, Matrai A et al 1991 Impaired blood rheology: a risk factor after stroke? J Intern Med 229: 457–462

Ernst E, Koenig W, Lowe G D O, Meade T W (eds) 1992 Fibrinogen: a 'new' cardiovascular risk factor. Blackwell-MZV, Vienna.

Evans A, Behague I, Poirier O et al 1995 Polymorphisms of the fibrinogen gene contributing to the degree of coronary atherosclerosis. Eur Heart J 16 (abstract suppl): 21

Fowkes F G R, Connor J M, Smith F B et al 1992 Fibrinogen genotype and risk of peripheral atherosclerosis. Lancet 339: 693–696

Fowkes F G R, Lowe G D O, Housley E et al 1993 Cross-linked fibrin degradation products, risk of coronary heart disease, and progression of peripheral arterial disease. Lancet 342: 84–86

Gaffney P J, Wong M Y 1992 Collaborative study of a proposed international standard for plasma fibrinogen measurements. Thromb Haemost 68: 428–432

Ginsburg K S, Liang M H, Newcomer L et al 1992 Anticardiolipin antibodies and the risk for ischaemic stroke and venous thrombosis. Ann Intern Med 117: 997–1002

Godsland F, Stevenson J C 1995 Insulin resistance: syndrome or tendency? Lancet 346: 100–103

Goldhaber S Z, Savage D D, Garrish R J et al 1983 Risk factors for pulmonary embolism. The Framingham Study. Am J Med 74: 1023–1028

Green F, Humphries S 1994 Genetic determinants of arterial thrombosis. Baillières Clin Haematol 7: 675–692

Green K G, Heady A, Oliver M F 1989 Blood pressure, cigarette-smoking and heart attack in the WHO Cooperative Trial of clofibrate. Int J Epidemiol 18: 355–360

Hamsten A, de Faire U, Walldius G et al 1987 Plasminogen activator inhibitor in plasma: risk factor for recurrent myocardial infarction. Lancet ii: 3–9

Harris E N, Baguley E, Asherson R A, Hughes G R V 1987 Clinical and serological features of the antiphospholipid syndrome. Br J Rheumatol 26: 19

Heinrich J, Balleisen L, Schulte H et al 1994 Fibrinogen and factor VII in the prediction of coronary risk. Results from the PROCAM study in healthy men. Arterioscler Thromb 14: 54–59

Heller R F, Chinn S, Tunstall-Pedoe H, Rose G 1984 How well can we predict coronary heart disease? Findings in the United Kingdom Heart Disease Prevention Project. Br Med J 288: 1409–1411

Hoffman C J, Burns P, Lawson W E et al 1993 Plasma fibrinogen level is elevated in young adults from families with premature ischaemic heart disease. Arterioscler Thromb 13: 800–803

Ibbotson S H, Davies J A, Grant P J 1992 The influence of infusion of 1-desamino-8-D-arginine vasopressin (DDAVP) in vivo on thrombin generation in vitro. Thromb Haemost 68: 37–39

Jansson J H, Nilsson T K, Johnson O 1991a von Willebrand factor in plasma: a novel risk factor for recurrent myocardial infarction and death. Br Heart J 66: 351–355

Jansson J H, Nilsson T K, Oloffson B O 1991b Tissue plasminogen activator and other risk factors as predictors of cardiovascular events in patients with severe angina pectoris. Eur Heart J 12: 157–161

Jansson J H, Oloffson B O, Nilsson T K 1993 Predictive value of tissue plasminogen activator mass concentration on long-term mortality in patients with coronary artery disease: a 7 year follow-up. Circulation 88: 2030–2034

Juhan-Vague I, Alessi M C 1993 Plasminogen activator inhibitor I and atherothrombosis Thromb Haemost 70: 138–143

Kannel W B, Dawber T R, Kagan A et al 1961 Factors of risk in the development of coronary heart disease – six-year follow-up experience. Ann Intern Med 55: 33–50

Kannel W B, D'Agostino R B, Belanger A J 1987 Fibrinogen, cigarette smoking, and risk of cardiovascular disease: insights from the Framingham Study. Am Heart J 113: 1006–1010

Kannel W B, D'Agostino R B, Wilson P W F et al 1990 Diabetes, fibrinogen and risk of cardiovascular disease: the Framingham experience. Am Heart J 120: 672–676

Koster T 1995 Deep-vein thrombosis. A population-based case-control study: Leiden Thrombophilia Study. Thesis, University of Leiden

Koster T, Rosendaal F R, de Ronde H et al 1993 Venous thrombosis due to poor anticoagulant response to activated protein C: Leiden Thrombophilia Study. Lancet 362: 1503–1506

Koster T, Rosendaal F R, Reitsma P H et al 1994a Factor VII and fibrinogen levels as risk factors for venous thrombosis. A case-control study of plasma levels and DNA polymorphisms. Leiden Thrombophilia Study (LETS). Thromb Haemost 71: 719–722

Koster T, Rosendaal F R, Briët E, Vandenbroucke J 1994b John Hageman's factor and deep vein thrombosis: Leiden Thrombophilia Study. Br J Haematol 87: 422–424

Koster T, Blann A D, Briët E et al 1995 Role of clotting factor VIII in effect of von Willebrand factor on occurrence of deep vein thrombosis. Lancet 345: 152–155

Law M R, Wald N J, Wu T et al 1994 Systematic underestimation of association between serum cholesterol concentration and ischaemic heart disease in observational studies: data from the BUPA study. Br Med J 308: 363–366

Lee A J, Smith W C S, Lowe G D O et al 1990 Plasma fibrinogen and coronary risk factors: the Scottish Heart Health Study. J Clin Epidemiol 43: 913–919

Lee A J, Lowe G D O, Woodward M, Tunstall-Pedoe H 1993a Fibrinogen in relation to personal history of prevalent hypertension, diabetes, stroke, intermittent claudication, coronary heart disease and family history: the Scottish Heart Health Study. Br Heart J 69: 338–342

Lee A J, Lowe G D O, Smith W C S, Tunstall-Pedoe H 1993b Plasma fibrinogen in women: relationships with oral contraception, the menopause and hormone replacement therapy. Br J Haematol 83: 616–621

Lee A J, Fowkes F G R, Lowe G D O, Rumley A 1995 Fibrin D-dimer, haemostatic factors and peripheral arterial disease. Thromb Haemost 74: 828–832

Levi M, Lensing A W A, Buller H R et al 1991 Deep vein thrombosis and fibrinolysis: defective urokinase plasminogen activator release. Thromb Haemost 66: 426–429

Lip G Y H, Lowe G D O 1995 Fibrin D-dimer: a useful clinical marker of thrombogenesis? Clin Sci 89: 205–214

Lip G Y H, Lowe G D O, Rumley A, Dunn F G 1995 Increased markers of thrombogenesis in chronic atrial fibrillation: effects of warfarin treatment. Br Heart J 73: 527–533

Lowe G D O 1984 Blood rheology and venous thrombosis. Clin Hemorheol 4: 571–588

Lowe G D O 1993a Laboratory investigation of pre-thrombotic states. In: Poller L,

Thomson J M (eds) Thrombosis and its management. Churchill Livingstone, Edinburgh, pp 31–46

Lowe G D O 1993b The impact of fibrinogen on arterial disease. Excerpta Medica, Amsterdam

Lowe G D O 1994a Blood rheology, haemostasis and vascular disease. In: Bloom A L, Forbes C D, Thomas D P, Tuddenham E G D (eds) Haemostasis and thrombosis, 3rd edn. Edinburgh, Churchill Livingstone, pp 1169–1188

Lowe G D O 1994b Should plasma viscosity replace the ESR? Br J Haematol 86: 6–11

Lowe G D O 1995 Haematology and risk – a neglected link? Issues in hyperlipidaemia, No. 12. Kluwer, Lancaster

Lowe G D O, Small M 1988 Stimulation of endogenous fibrinolysis. In: Kluft C (ed) Tissue-type plasminogen activator (t-PA): physiological and clinical aspects. CRC Press, Boca Raton, vol II, p 129

Lowe G D O, Osborne D H, McArdle B M et al 1982 Prediction and selective prophylaxis of venous thrombosis in elective gastrointestinal surgery. Lancet i: 409–412

Lowe G D O, Fowkes F G R, Dawes J et al 1993 Blood viscosity, fibrinogen and activation of coagulation and leukocytes in peripheral arterial disease and the normal population in the Edinburgh Artery Study. Circulation 87: 1915–1920

Lowe G D O, Rumley A, Woodward M et al 1994 Plasma fibrinogen and blood rheology in the Third Glasgow MONICA Study: reference ranges using the International Fibrinogen Standard. Blood Coagulat Fibrinol 5 (suppl 2): 38

Lowe G D O, Fowkes F G R, Koenig W, Mannucci P M (eds) 1995a Fibrinogen and cardiovascular disease. Eur Heart J 16 (suppl A)

Lowe G D O, Rumley A, Yarnell J W G, Sweetnam P M 1995b Fibrin D-dimer, von Willebrand factor, tissue plasminogen activator antigen, and plasminogen activator inhibitor activity are primary risk factors for ischaemic heart disease: the Caerphilly Study. Thromb Haemost 73: 950

Macfarlane R G 1977 Introduction. Br Med Bull 33: 183–185

MacMahon S, Peto R, Cutler J et al 1990 Blood pressure, stroke and coronary heart disease. I. Prolonged differences in blood pressure: prospective observational studies corrected for the regression dilution bias. Lancet 335: 765–774

Martin J F, Bath P M W, Burn M L 1991 Influence of platelet size on outcome after myocardial infarction. Lancet 338: 1409–1411

Meade T W 1995 Haemostatic variables, thrombosis and ischaemic heart disease. Excerpta Medica, Amsterdam

Meade T W, North W R S, Chakrabarti R et al 1980 Haemostatic function and cardiovascular death: early results of a prospective study. Lancet i: 1050–1054

Meade T W, Mellows S, Brozovic M et al 1986 Haemostatic function and ischaemic heart disease: principal results of the Northwick Park Heart Study. Lancet ii: 533–537

Meade T W, Imeson J, Stirling Y 1987 Effects of changes in smoking and other characteristics on clotting factors and the risk of ischaemic heart disease. Lancet ii: 986–988

Meade T W, Wilkes H C, Stirling Y et al 1988 Randomized controlled trial of low dose warfarin in the primary prevention of ischaemic heart disease in men at high risk: design and pilot study. Eur Heart J 9: 836–843

Meade T W, Cooper J, Miller G J et al 1991 Antithrombin III and arterial disease. Lancet 337: 850–851

Meade T W, Ruddock V, Stirling Y et al 1993 Fibrinolytic activity, clotting factors and long-term incidence of ischaemic heart disease in the Northwick Park Heart Study. Lancet 342: 1076–1079

Meade T W, Cooper J C, Stirling Y et al 1994a Factor VIII, ABO blood group and the incidence of ischaemic heart disease. Br J Haematol 88: 601–607

Meade T W, Howarth D J, Cooper J et al 1994b Fibrinolytic activity and arterial disease. Lancet 343:1442

Meilahn E N, Kuller L H, Matthews K A, Kiss J E 1992 Variation in plasma fibrinogen levels by menopausal status and use of hormone replacement therapy: the Healthy Women Study. In: Ernst E, Koenig W, Lowe G D O, Meade T W (eds) Fibrinogen: a 'new' cardiovascular risk factor. Blackwell-MZV, Vienna, pp 338–343

Miller G J, Stirling Y, Esnouf M P et al 1994 Factor VII-deficient substrate plasma depleted of protein C raises the sensitivity of the factor VII bio-assay to activated factor

VII. An international study. Thromb Haemost 71: 38–48

Muir K W 1995 Anticardiolipin antibodies and cardiovascular disease. J R Soc Med 88: 433–436

Nabulsi A A, Folson A R, White A et al 1993 Association of hormone replacement therapy with various cardiovascular risk factors in postmenopausal women. N Engl J Med 328: 1069–1075

Nieuwenhuizen W 1991 The formation, measurement and clinical value of fibrinogen derivatives. In: Thomson J M (ed) Blood coagulation and haemostasis: A practical guide, 3rd edn. Churchill Livingstone, Edinburgh, pp 151–176

Nilsson T, Mellbring G, Hedner U 1986 Relationship between factor XII, von Willebrand factor and postoperative deep vein thrombosis. Acta Chir Scand 152: 347–349

Paramo J A, Alfaro M J, Rocha E 1985 Postoperative changes in the plasmatic levels of tissue-type plasminogen activator and its fast-acting inhibitor. Relationship to deep vein thrombosis and influence of prophylaxis. Thromb Haemost 53: 713–716

Parish S, Collins R, Peto S et al 1995 Cigarette smoking, tar yields, and non-fatal myocardial infarction: 14000 cases and 32000 controls in the United Kingdom. Br Med J 311: 471–477

Pearson J D 1994 Endothelial cell function and thrombosis. Baillières Clin Haematol 7: 441–452

PEPI Trial 1995 Effects of estrogen or estrogen/progestin regimes on heart disease risk factors in postmenopausal women: the Postmenopausal Estrogen/Progestin Interventions (PEPI) Trial. JAMA 273: 199–208

Prins M H, Hirsh J 1991 A critical review of the evidence supporting a relationship between impaired fibrinolytic activity and venous thromboembolism. Arch Intern Med 151: 1721–1731

Reid D 1991 The clinical role of fibrinogen and fibrin in peripheral arterial disease. MD Thesis, University of Glasgow

Resch K L, Ernst E 1995 The complex impact of fibrinogen on atherosclerosis-related diseases. In: Koenig W, Hombach V, Bond M G, Kramsch D M (eds) Progression and regression of atherosclerosis. Blackwell-MZV, Vienna, pp 36–40

Ridker P M, Vaughan D E, Stampfer M J et al 1992a A prospective study of plasminogen activator inhibitor and the risk of future myocardial infarction. Circulation 86 (suppl I): I-325

Ridker P M, Vaughan D E, Stampfer M J et al 1992b Baseline fibrinolytic state and the risk of future venous thrombosis. A prospective study of endogenous tissue-type plasminogen activator and plasminogen activator inhibitor. Circulation 85: 1822–1827

Ridker P M, Vaughan D E, Stampfer M J et al 1993 Endogenous tissue-type plasminogen activator and risk of myocardial infarction. Lancet 341: 1165–1168

Ridker P M, Hennekens C H, Stampfer M J et al 1994a Prospective study of endogenous tissue plasminogen activator and risk of stroke. Lancet 343: 940–943

Ridker P M, Hennekens C H, Cerskus A, Stampfer M H 1994b Plasma concentration of cross-linked fibrin degradation products (D-dimer) and the risk of future myocardial infarction among apparently healthy men. Circulation 90: 2236–2240

Ridker P M, Hennekens C H, Lindpaintner K et al 1995 Mutation in the gene coding for coagulation factor V and the risk of myocardial infarction, stroke, and venous thrombosis in apparently healthy men. N Engl J Med 332: 912–917

Rosendaal F R, Varekamp I, Smit C et al 1989 Mortality and causes of death in Dutch haemophiliacs, 1973–86. Br J Haematol 71: 71–76

Rosenson R S, Tangrey C C, Hafner J M 1994 Intra-individual variability of fibrinogen levels and cardiovascular risk profile. Arterioscler Thromb 14: 1928–1932

Rössle R 1937 Über die Bedeutung und Entstehung der Wadenvenenthrombosen. Virchows Arch Pathol Anat 300: 180

Rowbotham B J, Whitaker A N, Harrison J et al 1992 Measurement of cross-linked fibrin derivatives in patients undergoing abdominal surgery: use in the diagnosis of post-operative venous thrombosis. Blood Coagulat Fibrinol 3: 25–31

Ruddock V, Meade T W 1994 Factor VII activity and ischaemic heart disease: fatal and non-fatal events. Q J Med 87: 403–406

Rumley A, Woodburn K R, Lowe G D O et al 1994 Correlation between plasma fibrinogen, fibrin degradation products, and the angiographic extent of peripheral arterial occlusive disease. Blood Coagulat Fibrinol 5 (suppl 2): 38

Shaper A G 1988 Coronary heart disease: risks and reasons. Current Medical Literature, London

Small M, Jack A S, Lowe G D O et al 1983 Coronary artery disease in severe haemophilia. Br Heart J 49: 604–607

Smith F B, Lowe G D O, Fowkes F G R et al 1993 Smoking, haemostatic factors and lipid peroxides in a population case-control study of peripheral arterial disease. Atherosclerosis 102: 155–162

Smith F B, Lee A J, Rumley A et al 1995 Tissue-plasminogen activator, plasminogen activator inhibitor and risk of peripheral arterial disease. Atherosclerosis 115: 35–43

Stone M C, Thorp M C 1983 Plasma fibrinogen – a major coronary risk factor. In: Lenzi S, Descovitch G C (eds) Atherosclerosis and cardiovascular diseases. Editrice Compositori, Bologna, p 3

Sudlow C M, Rodgers H, Kenney R A, Thomson R G 1995 Service provision and use of anticoagulants in atrial fibrillation. Br Med J 311: 558–601

Sue-Ling H M, Johnston D, McMahon M J et al 1986 Preoperative identification of patients at high risk of deep venous thrombosis after elective major abdominal surgery. Lancet i: 1173–1176

Sweetnam P M, Thomas H F, Yarnell J W G, Elwood P C 1994 Fibrinogen is a good predictor of cardiovascular disease. The ten year follow-up of the Caerphilly and Speedwell studies. Blood Coagulat Fibrinol 5 (suppl 2): 1

Thaulow E, Erikssen J, Sandrik L et al 1991 Blood platelet count and function are related to total and cardiovascular death in apparently healthy men. Circulation 84: 613–617

Thompson S G, Martin J C, Meade T W 1987 Sources of variability in coagulation factor assays. Thromb Haemost 58: 1073–1077

Thompson S G, Kienast J, Pyke S D M et al 1995 Haemostatic factors and the risk of myocardial infarction or sudden death in patients with angina pectoris. N Engl J Med 332: 635–641

Thromboembolic Risk Factor (THRIFT) Consensus Group 1992 Risks of and prophylaxis for venous thromboembolism in hospital patients. Br Med J 305: 567–574

Trip M D, Manger Cats V, van Capell F J L, Vreeken J 1990 Platelet hyperreactivity and prognosis in survivors of myocardial infarction. N Engl J Med 322: 1549–1554

Tunstall-Pedoe H, Woodward M, A'Brook R et al 1994 Plasma fibrinogen and coronary events in the Scottish Heart Health Study. Blood Coagulat Fibrinol 5 (suppl 2): 15

Vandenbroucke J P, Koster T, Briët E et al 1994 Increased risk of venous thrombosis in oral-contraceptive users who are carriers of factor V Leiden mutation. Lancet 344: 1453–1457

Vickers M V, Thompson S G 1985 Sources of variability in dose response platelet aggregometry. Thromb Haemost 53: 216–218

Wilhelmsen L 1991 Thrombocytes and coronary heart disease. Circulation 84: 936–938

Wilhelmsen L, Svardsudd K, Korsan-Bengtsen K et al 1984 Fibrinogen as a risk factor for stroke and myocardial infarction. N Engl J Med 311: 501–505

Wiman B, Hamsten A 1990 The fibrinolytic enzyme system and its role in the etiology of thromboembolic disease. Semin Thromb Hemost 16: 207–216

Wissler R W, Robertson A L, Cornhill J F et al 1993 Natural history of aortic and coronary atherosclerotic lesions in youth: findings from the PDAY study. Arterioscler Thromb 13: 1291–1298

Woodburn K R, Rumley A, Lowe G D O et al 1994 Predictive value of preoperative plasma fibrinogen, fibrin degradation products, and von Willebrand factor for graft occlusion or death following infra-inguinal revascularization surgery for peripheral arterial disease. Blood Coagulat Fibrinol 5 (suppl 2): 13

Woodward M, Tunstall-Pedoe H, A'Brook R et al 1994 Plasma fibrinogen and all causes of mortality in the Scottish Heart Health Study. Blood Coagulat Fibrinol 5 (suppl 2): 41

Yarnell J W G, Baker I A, Sweetnam P M et al 1991 Fibrinogen, viscosity and white blood cell count are major risk factors for ischaemic heart disease. The Caerphilly and Speedwell Collaborative Heart Disease Studies. Circulation 83: 836–844

6. Thromboembolism in pregnancy and its prevention

J. G. Ray   J. S. Ginsberg

Thromboembolic disease (TED) during pregnancy is of major clinical importance to the haematologist. Often, there is a request to assist in the management of a pregnant woman with clinically suspected TED or who is at increased risk for the development of TED. Deep vein thrombosis (DVT) complicates between 0.1 and 0.7 cases per 1000 pregnancies (Bergqvist et al 1983, Kierkegaard 1983), yet data from Canada, America, England and Wales demonstrate that pulmonary embolism (PE) follows hypertensive diseases as the second leading cause of maternal mortality (Kaunitz et al 1985, Steinberg & Farine 1985, Department of Health and Social Security 1986). Since effective methods exist for the prevention and treatment of pregnant women with TED, it is important to be vigilant in those with an increased risk of TED or clinically suspected DVT or PE.

In this chapter we review the management of thromboembolism during pregnancy. Emphasis is placed on the diagnosis of DVT and PE, as well as on the safety of anticoagulants for mother and fetus. Valvular heart disease during pregnancy is also discussed.

PATHOPHYSIOLOGY OF VENOUS THROMBOEMBOLISM (VTE) DURING PREGNANCY

There appears to be a relatively equal distribution for DVT during the three trimesters (Bergqvist et al 1983, Ginsberg et al 1991). There are several explanations for how and why pregnancy increases the risk of DVT formation. External venous compression by the gravid uterus and the engaged fetal head leads to venous stasis. The preponderance for DVT in the left leg may occur from compression of the left internal iliac vein by the right iliac artery (Bergqvist et al 1983, Hull et al 1990a, Ginsberg et al 1991). This mechanism may also explain the possible increase in the incidence of isolated iliac vein thrombosis during pregnancy (Bergqvist 1983). Diminished venomotor tone from the effects of elevated progestin levels further contributes to stasis. Hypercoagulability arises secondary to increased levels of clotting factors I (fibrinogen), II (prothrombin), VII, VIII, IX and X, as well as a decrease in plasma fibrinolytic activity (Stirling et al 1984). This combination of stasis and hypercoagulability places the pregnant woman at higher risk for DVT.

DIAGNOSING VENOUS THROMBOEMBOLISM (VTE)

Deep vein thrombosis (DVT)

The formation of thrombus within the proximal deep venous system – the popliteal, femoral and iliac veins, or the inferior vena cava – poses a high risk for major embolization to the lungs, and patients with such disease should be treated. Calf-vein thrombosis, on the other hand, denotes the presence of clot distal to the popliteal venous trifurcation, and poses a negligible risk of embolization provided it remains confined to the calf (Moser & LeMoine 1981). However, in non-pregnant patients, approximately 30% of calf-vein thrombi extend into the proximal veins within 2 weeks of presentation and, therefore, must be identified and treated (Hull et al 1985).

Clinical suspicion of DVT

The possibility of leg DVT is raised when a pregnant woman presents with persistent leg swelling and/or pain. Since non-thrombotic leg swelling is common in pregnancy, however, these symptoms are non-specific. The physical examination may help to explore other processes in the differential diagnosis of DVT: ruptured Baker's cyst, muscle strain or haematoma, myositis, neurogenic pain, arthritis, bone disease, lymphangitis, and varicose veins (Weiner 1985).

Several studies have demonstrated a higher tendency for DVT in the left leg throughout pregnancy, as alluded to above. In a prospective study by Ginsberg et al (1991), of 60 consecutive gravidas with documented gestational DVT, 58 were isolated to the left leg and two were bilateral. Hence, the presence of clinical signs or symptoms of clot in the left leg in a pregnant woman appears to be a sensitive clinical marker for the presence of DVT. If signs or symptoms are isolated to the right leg, then the likelihood of DVT is reduced, but by no means excluded.

Venography and DVT

Contrast venography is the 'gold standard' for the diagnosis of DVT. Complete visualization of the calf, thigh and external iliac veins is possible. The adverse effects of venography include pain associated with the examination, as well as risks associated with radiation exposure and intravenous contrast, including allergic reactions and nephrotoxicity. As Table 6.1 illustrates, lead-apron abdominal and pelvic shielding markedly reduces the radiation dose, while permitting adequate visualization of the calf, popliteal and superficial femoral veins (Ginsberg et al 1989). The downside to shielding is the inability to visualize the iliac vein, resulting in insensitivity to isolated iliac vein thrombosis. Venography is also relatively expensive.

Impedance plethysmography and DVT

Impedance plethysmography (IPG) is an inexpensive, non-invasive bed-side test that is sensitive to obstruction of venous outflow, as occurs with DVT. A randomized controlled trial involving 645 non-pregnant patients with clinically suspected DVT demonstrated the approach of using serial IPG (if the initial IPG was negative) and safely withholding anticoagulants if the IPG results remained normal (Hull et al 1985). Similar results were obtained from a community hospital outpatient cohort study (Huisman et al 1989). These studies indicate that, because of its sensitivity to proxi-mal DVT, serially negative IPG essentially rules out the presence of clini-cally important DVT.

A prospective study was performed by Hull et al (1990a) using serial IPG on 152 consecutive pregnant women with clinically suspected DVT. They reported that, among those 139 women with normal serial IPG, an-ticoagulants were withheld safely.

For women being evaluated with IPG in the 2nd and 3rd trimesters, it is recommended that they lie in the lateral decubitus position for 20 min before testing. This manoeuvre reduces compression of the deep veins by the gravid uterus and fetal head, thus lessening the chance of false-positive results (Hull et al 1990).

Ultrasonography and DVT

The availability of real-time B-mode compression ultrasonography and Doppler flow technology has enabled non-invasive imaging for DVT to be carried a step further. Not only does ultrasound aid in the diagnosis of proximal DVT, but it can also help identify other causes of leg swelling, such as muscle haematoma or Baker's cyst.

Prospective studies clearly support the use of B-mode ultrasonography for diagnosing DVT in non-pregnant patients (Dauzat et al 1986, Monreal et al 1989). Unlike IPG, however, ultrasonography cannot accurately rule out isolated iliac DVT, due to technical limitations (Comerota et al 1993). Prospective studies on the use of ultrasound in pregnant women with sus-pected DVT are pending.

Diagnosis of DVT: summary

There is now high-quality evidence that ultrasound is better than IPG in non-pregnant subjects (Heijboer et al 1993), yet it has not been validated in pregnant patients. However, we believe that either test is reasonable in pregnant women with suspected DVT, provided the limitations of each are understood. Regardless of which investigation is chosen, at a minimum, repeat testing should be performed in patients whose initial test is negative. Other practical issues exist: Are both tests available at one's facility? What are the comparative diagnostic skills of the ultrasonographer versus the IPG technician, since both depend upon the user's training and experience? Figure 6.1 summarizes a diagnostic approach to DVT using IPG, while Figure 6.2 outlines an approach using ultrasonography.

Pulmonary embolism

Clinical suspicion of pulmonary embolism

The possibility of pulmonary embolism (PE) is raised in a gravida with sudden-onset dyspnoea, tachypnoea, or pleuritic chest pain. Hypotension, with evidence of elevated jugular venous pressure, and hypoxia are quite rare, but certainly heighten one's diagnostic suspicion. Overall, however, the clinical diagnosis of PE is not reliable enough to direct decisions about therapy (Dalen 1991). The plain chest radiograph cannot be used to diagnose or rule out PE, but is essential in excluding other disease processes and interpreting the ventilation/perfusion (V/Q) lung scan (Worsley et al 1993).

Diagnostic testing for PE

The 'gold standard' for diagnosing PE is pulmonary angiography (Goodman 1984). The downside to this technique is its degree of invasiveness, the associated reactions to intravenous contrast (Perrier et al 1994), the relatively high levels of radiation exposure (Table 6.1), and its expense. If pulmonary angiography is necessary, then the combination of brachial vein cannulation plus abdominal and pelvic lead shielding can help to minimize radiation exposure of the fetus.

Table 6.1 Fetal radiation exposure from various techniques used in the diagnosis of DVT and PE

Technique	Estimated fetal radiation exposure (rad)
Bilateral venography (without shielding)	0.628
Unilateral venography (without shielding)	0.314
Venography (with pelvic shielding)	<0.050
Pulmonary angiography via femoral route	0.221–0.374
Pulmonary angiography via brachial route	<0.050
Perfusion lung scan	0.0060–0.018
Ventilation lung scan	0.001–0.035
[125]I-fibrinogen leg scanning	2.000
Plain chest X-ray	<0.001

Based on Ginsberg et al (1989).

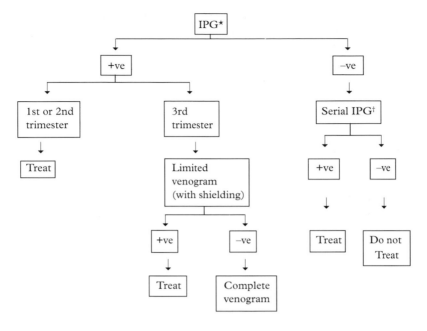

Fig. 6.1 An approach to the diagnosis of clinically suspected isolated DVT during pregnancy using impedance plethysmography (IPG). *Women tested with IPG in the second or third trimester of pregnancy should lie in the lateral decubitus position for 20 min before and during the test. †Serial IPG are repeated on days 2, 5, and 7, and between days 10–14.

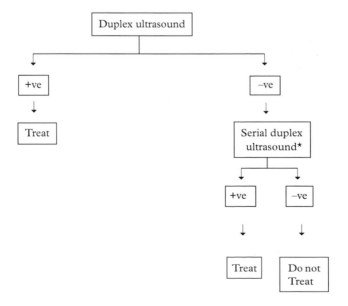

Fig. 6.2 Diagnosis of clinically suspected isolated DVT during pregnancy using duplex ultrasonography. *Serial duplex ultrasounds are repeated on days 2 and 7.

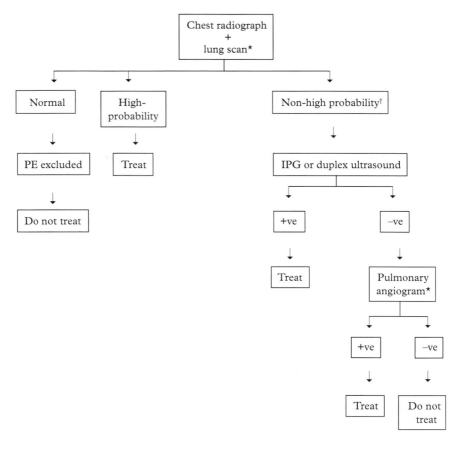

Fig. 6.3   Diagnosis of clinically suspected PE during pregnancy. *Abdominal and pelvic shielding with a lead apron is suggested. †A 'non-high-probability' V/Q scan is sometimes called 'intermediate probability', 'indeterminate' or 'inconclusive'.

Because of the safety limitations of pulmonary angiography, the V/Q lung scan is the pivotal test for diagnosing PE in pregnancy. A prospective study of 515 non-pregnant patients with suspected PE demonstrated that a normal V/Q scan had very high negative predictive value for PE, and that withholding treatment in such cases was safe (Hull et al 1990b). Likewise, a 'high-probability' lung scan, as defined by a segmental or large subsegmental perfusion defect with normal ventilation, strongly supports the diagnosis of PE (PIOPED Investigators 1990). Exactly how the pregnant state might modify these results is unclear, since prospective studies of PE during pregnancy are quite limited.

A common diagnostic dilemma occurs in patients with suspected PE who have a V/Q scan that is 'non-high-probability' (sometimes also called 'intermediate probability', 'indeterminate' or 'inconclusive'), because 10–40% of such patients have PE. In a large study, this scenario occurred in about

50% of non-pregnant patients with suspected PE (PIOPED Investigators 1990). Although one may opt to perform pulmonary angiography, there are the associated risks, as outlined above. Other clinical strategies have been developed in an attempt to resolve this issue 'less invasively'.

Ultrasonography or IPG is helpful in the pregnant patient with a 'non-high-probability' lung scan because a positive test result provides sufficient grounds for initiating anticoagulation. However, in the remainder of patients with a normal IPG or ultrasound, strong consideration should be given to performing pulmonary angiography, since a normal IPG or ultrasound cannot reliably exclude PE (Perrier et al 1994).

Diagnosis of PE: summary

Figure 6.3 provides an outline for the diagnosis of PE. A high-probability or normal lung scan result rules in or rules out PE, respectively. A non-high-probability scan should be followed by IPG or duplex ultrasonography; if the results are positive, anticoagulants can be started, whereas, if they are negative, pulmonary angiography should be considered.

TREATMENT OF PATIENTS WITH VTE

Heparin

Both subcutaneous and intravenous heparin have been used effectively and safely in the treatment of TED in non-pregnant patients. The drug has also been studied prospectively among several hundred pregnant women being treated for TED. Heparin does not cross the placenta or into breast milk, nor does the evidence suggest that there are any adverse fetal effects with maternal administration (Ginsberg & Hirsh 1992). Long-term administration of heparin has been associated with loss of maternal trabecular bone density (Ginsberg et al 1990).

The currently recommended treatment of patients with VTE in pregnancy is full-dose intravenous heparin for 5–10 days, with a therapeutic end-point of an activated partial thromboplastin time (APTT) approximately twice control. Full-dose subcutaneous heparin (to achieve a mid-interval APTT twice control) is then begun for the remainder of the pregnancy, and should be discontinued approximately 24 h before elective induction of labour. In high-risk patients, intravenous heparin can then be resumed, and stopped about 4–6 h prior to anticipated time of delivery (Anderson et al 1991). If the onset of labour is sudden, the effect of heparin can be reversed using intravenous protamine sulphate.

Immediately postpartum, both full-dose subcutaneous heparin and oral warfarin are begun. Once a therapeutic international normalized ratio (INR) of 2.0–3.0 is achieved, the heparin is discontinued, and the warfarin is maintained for at least 2 weeks postpartum (Ginsberg & Hirsh 1992).

Warfarin

Warfarin (coumadin) is believed to be teratogenic during the embryonic and fetal periods, especially in the first 6–12 weeks of gestation (Iturbe-Alessio et al 1986). Warfarin crosses the placenta and is thought to cause the syndrome of warfarin embryopathy, which includes mid-face and nasal hypoplasia, optic atrophy, digital hypoplasia, stippled epiphyses (chondrodysplasia punctata) and mental retardation (Holzgreve et al 1976, Stevenson et al 1980, Iturbe-Alessio et al 1986).

Based on case reviews and case-control studies, some authors have challenged whether warfarin is more harmful to the fetus than heparin (Hall et al 1980, Chong et al 1984). However, the quality of the data is too poor to demonstrate warfarin's safety during the first trimester reliably, and hence the administration of warfarin during early pregnancy cannot be endorsed. The use of warfarin among breast-feeding women appears to be safe, with no detectable drug levels or anticoagulant effects on the infant with long-term administration (Ginsberg & Hirsh 1992).

Alternatives to anticoagulation

When there is a contraindication to the use of anticoagulation such as intracranial haemorrhage or active bleeding in a patient with DVT, an inferior vena cava filter should be inserted. Such filters prevent the transmission of large venous emboli to the pulmonary circulation. Although the experience with such devices among pregnant patients is limited to small case series, they appear to be safe for both mother and fetus (Narayan et al 1992).

PRIOR VTE AND PREGNANCY

The true risk of VTE recurrence among pregnant women with a history of a previous DVT or PE is unknown, but has been estimated at 4–12% (Ginsberg & Hirsh 1992). In women who are receiving long-term warfarin prior to pregnancy, either because of recurrent VTE or the presence of a thrombophilic state (deficiency of protein C, protein S or antithrombin III, or resistance to activated protein C or the presence of antiphospholipid antibodies), full-dose subcutaneous heparin should be substituted for warfarin. This can either be done prior to attempted conception or as soon as a pregnancy test becomes positive (Ginsberg & Hirsh 1992).

At present, there are two options for management of women with previous VTE who are not on long-term anticoagulants. The first is to administer prophylactic subcutaneous heparin at a dose of between 5000 and 10 000 IU twice daily at the start of pregnancy (Howell et al 1983). The APTT does not need to be monitored at these doses.

Besides the great inconvenience of subcutaneous dosing, the major disadvantages of long-term heparin prophylaxis include the risk of heparin-induced thrombocytopenia, as well as osteoporosis (Barbour et al 1994, Dahlman 1994). Substitution of heparin with subcutaneous low-molecular-weight heparin (LMWH) for thromboprophylaxis may lessen these risks, and is currently raising interest as an alternative to heparin for the prevention of recurrent VTE, even though it remains very expensive at present (Gillis 1992, Nelson-Piercy 1994, Sturridge et al 1994).

An alternative option in the management of a gravida with prior VTE is to withhold prophylaxis, and combine vigilance by the patient with periodic surveillance using IPG or ultrasonography. The goal is to monitor for the development of proximal leg DVT. Choosing the 'better' option depends on several factors. Following the route of surveillance depends on the local availability of non-invasive testing and the reliability of the patient to report new symptoms and follow-up regularly for testing. If IPG or ultrasonography is available, then it is necessary to sit down with the patient and present the benefits and downside of either choice. Ultimately, if she is properly informed, then the decision is hers to make.

PREGNANT WOMEN WITH VALVULAR HEART DISEASE

The management of a pregnant woman with a prosthetic heart valve poses an even greater challenge for the clinician – there is a paucity of data on this subject, and no controlled clinical trials have been done. Mechanical heart valves last much longer than those derived from tissue, yet the former also carry a much higher risk of embolization (Ben-Ismail et al 1986), thereby necessitating thromboprophylaxis (Edmunds 1982). Anticoagulation is unnecessary in those with bioprosthetic valves, unless there is associated atrial fibrillation (Born et al 1992).

The only prospective study was of 72 pregnancies among 63 women with either tissue or mechanical heart valves and employed a high warfarin dose regimen. Warfarin exposure during the first 6–12 weeks of gestation was unsafe for the fetus, with high rates of teratogenicity (25%) and spontaneous abortion (16.2%) (Iturbe-Alessio et al 1986). Among women with either a mechanical valve, or a bioprosthetic valve and associated atrial fibrillation, warfarin with a target INR of 3.0–3.5 is reasonable after the 12th week of pregnancy, until 2 weeks prior to delivery. Before the 12th and after the 36–37th week of pregnancy, it seems reasonable to administer a high dose of subcutaneous heparin (e.g. 17 500 U every 12 h) for a target mid-dosing APTT of at least twice control, to be followed with judicious monitoring. This switch to heparin lessens the likelihood of teratogenicity and fetal haemorrhage associated with early and late warfarin use, respectively. Lower doses of heparin (e.g. 5000 U every 12 h) do not appear to provide adequate protection against thromboembolic complications (Caruso et al 1994).

Another approach to thromboprophylaxis of pregnant women with prosthetic heart valves is the administration of a therapeutic dose of subcutaneous heparin (mid-dosing APTT of at least twice control) throughout pregnancy. This eliminates the small risk of central nervous system and optic tract abnormalities described with warfarin exposure after the 1st trimester. Again, a decision should be made by the patient after she has been properly informed of the advantages and disadvantages of each option.

Among non-pregnant patients with mechanical heart valves, the addition of low-dose aspirin (80–100 mg once daily) to therapeutic warfarin was shown to lower the rate of embolic stroke without significantly increasing haemorrhagic complications (Turpie et al 1993). Several randomized control trials of aspirin for the prevention of pregnancy-induced hypertension have shown that its use during pregnancy is safe for the fetus. Therefore, by way of extrapolation, we endorse the addition of low-dose aspirin to anticoagulants for the treatment of pregnant women with mechanical heart valves. This opinion is based largely upon the benefit demonstrated in non-pregnant patients.

All women of childbearing age who require valve replacement, or who are taking long-term warfarin, must be informed about the risks associated with fetal warfarin exposure, as well as the effects of pregnancy and delivery on cardiac function. With proper contraception, careful planning, and pregnancy testing, most women with prosthetic cardiac valves can carry a child to term while reducing the risk of harm to themselves and their fetuses.

FUTURE CONSIDERATIONS IN VTE

D-dimer assay is a fibrin degradation product that can be quantified in plasma using enzyme-linked immunosorbent assays, latex agglutination, and whole-blood red-cell agglutination assays. Recent data from studies of non-pregnant patients (Goldhaber et al 1993, Ginsberg et al 1995) suggest that a low D-dimer blood level among those with suspected PE rules out PE. Studies among pregnant women will likely be done as the test gains acceptance in the general population.

LMWH offer a promising alternative in the treatment of patients with VTE. The pharmacokinetic behaviour of these agents is more predictable than heparin, with a more direct dose–response relationship. LMWH also appear to have fewer adverse effects, such as haemorrhage, heparin-induced thrombocytopenia, and osteoporosis (Nelson-Piercy 1994). They also have the potential for once-daily dosing.

LMWH are safe during pregnancy, since they do not appear to cross the placenta (Forestier et al 1984, Melissari et al 1992). Melissari et al's (1992) study of LMWH in 11 pregnancies complicated by VTE found no demonstrable adverse outcomes to mother or child. Future controlled studies might prove that LMWH are safer and more efficacious than unfractionated heparin during pregnancy.

KEY POINTS FOR CLINICAL PRACTICE

- PE follows hypertensive disease as the second leading cause of maternal mortality during pregnancy.

- Pregnancy increases the risk of thromboembolic disease due to venous stasis and hypercoagulability.

- Although contrast venography is the 'gold standard' for the diagnosis of DVT, there are several associated adverse effects.

- Serial IPG or duplex ultrasonography is reasonable in pregnant women with suspected DVT.

- The 'gold standard' for diagnosing PE is pulmonary angiography, but it is invasive.

- The V/Q lung scan is the pivotal test for diagnosing PE during pregnancy. A high-probability or normal lung scan essentially rules in or rules out PE, respectively. A non-high-probability scan should be followed by further testing.

- The recommended treatment of VTE in pregnancy is full-dose intravenous heparin for 5–10 days, with a therapeutic end-point of an APTT approximately twice control. Full-dose subcutaneous heparin is then given for the remainder of the pregnancy. Postpartum, oral warfarin is begun.

- Warfarin is believed to be teratogenic during embryogenesis, leading to the syndrome of warfarin embryopathy. The administration of warfarin appears to be safe during breastfeeding.

- Among pregnant women with a history of a previous DVT or PE who are not receiving long-term warfarin, the two main options are either to administer prophylactic subcutaneous heparin at a dose of between 5000 and 10 000 IU twice daily, or to withhold prophylaxis and perform periodic surveillance using IPG or ultrasonography. In women receiving long-term warfarin, adjusted-dose subcutaneous heparin should be used.

- The management of pregnant women with mechanical heart valves includes either warfarin after the 12th week of pregnancy, until 2 weeks prior to delivery, with therapeutic doses of subcutaneous heparin at other times, or therapeutic doses of subcutaneous heparin throughout. Low-dose aspirin should be added to anticoagulation. All women of childbearing age with valvular heart disease require extensive counselling and planning of their pregnancy.

REFERENCES

Anderson D R, Ginsberg J S, Burrows R et al 1991 Subcutaneous heparin therapy during pregnancy: a need for concern at the time of delivery. Thromb Haemost 65: 248–250

Barbour L A, Kick S D, Steiner J F et al 1994 A prospective study of heparin-induced osteoporosis in pregnancy using bone densitometry. Am J Obstet Gynecol 170: 862–869

Ben-Ismail M, Abid F, Trabelsi S et al 1986 Cardiac valve prostheses, anticoagulation and pregnancy. Br Heart J 55: 101–105

Bergqvist A, Bergqvist D, Hallbook T 1983 Deep vein thrombosis during pregnancy: a prospective study. Acta Obstet Gynecol Scand 62: 443–448

Born D, Martinez E E, Almeida P A M et al 1992 Pregnancy in patients with prosthetic heart valves: the effects of anticoagulation on mother, fetus, and neonate. Am Heart J 124: 413–417

Caruso A C, Carolis S D, Ferrazzani S 1994 Pregnancy outcome in women with cardiac valve prosthesis. Eur J Obstet Gynecol 54: 7–11

Chong M K B, Harvey D, de Swiet M 1984 Follow-up study of children whose mothers were treated with warfarin during pregnancy. Br J Obstet Gynaecol 91: 1070–1073

Comerota A J, Katz M L, Hashemi H A 1993 Venous duplex imaging for the diagnosis of acute deep venous thrombosis. Haemostasis 23 (suppl 1): 61–71

Dahlman T C, Sjoberg H E, Ringertz H 1994 Bone mineral density during long-term prophylaxis with heparin in pregnancy. Am J Obstet Gynecol 170: 1315–1320

Dalen J E 1991 Clinical diagnosis of acute pulmonary embolism: when should a V/Q scan be ordered? Chest 100: 1185–1186

Dauzat M M, Laroche J P, Charras C et al 1986 Real-time B-mode ultrasonography for better specificity in the non-invasive diagnosis of deep vein thrombosis. J Ultrasound Med 5: 625–631

Department of Health and Social Security 1986 Report on confidential inquiries into maternal deaths for England and Wales 1979–1981. HMSO, London

Edmunds L H Jr 1982 Thromboembolic complications of current cardiac valvular prostheses. Ann Thorac Surg 34: 96–106

Forestier F, Daffos E, Cappella-Pavlovsky M 1984 Low molecular weight heparin (PK 10169) does not cross the placenta during the second trimester of pregnancy: study by direct fetal blood sampling under ultrasound. Thromb Res 34: 557–560

Gillis S, Shushan A, Eldor A 1992 Use of low molecular weight heparin for prophylaxis and treatment of thromboembolism in pregnancy. Int J Gynecol Obstet 39: 297–301

Ginsberg J S, Hirsh J 1992 Use of antithrombotic agents during pregnancy. Chest 102 (suppl): 385S–390S

Ginsberg S, Hirsh J, Rainbow A J et al 1989 Risks to the fetus of radiologic procedures used in the diagnosis of maternal venous thromboembolic disease. Thromb Haemost 61: 189–196

Ginsberg J S, Kowalchuk G, Hirsh J et al 1990 Heparin effect on bone density. Thromb Haemost 64: 286–289

Ginsberg J S, Brill-Edwards P, Bona R et al 1991 Deep vein thrombosis (DVT) during pregnancy: leg and trimester of presentation. Thromb Haemost 65: 720a

Ginsberg J S, Wells P S, Brill-Edwards et al 1995 Application of a novel and rapid whole blood assay for D-dimer in patients with clinically suspected pulmonary embolism. Thromb Haemost 73: 35–38

Goldhaber S Z, Simons G R, Eliott C G et al 1993 Quantitative plasma D-dimer levels among patients undergoing pulmonary angiography for suspected pulmonary embolism. JAMA 270: 2819–2822

Goodman P C 1984 Pulmonary angiography. Clin Chest Med 5: 465–477

Hall J G, Pauli R M, Wilson K M 1980 Maternal and fetal sequelae of anticoagulation during pregnancy. Am J Med 68: 122–140

Heijboer H, Buller H R, Lensing A W A et al 1993 A comparison of real-time compression ultrasonography with impedance plethysmography for the diagnosis of deep-vein thrombosis in symptomatic outpatients. N Engl J Med 329: 1365–1369

Holzgreve W, Carey J C, Hall B D 1976 Warfarin-induced fetal abnormalities. Lancet ii: 914–915

Howell R, Fidler J, Letsky E et al 1983 The risks of antenatal subcutaneous heparin prophylaxis: a controlled trial. Br J Obstet Gynaecol 90: 1124–1128

Huisman M V, Buller H R, ten Cate J W et al 1989 Management of clinically suspected acute venous thrombosis in outpatients with serial impedance plethysmography in a community hospital setting. Arch Intern Med 149: 511–513

Hull R D, Hirsh J, Carter C J et al 1985 Diagnostic efficacy of impedance plethysmography for clinically suspected deep-vein thrombosis. Ann Intern Med 102: 21–28

Hull R D, Raskob G E, Carter C J 1990a Serial impedance plethysmography in pregnant patients with clinically suspected deep-vein thrombosis: clinical validity of negative findings. Ann Intern Med 112: 663–667

Hull R D, Raskob G E, Coates G et al 1990b Clinical validity of a normal perfusion lung scan in patients with suspected pulmonary embolism. Chest 97: 23–26

Iturbe-Alessio I, del Carmen Fonseca M, Mutchinik O et al 1986 Risks of anticoagulant therapy in pregnant women with artificial heart valves. N Engl J Med 315: 1390–1393

Kaunitz A M, Hughes J M, Grimes D A et al 1985 Causes of maternal mortality in the United States. Obstet Gynecol 65: 605–612

Kierkegaard A 1983 Incidence and diagnosis of deep vein thrombosis associated with pregnancy. Acta Obstet Gynecol Scand 62: 239–243

Melissari E, Parker C, Wilson N V et al 1992 Use of low molecular weight heparin in pregnancy. Thromb Haemost 68: 652–656

Monreal M, Montserrat E, Salvador R et al 1989 Real-time ultrasound for diagnosis of symptomatic venous thrombosis and for screening patients at risk: correlation with ascending conventional venography. Angiology 40: 527–533

Moser K M, LeMoine J R 1981 Is embolic risk conditioned by location of deep venous thrombosis? Ann Intern Med 94: 439–444

Narayan H, Krarup K, Thurston H et al 1992 Experience with the Cardial inferior vena cava filter as prophylaxis against pulmonary embolism in pregnant women with extensive deep venous thrombosis. Br J Obstet Gynaecol 99: 637–640

Nelson-Piercy C 1994 Low molecular weight heparin for obstetric thromboprophylaxis. Br J Obstet Gynaecol 101: 6–8

Perrier A, Bounameaux H, Morabia A et al 1994 Contribution of D-dimer plasma measurement and lower-limb venous ultrasound to the diagnosis of pulmonary embolism: a decision analysis model. Am Heart J 127: 624–635

PIOPED Investigators 1990 Value of the ventilation/perfusion scan in acute pulmonary embolism. Results of the prospective investigation of pulmonary embolism diagnosis (PIOPED). JAMA 263: 2753–2759

Steinberg W M, Farine D 1985 Maternal mortality in Ontario from 1970 to 1980. Obstet Gynecol 66: 510–512

Stevenson R E, Burton O M, Ferlauto G J, Taylor H A 1980 Hazards of oral anticoagulation during pregnancy. JAMA 243: 1549–1551

Stirling Y, Woolf L, North W R S et al 1984 Haemostasis in normal pregnancy. Thromb Haemost 52: 176–183

Sturridge F, de Swiet M, Letsky E 1994 The use of low molecular weight heparin for thromboprophylaxis in pregnancy. Br J Obstet Gynaecol 101: 69–71

Turpie A G G, Gent M, Laupacis A 1993 A comparison of aspirin with placebo in patients treated with warfarin after heart valve replacement. N Engl J Med 329: 524–529

Weiner C P 1985 Diagnosis and management of thromboembolic disease during pregnancy. Clin Obstet Gynecol 28: 107–118

Worsley D F, Alavi A, Aronchick J M et al 1993 Chest radiographic findings in patients with acute pulmonary embolism: observations from the PIOPED study. Radiology 189: 133–136

7. Plasma factor VIIa

J. H. Morrissey

Coagulation factor VII, or, more correctly, the activated form (VIIa), oc-
cupies a unique position as the first enzyme in the blood-clotting cascade.
As such, it may play an important role in hypercoagulable states. In fact,
certain epidemiologic studies have found elevated plasma factor VII coagulant activity (VII:C) to be an independent risk factor for heart disease.
However, factor VII exists in at least two, and possibly more, forms in plasma,
and factor VII:C assays measure an aggregate of all of them. Therefore,
there has been considerable controversy concerning which plasma forms of
factor VII, if any, represent actual risk factors for thrombotic disease. Several years ago it was proposed that low levels of factor VIIa might circulate
normally in the plasma, and that such trace levels of pre-existing factor VIIa
may be essential in priming the coagulation cascade. Accordingly, elevated
levels of plasma factor VIIa per se have been proposed by some to be the
actual risk factor being measured in epidemiologic studies employing factor VII:C assays. New assay techniques based on genetically engineered
mutants of tissue factor (TF) now permit measurement of plasma factor
VIIa without interference from the large excess of zymogen factor VII. This
has enabled direct examination of the role of plasma factor VIIa in disease.
The present review focuses on plasma forms of factor VII, current assay
techniques for measuring plasma factor VII and factor VIIa levels, and the
possible roles of plasma factor VIIa in hypercoagulable states and thrombotic disease.

BRIEF BACKGROUND: FACTOR VII AND TISSUE FACTOR

It is now widely accepted that the cell-surface complex of TF and factor
VIIa is the physiologic triggering agent of blood clotting, both in normal
hemostasis as well as in a variety of thrombotic diseases. (For an excellent
review of the biology of TF and its role in the generation of thrombin, see
Carson & Brozna 1993.) Unlike other protein cofactors of the clotting
system, TF is fully functional as a single-chain protein and does not undergo proteolytic activation. TF has high affinity for both factor VII and
factor VIIa, and serves as the essential protein cofactor for factor VIIa
enzymatic activity; in short, this is how TF triggers the clotting cascade.

Because TF is an integral membrane protein, the factor VIIa–TF complex is always tethered to the membrane surface.

Although TF is present throughout the body, its distribution is highly cell type-specific. Thus, TF is prominent in adventitial cells surrounding blood vessels larger than capillaries, in epidermal keratinocytes, in a variety of epithelia surrounding organs and organ structures, and in certain other cell types. Under normal conditions, TF is completely undetectable in all cell types in direct contact with the plasma (Drake et al 1989, Wilcox et al 1989, Fleck et al 1990). This tissue distribution has been likened to a 'hemostatic envelope' surrounding the vasculature, organ structures, and the entire organism (Drake et al 1989).

Factor VII is a vitamin K-dependent protein which is synthesized in the liver. It circulates in the plasma at about 400–500 ng/ml (approximately 10 nM; Fair 1983). The vast majority of plasma factor VII is in the inert precursor, or zymogen, form which consists of a single polypeptide chain of about 50 kDa (Hagen et al 1986). The enzymatically active form, factor VIIa, is generated from factor VII by limited proteolysis – specifically, through cleavage of a single arginine-isoleucine peptide bond located between the second growth factor-like domain and the serine proteinase domain. The resulting factor VIIa molecule consists of two polypeptide chains held together by a single disulfide bond. Unlike the activation of other coagulation serine proteinases, conversion of factor VII to factor VIIa is not accompanied by release of an activation peptide.

Although factor VIIa has measurable proteinase activity on its own, its enzymatic activity is enhanced tremendously upon binding to TF. Thus, the 1:1 complex of TF and factor VIIa can be thought of as a two-subunit enzyme, with factor VIIa representing the catalytic subunit and TF the regulatory subunit. The natural substrates of factor VIIa–TF are factor IX and factor X.

Due to a number of circulating proteinase inhibitors present in plasma, most active serine proteinases have plasma half-lives measured in seconds to minutes. However, the in vivo half-life of factor VIIa is about 2 h (Seligsohn et al 1978a). This unique stability of factor VIIa in plasma led Miller et al (1985) to propose that trace levels of factor VIIa are present in plasma at all times. They and others have speculated that these low levels of plasma factor VIIa may play an important role in priming the clotting cascade (Seligsohn et al 1978a, Miller et al 1985, Nakagaki et al 1991, Rapaport 1991, Neuenschwander & Morrissey 1992). According to this view, when TF is exposed to plasma it captures trace levels of circulating factor VIIa, initially resulting in the formation of small amounts of factor VIIa–TF complexes. These initial factor VIIa–TF complexes are then thought to convert neighboring factor VII–TF to factor VIIa–TF either directly by autoactivation (Nakagaki et al 1991), or indirectly by generation of a burst of factor IXa and/or factor Xa which in turn back-activates factor VII bound to TF (Nemerson & Repke 1985). If trace levels of plasma factor

VIIa represent the very first active proteinase in the clotting cascade, then elevated plasma factor VIIa levels might reasonably be expected to contribute to hypercoagulable states.

TF FUNCTION: INSIGHTS FROM SITE-DIRECTED MUTANTS

From the original cDNA cloning of TF it was clear that the protein consisted of three regions: an extracellular domain constituting the bulk of the protein mass, a single membrane-spanning domain, and a short cytoplasmic tail (Fisher et al 1987, Scarpati et al 1987, Morrissey et al 1987, Spicer et al 1987). The membrane-spanning and cytoplasmic domains of TF have been deleted to yield a truncated form which, unlike the wild-type molecule, is highly water-soluble (soluble TF, or sTF; Paborsky et al 1991, Ruf et al 1991, Rezaie et al 1992, Shigematsu et al 1992, Waxman et al 1992, 1993). Recently, the X-ray crystal structure of sTF has been solved (Harlos et al 1994, Muller et al 1994). This confirmed the earlier proposal that TF belongs to the cytokine receptor superfamily, and that its extracellular region is composed of two fibronectin type III domains (Bazan 1990). The putative factor VIIa binding site on TF has been mapped using site-directed mutagenesis in several studies (Gibbs et al 1994, Ruf et al 1994, Schullek et al 1994, Martin et al 1995).

sTF binds to factor VIIa with high affinity (Paborsky et al 1991, Ruf et al 1991, Rezaie et al 1992, Shigematsu et al 1992, Waxman et al 1992, 1993, Neuenschwander & Morrissey 1992, 1994). sTF was initially reported to be equivalent to wild-type TF in promoting the cleavage of small amide substrates by factor VIIa, somewhat deficient in promoting factor X activation by factor VIIa, and severely deficient in procoagulant activity (Paborsky et al 1991, Ruf et al 1991, Rezaie et al 1992, Shigematsu et al 1992, Waxman et al 1992, 1993, Neuenschwander & Morrissey 1992, 1994). Subsequently, the extremely low procoagulant activity of sTF was shown to result from a selective deficiency in the conversion of TF-bound factor VII to factor VIIa (Neuenschwander & Morrissey 1992). This in turn was shown to be a direct consequence of increasing the dimensionality of the factor VIIa–sTF interaction with macromolecular substrates, compared to wild-type factor VIIa–TF where movement of both enzyme and substrate are constrained to the plane of the membrane (Fiore et al 1994). The selective deficiency of sTF in promoting conversion of factor VII to factor VIIa has been exploited to develop an activity assay for plasma factor VIIa that is free from interference from the vast excess of zymogen factor VII (see below).

FORMS OF FACTOR VII IN PLASMA

In normal individuals, about 99% of plasma factor VII exists in the zymogen form, while about 1% is in the form of factor VIIa (Morrissey & Macik

1991, Wildgoose et al 1992, Morrissey et al 1993, Kario et al 1994). An apparent third form of factor VII was proposed to exist in plasma, based on the finding that treating plasma with phospholipase C reduced the level of factor VII:C (Østerud et al 1972, Dalaker & Prydz 1984, Dalaker et al 1985, 1987). This was interpreted to mean that some factor VII or factor VIIa molecules might be in association with lipoprotein particles. The physical basis of this apparently novel form of factor VII has not been demonstrated, and recently doubt has been cast on its existence. Hubbard & Parr (1991) found that the loss of plasma factor VII:C activity following phospholipase treatment could be prevented or reversed by treating the plasma with detergent. They proposed that when phospholipase C removes phospholipid head groups from lipoprotein particles, it generates a hydrophobic surface that can adsorb factor VII from the plasma. They further propose that detergent treatment of plasma releases the adsorbed factor VII, whereupon it becomes measurable again in factor VII:C assays. Hayes et al (1993) arrived at similar conclusions. The authors of these two studies conclude that phospholipase-sensitive factor VII:C activity does not reflect a separate form of factor VII in plasma (Hubbard & Parr 1991, Hayes et al 1993).

In individuals being treated with warfarin, there can be a discrepancy between factor VII antigen (VII:Ag) and factor VII:C levels (see, for example, Fair 1983). This has been interpreted to mean that the plasma of such individuals contains under-carboxylated factor VII.

ASSAY METHODS FOR PLASMA FACTOR VII AND FACTOR VIIa

A variety of different methods have been developed for measuring plasma levels of factor VII, factor VIIa, or both. One useful measure is the overall concentration of factor VII mass in plasma (i.e. factor VII + factor VIIa). This is routinely accomplished by quantifying factor VII:Ag using immunologic methods that do not discriminate between factor VII and factor VIIa (Fair 1983, Broze et al 1985, Bom et al 1986, Takase et al 1988). These assays can be standardized against purified factor VII or against pooled normal plasma (the latter being more common). Such methods have been reviewed recently by Kitchen et al (1992). A non-immunologic method for quantifying factor VII mass is the coupled amidolytic assay (factor VII:Am). In the first stage of this assay, factor X, thromboplastin, and a dilution of the test plasma are mixed together to allow factor Xa to be generated for a defined period of time. In the second stage, the newly generated factor Xa is quantified by measuring the cleavage of a factor Xa specific amide substrate under conditions that block further factor X activation (Seligsohn et al 1978b). Owing to the very rapid back-activation of TF-bound factor

VII in this setting, the factor VII:Am assay is insensitive to the prior activation state of plasma factor VII/VIIa. Unless the plasmas to be assayed contain significant levels of inactive factor VIIa or unactivatable factor VII, assays of factor VII:Am and factor VII:Ag should give comparable results (Kitchen et al 1992).

Another approach to quantifying factor VII is the factor VII:C assay. In a typical factor VII:C assay, a dilution of test plasma is mixed with thromboplastin, factor VII deficient plasma, and a source of Ca^{2+}. The time to clot formation is measured, and the activity of the plasma sample is derived from a standard curve prepared using various dilutions of pooled normal plasma. In this setting there is some conversion of factor VII to factor VIIa during the course of the assay, but unlike the factor VII:Am assay the conversion is not complete. Thus, factor VII:C assays measure an aggregate of both factor VII zymogen and preformed factor VIIa in the test plasma.

Factor VII:C assays are performed differently in different laboratories, which results in varying relative sensitivities to factor VII versus factor VIIa. One important variable is the nature of the thromboplastin. In particular, factor VII:C assays employing bovine brain thromboplastin are more sensitive to preformed factor VIIa (compared to zymogen factor VII) than are comparable assays employing thromboplastins of human or rabbit origin (Hemker et al 1976, Van Deijk et al 1983, Kitchen et al 1988, Poggio et al 1991, Kario et al 1995a). In some studies, the ratio of factor VII:C to factor VII mass (factor VII:Ag or factor VII:Am) has been used as an indirect measure of the activity state of factor VII in plasma (Hemker et al 1976, Seligsohn et al 1978b, Kitchen et al 1988).

Another important variable governing the relative sensitivity of factor VII:C assays to the level of preformed factor VIIa is the nature of the factor VII deficient plasma employed. A recent study comparing factor VII:C assays demonstrated that the method used by the Northwick Park Heart Study (NPHS) had greater sensitivity to factor VIIa than more commonly used factor VII:C assays (Miller et al 1994). In the NPHS the method for preparing the factor VII deficient plasma (making it also deficient in protein C) was shown to be responsible for increasing the sensitivity to pre-existing plasma factor VIIa (Miller et al 1994).

Even factor VII:C assays with enhanced sensitivity to factor VIIa are still sensitive to both factor VII and factor VIIa. About 8–30% of the factor VII:C activity of assays based on rabbit or bovine thromboplastin can be attributed to preformed factor VIIa, while the remaining 70–92% of the activity is apparently due to zymogen factor VII (Morrissey et al 1996 unpublished observations). Therefore, even using factor VII:C assays with increased sensitivity to preformed factor VIIa, elevated factor VII:C in a given individual can be due to increased zymogen factor VII, pre-existing factor VIIa, or both (Mann 1989, Hultin 1991).

DIRECT MEASUREMENT OF FACTOR VIIa IN PLASMA

Once the selective deficiency in sTF function was demonstrated (i.e. retention of factor VIIa cofactor function but not activation of factor VII to factor VIIa; Neuenschwander & Morrissey 1992), this property was exploited to create a highly sensitive, clot-based method for quantifying trace levels of factor VIIa in plasma without interference from zymogen factor VII (Morrissey & Macik 1991, Morrissey et al 1993). The sTF-based assay is performed almost exactly like the factor VII:C assay, except that a mixture of sTF and phospholipid vesicles is used in place of thromboplastin. The assay is calibrated against factor VII deficient plasma to which varying concentrations of purified factor VIIa have been added, and the results are typically expressed as ng/ml factor VIIa.

Hubbard & Barrowcliffe (1994) have pointed out that purified factor VIIa from different laboratories will have different specific activities, and this will make direct comparisons of factor VIIa levels between laboratories difficult. They propose using the 1st International Standard Factor VIIa Concentrate (89/688), established by the World Health Organization in October 1993 and available from the National Institute for Biological Standards and Control in the UK, as a standard for calibrating the new sTF-based assay. In this case, the assay would report factor VIIa levels in international units of factor VII rather than ng/ml factor VIIa. A commercial sTF-based assay of plasma factor VIIa in kit form is now being marketed (Diagnostica Stago) which follows this proposal; it is calibrated against the 1st International Standard Factor VIIa Concentrate.

In an initial study employing the new sTF-based assay, plasma factor VIIa levels were measured in 188 normal volunteers (Morrissey et al 1993). The plasma of all individuals tested had detectable levels of factor VIIa, with a very broad normal range (0.5–8.4 ng/ml). Mean factor VIIa levels were 3.6 ng/ml, or about 0.8% of the total factor VII mass being in the form of factor VIIa. There was no relationship between factor VIIa and fibrinogen levels, nor were there significant differences in factor VIIa levels between men versus women, smokers versus non-smokers, or users versus non-users of oral contraceptives. Plasma factor VIIa levels were found to increase during pregnancy and decrease dramatically as deep vein thrombosis patients underwent oral anticoagulant therapy (Morrissey et al 1993). Recent studies have demonstrated that the sTF-based factor VIIa assay represents a highly sensitive means of measuring the effect of oral anticoagulant therapy (Raskob et al 1995, Sakata et al 1995).

Wildgoose et al (1992) employed the sTF-based clotting assay to measure plasma factor VIIa in hemophiliacs, reporting that hemophilia A patients had factor VIIa levels about 60% of normal controls while hemophilia B patients had factor VIIa levels only about 10% of normal. The implication of this finding is that factor IXa is involved in the generation of much (but not all) of the pre-existing plasma factor VIIa. The sTF assay has been adapted to use a fluorogenic substrate method to detect thrombin generation instead of clotting (Kario et al 1994). Using this form of the assay, Kario et al (1994) showed that plasma factor VIIa levels were not correlated with serum cholesterol or triglyceride levels. This differs dramatically from the results of several studies showing a relationship between factor VII:C activity and serum lipid content (see Hultin 1991 for review). Finally, measurement of factor VIIa levels in commercial clotting factor concentrates has been proposed as one method to screen for contamination by potentially thrombogenic materials (Limentani et al 1995).

SIGNIFICANCE OF PLASMA FACTOR VII AND/OR FACTOR VIIa LEVELS

A number of population studies have looked for relationships between thrombotic disease and markers of the hemostatic system (including factor VII). Some of these studies have reported significantly higher factor VII levels in various diseases such as myocardial infarction, stable or unstable angina pectoris, transient ischemic attacks, diabetes, uremia, and peripheral vascular disease (Meade et al 1986, Balleisen et al 1987, Orlando et al 1987, Carvalho de Sousa et al 1988, Hoffman et al 1988, 1989, Broadhurst et al 1990, Suzuki et al 1991, Cortellaro et al 1992, Kario et al 1993, 1994, 1995b, Heinrich et al 1994, Ruddock & Meade 1994). A notable example is the NPHS, a large prospective study of the role of several hemostatic parameters in ischemic heart disease. In that study a significant correlation was found between elevated plasma factor VII:C levels and risk of heart disease (Meade et al 1986). More recently, a long-term follow-up study of the NPHS participants reported a strong correlation between factor VII:C and fatal events of ischemic heart disease but not non-fatal events (Ruddock & Meade 1994). Another large prospective study, the Prospective Cardiovascular Münster (PROCAM) study, also reported a correlation between plasma factor VII:C and coronary events, but with less significance than the NPHS (Balleisen et al 1987). Long-term follow-up of participants enrolled in the PROCAM study has recently shown no statistically significant difference in factor VII:C levels among men who had or had not experienced coronary events (Heinrich et al 1994). However, as with the long-term follow-up to the NPHS, when only fatal coronary events were analysed there was a relationship between factor VII:C levels and coronary events. Unlike the NPHS, however, the relationship in the PROCAM study barely reached statistical significance ($P = 0.06$).

Because factor VII:C assays measure both factor VII and factor VIIa, there has been substantial debate for a number of years as to whether factor VIIa or zymogen factor VII were actual risk factors for thrombotic disease. This has included speculation that the level of pre-existing factor VIIa might be a better risk predictor than factor VII mass or factor VII:C (ARIC Investigators 1989, Heinrich et al 1994, Miller et al 1994, Ruddock & Meade

1994). On the other hand, some investigators have argued that elevated factor VII mass may be a more important risk factor for thrombotic disease than elevated plasma factor VIIa (the latter being estimated using indirect methods only; Hoffman et al 1988, 1989, Hultin 1991). Finally, some studies have failed to find a significant relationship between various types of thrombotic disease and factor VII levels altogether (Vaziri et al 1992, Bara et al 1994, Koster et al 1994, Sosef et al 1994, Moor et al 1995).

How might one explain the relationship between elevated levels of plasma factor VII:C and fatal (but not non-fatal) coronary episodes reported in the NPHS and PROCAM studies cited above? Current understanding of the precipitating event in myocardial infarction is that thrombosis is triggered by rupture or fissure of atherosclerotic plaques, exposing TF to blood in the vessel lumen and thereby initiating the clotting cascade (Forrester et al 1987, Wilcox et al 1989). Ruddock & Meade (1994) have proposed that elevated plasma factor VIIa levels may facilitate the growth of more extensive thrombi following plaque rupture, making it more likely that an occlusive thrombus will form in a given event. This proposal echoes a similar idea proposed a number of years ago by Hemker et al (1976). According to this view, factor VIIa might not be involved in the development of atherosclerosis per se, and therefore might not necessarily correlate with degree of intima-medial thickening, overall frequency of coronary events, and so forth. Correlation between factor VII:C (or factor VIIa) and only fatal coronary events in the NPHS and PROCAM studies may explain why factor VII has failed, in some population studies, to show an association with carotid artery thickness, non-fatal coronary events, or other manifestations of vascular disease (Vaziri et al 1992, Folsom et al 1993, Koster et al 1994, Sosef et al 1994, Moor et al 1995).

CLINICAL PERSPECTIVES

Factor VII:C was found to be a highly significant risk predictor for fatal coronary events in a major prospective study and has been linked to heart disease in a number of other population-based studies. These findings have generated considerable interest in factor VII as a possible independent risk factor for thrombotic disease. However, lack of standardization of factor VII:C assay technology between laboratories, and the complicating relationship between factor VII:C and dietary fat and serum lipid levels, has raised a number of questions about the clinical significance of elevated factor VII:C as a reliable, independent predisposing factor for heart disease and other thrombotic diseases. This has probably tempered enthusiasm somewhat for employing factor VII:C assays in clinical studies. The availability of new assay technologies permitting highly specific measurement of pre-existing factor VIIa in plasma now makes it possible to enquire into the relationship between factor VIIa levels per se and thrombotic disease. The extremely broad range of factor VIIa among normal individuals (variation of about 17-fold from lowest to highest among 188 normals) is remarkable. The finding that the factor VII:C assay employed in the NPHS has increased sensitivity to plasma factor VIIa is consistent with the idea that factor VIIa levels are the actual risk factor being measured, although this finding alone certainly does not prove this point. It will therefore be of interest to examine plasma factor VIIa levels as a potential risk factor in future prospective studies of thrombotic diseases.

Some additional important questions to be answered include the relationship between factor VIIa levels and other new methods for measuring ongoing activation of the clotting system (circulating levels of serine proteinase activation peptides and proteinase-inhibitor complexes; see Bauer 1993). In this way it should be possible to find out if factor VIIa levels reflect overall turnover of the clotting system, or alternatively represent an independent contribution to hypercoagulable states. The sTF-based assay for plasma factor VIIa has some advantages over other measures of turnover of the clotting system in that it is easy to perform, does not require exotic anticoagulants, and is remarkably free from phlebotomy artefacts (Bauer 1993, Morrissey et al 1993).

Another important question to be answered is the effect of dietary fat and serum lipid levels on plasma factor VIIa. If, for example, factor VIIa were highly correlated with triglyceride levels then its significance as an independent risk factor for heart disease would be diminished. However, unlike the case for factor VII:C levels, little or no correlation between factor VIIa and serum lipid levels has been found (Kario et al 1994, Moor et al 1995). Not all studies have examined factor VII:C in fasting individuals and the possible confounding effects of postprandial lipemia on factor VII:C is another concern in interpreting such results. Early results using the factor VIIa assay indicate that plasma factor VIIa levels may be much less sensitive to postprandial lipemia than factor VII:C assays. However, additional studies are clearly warranted.

A number of studies are currently underway to investigate the possible relationship between plasma factor VIIa levels and various thrombotic diseases. The availability of new assay technologies for measuring factor VIIa without interference from zymogen factor VII now permits such highly specific experimental questions to be asked. The proposal to calibrate the assay using an international factor VIIa reference standard has merit and should greatly facilitate comparison of results between laboratories.

KEY POINTS FOR CLINICAL PRACTICE

- Plasma factor VIIa levels can now be measured using a simple clotting test based on a soluble mutant form of tissue factor (TF). The test has been commercialized in kit form but is currently available only for research purposes.

- A number of clinical studies are currently evaluating plasma factor VIIa as a risk factor for cardiovascular disease and a variety of other thrombotic diseases.

- Plasma factor VIIa shows promise as a very sensitive way to monitor low-dose oral anticoagulant therapy.

- Another potential use of the soluble TF-based assay is to monitor plasma factor VIIa levels in hemophilic patients receiving recombinant factor VIIa therapy.

REFERENCES

ARIC Investigators 1989 The atherosclerosis risk in communities (ARIC) study: design and objectives. Am J Epidemiol 129: 687–702

Balleisen L, Schulte H, Assmann G et al 1987 Coagulation factors and the progress of coronary heart disease. Lancet ii: 461

Bara L, Nicaud V, Tiret L et al 1994 Expression of a paternal history of premature myocardial infarction on fibrinogen, factor VII:C and PAI-1 in European offspring – The EARS study. Thromb Haemost 71: 434–440

Bauer K A 1993 Laboratory markers of coagulation activation. Arch Pathol Lab Med 117: 71–77

Bazan J F 1990 Structural design and molecular evolution of a cytokine receptor superfamily. Proc Natl Acad Sci USA 87: 6934–6938

Bom V J J, van Tilburg N H, Krommenhoek-van Es C et al 1986 Immunoradiometric assays for human coagulation factor VII using polyclonal antibodies against the Ca(II)-dependent and Ca(II)-independent conformation. Thromb Haemost 56: 343–348

Broadhurst P, Kelleher C, Hughes L et al 1990 Fibrinogen, factor VII clotting activity and coronary artery disease severity. Atherosclerosis 85: 169–173

Broze G J Jr, Hickman S, Miletich J P 1985 Monoclonal anti-human factor VII antibodies. J Clin Invest 76: 937–946

Carson S D, Brozna J P 1993 The role of tissue factor in the production of thrombin. Blood Coagulat Fibrinol 4: 281–292

Carvalho de Sousa J, Azevedo J, Soria C et al 1988 Factor VII hyperactivity in acute myocardial thrombosis: a relation to the coagulation activation. Thromb Res 51: 165–173

Cortellaro M, Boschetti C, Cofrancesco E et al 1992 The PLAT study: hemostatic function in relation to atherothrombotic ischemic events in vascular disease patients: principal results. Arterioscler Thromb 12: 1063–1070

Dalaker K, Hjermann I, Prydz H 1985 A novel form of factor VII in plasma from men at risk for cardiovascular disease. Br J Haematol 61: 315–322

Dalaker K, Prydz H 1984 The coagulation factor VII in pregnancy. Br J Haematol 56: 233–241

Dalaker K, Smith P, Arnesen H et al 1987 Factor VII–phospholipid complex in male survivors of acute myocardial infarction. Acta Med Scand 222: 111–116

Drake T A, Morrissey J H, Edgington T S 1989 Selective cellular expression of tissue factor in human tissues: implications for disorders of hemostasis and thrombosis. Am J Pathol 134: 1087–1097

Fair D S 1983 Quantitation of factor VII in the plasma of normal and warfarin-treated individuals by radioimmunoassay. Blood 62: 784–791

Fiore M M, Neuenschwander P F, Morrissey J H 1994 The biochemical basis for the apparent defect of soluble mutant tissue factor in enhancing the proteolytic activities of factor VIIa. J Biol Chem 269: 143–149

Fisher K L, Gorman C M, Vehar G A et al 1987 Cloning and expression of human tissue factor. Thromb Res 48: 89–99

Fleck R A, Rao L V M, Rapaport S I et al 1990 Localization of human tissue factor antigen by immunostaining with monospecific, polyclonal anti-human tissue factor antibody. Thromb Res 59: 421–437

Folsom A R, Wu K K, Shahar E et al 1993 Association of hemostatic variables with prevalent cardiovascular disease and asymptomatic carotid artery atherosclerosis. Arterioscler Thromb 13: 1829–1836

Forrester J S, Litvack F, Grundfest W et al 1987 A perspective of coronary disease seen through the arteries of living man. Circulation 75: 505–513

Gibbs C S, McCurdy S N, Leung L L K et al 1994 Identification of the factor VIIa binding site on tissue factor by homologous loop swap and alanine scanning mutagenesis. Biochemistry 33: 14003–14010

Hagen F S, Gray C L, O'Hara P et al 1986 Characterization of a cDNA coding for human factor VII. Proc Natl Acad Sci USA 83: 2412–2416

Harlos K, Martin D M A, O'Brien D P et al 1994 Crystal structure of the extracellular region of human tissue factor. Nature 370: 662–666

Hayes T E, Pike J, Tracy R P 1993 Factor VII assays. Arch Pathol Lab Med 117: 52–57

Heinrich J, Balleisen L, Schulte H et al 1994 Fibrinogen and factor VII in the prediction of coronary risk. Results from the PROCAM study in healthy men. Arterioscler Thromb 14: 54–59

Hemker H C, Muller A D, Gonggrup R 1976 The estimation of activated human blood coagulation factor VII. J Mol Med 1: 127–134

Hoffman C, Shah A, Sodums M et al 1988 Factor VII activity state in coronary artery disease. J Lab Clin Med 111: 475–481

Hoffman C J, Miller R H, Lawson W E et al 1989 Elevation of factor VII activity and mass in young adults at risk of ischemic heart disease. J Am Coll Cardiol 14: 941–946

Hubbard A R, Barrowcliffe T W 1994 Measurement of activated factor VII using soluble mutant tissue factor – proposal for standardization. Thromb Haemost 72: 643–651

Hubbard A R, Parr L J 1991 Phospholipase C mediated inhibition of factor VII requires triglyceride-rich lipoproteins. Thromb Res 62: 335–344

Hultin M B 1991 Fibrinogen and factor VII as risk factors in vascular disease. Prog Haemost Thromb 10: 215–241

Kario K, Sakata T, Matsuo T et al 1993 Factor VII in non-insulin-dependent diabetic patients with microalbuminuria. Lancet 342: 1552

Kario K, Miyata T, Sakata T et al 1994 Fluorogenic assay of activated factor VII. Plasma factor VIIa levels in relation to arterial cardiovascular diseases in Japanese. Arterioscler Thromb 14: 265–274

Kario K, Matsuo T, Asada R et al 1995a The strong positive correlation between factor VII clotting activity using bovine thromboplastin and the activated factor VII level. Thromb Haemost 73: 429–434

Kario K, Matsuo T, Matsuo M et al 1995b Marked increase of activated factor VII in uremic patients. Thromb Haemost 73: 763–767

Kitchen S, Malia R G, Greaves M et al 1988 A method for the determination of activated factor VII using bovine and rabbit brain thromboplastins: demonstration of increased levels in disseminated intravascular coagulation. Thromb Res 50: 191–200

Kitchen S, Malia R G, Preston F E 1992 A comparison of methods for the measurement of activated factor VII. Thromb Haemost 68: 301–305

Koster T, Rosendaal F R, Reitsma P H et al 1994 Factor VII and fibrinogen levels as risk factors for venous thrombosis. Thromb Haemost 71: 719–722

Limentani S A, Gowell K P, Deitcher S R 1995 In vitro characterization of high purity factor IX concentrates for the treatment of hemophilia B. Thromb Haemost 73: 584–591

Mann K G 1989 Factor VII assays, plasma triglyceride levels, and cardiovascular disease risk. Arteriosclerosis 9: 783–784

Martin D M A, Boys C W G, Ruf W 1995 Tissue factor: molecular recognition and cofactor function. FASEB J 9: 852–859

Meade T W, Mellows S, Brozovic M et al 1986 Haemostatic function and ischaemic heart disease: principal results of the Northwick Park Heart Study. Lancet ii: 533–537

Miller B C, Hultin M B, Jesty J 1985 Altered factor VII activity in hemophilia. Blood 65: 845

Miller G J, Stirling Y, Esnouf M P et al 1994 Factor VII-deficient substrate plasmas depleted of protein C raise the sensitivity of the factor VII bio-assay to activated factor VII: an international study. Thromb Haemost 71: 38–48

Moor E, Silveira A, van't Hooft F et al 1995 Coagulation factor VII mass and activity in young men with myocardial infarction at a young age: Role of plasma lipoproteins and factor VII genotype. Arterioscler Thromb Vasc Biol 15: 655–664

Morrissey J H, Fakhrai H, Edgington T S 1987 Molecular cloning of the cDNA for tissue factor, the cellular receptor for the initiation of the coagulation protease cascade. Cell 50: 129–135

Morrissey J H, Macik B G, Neuenschwander P F et al 1993 Quantitation of activated factor VII levels in plasma using a tissue factor mutant selectively deficient in promoting factor VII activation. Blood 81: 734–744

Morrissey J H, Macik B G (1991). Novel clotting assay for factor VIIa in plasma using a tissue factor mutant that does not support activation of factor VII. Arterioscler Thromb 11: 1544A (Abstract)

Muller Y A, Ultsch M H, Kelley R F et al 1994 Structure of the extracellular domain of human tissue factor: location of the factor VIIa binding site. Biochemistry 33: 10864–10870

Nakagaki T, Foster D C, Berkner K L et al 1991 Initiation of the extrinsic pathway of blood coagulation: evidence for the tissue factor dependent autoactivation of human coagulation factor VII. Biochemistry 30: 10819–10824

Nemerson Y, Repke D 1985 Tissue factor accelerates the activation of coagulation factor VII: the role of a bifunctional coagulation cofactor. Thromb Res 40: 351

Neuenschwander P F, Morrissey J H 1992 Deletion of the membrane-anchoring region of tissue factor abolishes autoactivation of factor VII, but not cofactor function: analysis of a mutant with a selective deficiency in activity. J Biol Chem 267: 14477–14482

Neuenschwander P F, Morrissey J H 1994 Roles of the membrane-interactive regions of factor VIIa and tissue factor: the factor VIIa Gla domain is dispensable for binding to tissue factor but important for activation of factor X. J Biol Chem 269: 8007–8013

Orlando M, Leri O, Macioce G et al 1987 Factor VII in subjects at risk for thromboembolism: activation or increased synthesis? Haemostasis 17: 340–343

Østerud B, Berre A, Otnaess B-A et al 1972 Activation of the coagulation factor VII by tissue thromboplastin and calcium. Biochemistry 11: 2853

Paborsky L R, Caras I W, Fisher K L et al 1991 Lipid association, but not the transmembrane domain, is required for tissue factor activity. Substitution of the transmembrane domain with a phosphatidylinositol anchor. J Biol Chem 266: 21911–21916

Poggio M, Tripodi A, Mariani G et al 1991 Factor VII clotting assay: influence of different thromboplastins and factor VII-deficient plasma. Thromb Haemost 65: 160–164

Rapaport S I 1991 Regulation of the tissue factor pathway. Ann N Y Acad Sci 614: 151

Raskob G E, Durica S S, Morrissey J H et al 1995 Effect of treatment with low-dose warfarin–aspirin on activated factor VII. Blood 85: 3034–3039

Rezaie A R, Fiore M M, Neuenschwander P F et al 1992 Expression and purification of a soluble tissue factor fusion protein with an epitope for an unusual calcium-dependent antibody. Protein Express Purif 3: 453–460

Ruddock V, Meade T W 1994 Factor VII activity and ischaemic heart disease: fatal and non-fatal events. Q J Med 87: 403–406

Ruf W, Rehemtulla A, Morrissey J H et al 1991 Phospholipid-independent and -dependent interactions required for tissue factor receptor and cofactor function. J Biol Chem 266: 2158–2166

Ruf W, Schullek J R, Stone M J et al 1994 Mutational mapping of functional residues in tissue factor: identification of factor VII recognition determinants in both structural modules of the predicted cytokine receptor homology domain. Biochemistry 33: 1565–1572

Sakata T, Kario K, Matsuo T et al 1995 Suppression of plasma-activated factor VII levels by warfarin therapy. Arterioscler Thromb Vasc Biol 15: 241–246

Scarpati E M, Wen D, Broze G J Jr et al 1987 Human tissue factor: cDNA sequence and chromosome localization of the gene. Biochemistry 26: 5234

Schullek J R, Ruf W, Edgington T S 1994 Key ligand interface residues in tissue factor contribute independently to factor VIIa binding. J Biol Chem 269: 19399–19403

Seligsohn U, Kasper C K, Østerud B et al 1978a Activated factor VII: presence in factor IX concentrate and persistence in the circulation after infusion. Blood 53: 828

Seligsohn U, Østerud B, Rapaport S I 1978b Coupled amidolytic assay for factor VII: its use with a clotting assay to determine the activity state of factor VII. Blood 52: 978–988

Shigematsu Y, Miyata T, Higashi S et al 1992 Expression of human soluble tissue factor in yeast and enzymatic properties of its complex with factor VIIa. J Biol Chem 267: 21329–21337

Sosef M N, Bosch J G, van Oostayen J et al 1994 Relation of plasma coagulation factor VII and fibrinogen to carotid artery intima-media thickness. Thromb Haemost 72: 250–254

Spicer E K, Horton R, Bloem L et al 1987 Isolation of cDNA clones coding for human tissue factor: primary structure of the protein and cDNA. Proc Natl Acad Sci USA 84: 5148–5152

Suzuki T, Yamauchi K, Matsushita T et al 1991 Elevation of factor VII activity and mass in coronary artery disease of varying severity. Clin Cardiol 14: 731–736

Takase T, Tuddenham E, Chand S et al 1988 Monoclonal antibodies to human factor VII: a one step immunoradiometric assay for VII:Ag. J Clin Pathol 41: 337–341

Van Deijk W A, van Dam-Mieras M C E, Muller A D et al 1983 Evaluation of a coagulation assay determining the activity state of factor VII in plasma. Haemostasis 13: 192–197

Vaziri N D, Kennedy S C, Kennedy D et al 1992 Coagulation, fibrinolytic, and inhibitory proteins in acute myocardial infarction and angina pectoris. Am J Med 93: 651–657

Waxman E, Ross J B A, Laue T M et al 1992 Tissue factor and its extracellular soluble domain: the relationship between intermolecular association with factor VIIa and enzymatic activity of the complex. Biochemistry 31: 3998–4003

Waxman E, Laws W R, Laue T M et al 1993 Human factor VIIa and its complex with soluble tissue factor: evaluation of asymmetry and conformational dynamics by ultracentrifugation and fluorescence anisotropy decay methods. Biochemistry 32: 3005–3012

Wilcox J N, Smith K M, Schwartz S M et al 1989 Localization of tissue factor in the normal vessel wall and in the atherosclerotic plaque. Proc Natl Acad Sci USA 86: 2839–2843

Wildgoose P, Nemerson Y, Hansen L L et al 1992 Measurement of basal levels of factor VIIa in hemophilia A and B patients. Blood 80: 25–28

8. Lipids and coagulation

G. J. Miller

The suggestion that a high blood cholesterol concentration causes atherosclerosis dates back to the pathological studies of Virchow (1856) and the experiments of Stuckey (1912) and Anitschow & Chatalow (1913) in the cholesterol-fed rabbit. The first clinical evidence for a role of plasma lipids in the human atherothrombotic disorders appears to be that of Weinhouse & Hirsch (1940). Subsequent reports linking hypercholesterolaemia with coronary heart disease (CHD) (Boas et al 1948, Gofman et al 1950, Barr et al 1951) took many years to gain widespread acceptance (Oliver 1987) and only recently has the causative role of a high plasma low-density lipoprotein (LDL) concentration in atherosclerotic heart disease become widely acknowledged (Law et al 1994, Scandinavian Simvastatin Survival Study Group 1994). Similarly, although the effects on blood cholesterol of a diet rich in saturated fatty acids became increasingly recognized after 1950 (Messinger et al 1950, Keys 1952, Bronte-Stewart et al 1955), evidence for the importance of diet in CHD remained unconvincing for many even beyond 1980 (Meade & Chakrabarti 1972, McMichael 1979). Only from the mid-1980s onwards has sufficient consensus been achieved to support widespread calls for a reduction in the fat content of the 'Western' diet for the primary prevention of CHD (Expert Panel 1988).

The early 1950s also saw the first tentative connections being made between dietary fat, the coagulability of blood and CHD (Duncan & Waldron 1949, Fullerton et al 1953, Manning & Walford 1954, Mustard 1957). Progress was hindered, however, by a very limited understanding of haemostasis in those years, and by restriction of measurements largely to clotting times of whole blood and recalcified plasma. Although the importance of phospholipids in membranes for surface-mediated coagulant reactions became increasingly recognized (Papahadjopolous & Hanahan 1964), research on dietary lipids, plasma lipoproteins and coagulation was overshadowed by advances in our understanding of cholesterol and CHD, and interest gradually waned (the extensive literature on lipids in relation to the fibrinolytic pathways and blood platelets is not considered in this review). Furthermore, even had this early work established a connection between a high-fat diet and hypercoagulability, its clinical relevance would still have been seriously questioned. As recently as the mid-1970s physicians generally doubted the significance of coronary thrombosis in myocardial infarction (Chandler et al 1974). Only since 1980, as a result of careful angiographic (De Wood et al 1980) and pathological (Bini et al 1989, Woolf & Davies 1992) studies has the central role of thrombosis in the acute coronary syndromes become generally accepted. Added to this, by the late 1970s the Northwick Park Heart Study was beginning to provide evidence for important changes in the coagulation system in men at high risk for CHD (Meade et al 1980) – changes which might predispose to thrombosis.

THE NORTHWICK PARK HEART STUDY AND FACTOR VII

In 1972, Meade et al (1977) commenced measurement of several haemostatic factors including factor VII coagulant activity (VII:C) in 1511 healthy men aged 40–64 years belonging to the Northwick Park Heart Study. After an average follow-up of 4 years, the mean factor VII:C in those who had died of CHD was found to have been 117% of standard at recruitment as compared with 102% of standard ($P < 0.01$) in those still alive (Meade et al 1980). This association has persisted through more than 16 years of follow-up, but, importantly, factor VII:C is not associated with the risk of non-fatal CHD (Ruddock & Meade 1994). More recently, factor VII:C has been included in prospective cardiovascular surveys in Germany (Heinrich et al 1994) and the USA (ARIC Investigators 1989), but definitive results are still awaited. Preliminary data for one study (Heinrich et al 1994) appeared to accord with those of Meade et al (1980), but the increase in factor VII:C in the small number of men dying from CHD up to the time of analysis was only of marginal statistical significance. Nevertheless, these epidemiological findings have prompted a search for the causes of a high factor VII:C.

FACTOR VII AND ITS MEASUREMENT (see also Chapter 7)

Factor VII circulates almost entirely as a single-chain zymogen at a plasma concentration of about 450 ng/ml (Fair 1983) and with a half-life of about 5 h (Hasselback & Hjort 1960). About 3 ng/ml circulates as the enzyme factor VIIa (Wildgoose et al 1992, Morrissey et al 1993) with a half-life of approximately 3 h (Seligsohn et al 1979a). Plasma factor VII zymogen is converted to factor VIIa by proteolytic cleavage at the peptide bond Arg152–Ile153 by factors IXa and Xa (Hagen et al 1986), but for expression of its coagulant activity factor VIIa must form a complex with a specific glycoprotein cofactor bound to subendothelial cell surfaces. This cofactor, known as tissue factor, also supports the autoactivation of factor VII zymogen (Yamamoto et al 1992) and its activation by factor Xa (Nemerson & Repke 1985).

Earlier measurements of factor VII concentration (zymogen and VIIa) were indirect and based upon preliminary activation by addition of thromboplastin and calcium to citrated test plasma, followed by estimation of the rate of conversion of factor X to factor Xa by factor VIIa. The rate of generation of factor Xa was measured either by employing tritiated factor X as substrate and recording the rate of release of the labelled activation peptide (Miller et al 1985), or by measuring factor Xa activity with an amidolytic substrate (Seligsohn et al 1978). These techniques have now been superseded by immunoassay of factor VII antigen (VII:Ag) (Fair 1983), which gives a very close approximation of factor VII (zymogen and VIIa).

The concentration of human factor VIIa in test plasma is measured with bioassays which employ types of tissue factor that have cofactor activity for human factor VIIa but which lack the ability to support the conversion of human factor VII zymogen to factor VIIa. Bovine tissue factor is frequently used for this purpose (Hemker et al 1976, Poggio et al 1991, Miller et al 1994). More recently, however, soluble recombinant human tissue factor preparations have been developed with the same properties (Neuenschwander & Morrissey 1992, Waxman et al 1992) and shown to be of value for the direct assay of preformed factor VIIa activity in test plasma (Wildgoose et al 1992, Morrissey et al 1993). Kario et al (1994) used such a mutant tissue factor in a modified bioassay for factor VIIa that employs a fluorogenic peptide as a substrate for thrombin generated in the assay system. These assays have proved useful in assessing the contributions of factor VII zymogen and factor VIIa to a high factor VII:C.

FACTOR VII AND PLASMA TRIGLYCERIDE

During the 1970s several clinical studies established that an increased factor VII:C was a frequent finding in diverse forms of hypertriglyceridaemia (Constantino et al 1977, Fuller et al 1979). Subsequently, factor VII:C (Miller et al 1985, Bruckert et al 1989, Wright et al 1993) and factor VII:Ag (Hoffman et al 1992) were shown to be positively associated with plasma triglyceride concentration in healthy normolipidaemic adults and to be raised in the physiological hypertriglyceridaemia of pregnancy (Stirling et al 1984, Hubbard et al 1990). Mitropoulos et al (1989) found that factor VII:C was more strongly correlated with the very-low-density (VLDL) and chylomicron (i.e. triglyceride-rich) fractions of the plasma lipoproteins than with LDL. The causal nature of this association was suggested by the decrease in factor VII:C following therapeutic restoration of normal triglyceride levels (Elkeles et al 1980, Simpson et al 1983, Bruckert et al 1989) and amelioration of the dyslipidaemia in obesity by weight loss (Baron et al 1989, Slabber et al 1992, Palareti et al 1994). Fasting serum triglyceride (the standard measurement of triglyceride in epidemiology) is frequently increased in adults at high risk of CHD (Bainton et al 1992, Stensvold et al 1993) although whether hypertriglyceridaemia has any causal role in the disease has been much debated (Hulley & Avins 1992). One possibility might be that the relation reflects in part a role for dietary fat intake in CHD, because fasting triglyceride levels are strongly correlated with non-fasting levels (Olefsky et al 1976), for which in turn fat consumption is a major determinant (Van Amelsvoort et al 1989). This line of reasoning, together with the effects on factor VII:C of a reduction in triglyceride concentration by dietary therapy as mentioned above, prompted study of the effects of diet on factor VII.

DIETARY FAT, POSTPRANDIAL LIPAEMIA AND FACTOR VII

Miller et al (1986) monitored fasting factor VII:C in six adults while they consumed in sequence their normal diet for 2 weeks, a low-fat diet for 2 weeks and a high-fat diet for 3 weeks. Mean factor VII:C was 16% of standard higher on the high-fat diet than on the low-fat diet ($P < 0.03$), but more striking was the way in which within individuals the peaks and troughs in the morning fasting factor VII:C mirrored those in fat intake during the previous day. Plasma factor VII concentration, measured by the tritiated factor X assay system, was not related to the subject's intake of dietary fat on the previous day, and neither fasting factor VII:C nor factor VII was associated with the fasting triglyceride concentration. In a later study, Miller et al (1991) examined the relations between factor VII and non-fasting triglyceride levels over 1 day within subjects while they ate three experimental meals. There was a clear tendency for factor VII:C to be associated positively with the plasma triglyceride concentration about 160 min earlier, whereas it was not related to that in the same blood sample. Plasma factor VII:Ag was not related to triglyceride concentration at any time of the day. These findings suggested that the increase in factor VII:C accompanying an increased fat intake and postprandial lipaemia was due to activation of factor VII zymogen rather than to an increase in factor VII concentration.

Salomaa et al (1993) followed factor VII after three single test meals rich, respectively, in saturated fatty acids, n-6 polyunsaturated fatty acids and carbohydrate. Six and 8 h postprandially, factor VII:C was significantly increased above the fasting level after the two fatty meals, but was lower than the fasting level after the carbohydrate meal. By contrast, factor VII:Ag declined postprandially irrespective of the meal's composition. Silveira et al (1994) took blood samples before and at 9 intervals after a fatty test meal. Substantial postprandial increases in factor VIIa were observed at times when factor VII:Ag was either unchanged or lower than the baseline level. Miller et al (1996) measured factor VIIa and factor VII:Ag in 14 healthy adults over 6.5 h on two occasions, first while consuming fat-rich meals for breakfast and lunch, and again when consuming isocaloric meals in which fat was exchanged for carbohydrate. As shown in Table 8.1, plasma factor VIIa increased postprandially only during the fat-rich regimen, while factor VII:Ag at 6.5 h did not differ significantly from the fasting level on either regimen. The magnitude of the postprandial rise in factor VIIa appears to be associated with the fat content of meal (Sanders et al 1996) and the magnitude of the postprandial triglyceridaemia (Silveira et al 1994).

Possible mechanisms underlying the postprandial increase in factor VIIa

On the basis of in vitro (Carvalho de Sousa et al 1988) and in vivo studies in hyperlipidaemic patients (Carvalho de Sousa et al 1989a,b), the increased factor VII:C in hypertriglyceridaemic patients was thought to be due possibly to attachment of factor VII zymogen, factor VIIa or both to the surface of triglyceride-rich particles with consequent impaired clearance. A similar mechanism could be proposed for the increase in the concentration of the other vitamin K-dependent clotting factors (Constantino et al 1977) in hyperlipidaemias types IIb, IV and V as classified by Fredrickson et al (1967). However, factor VII:C and factor VII:Ag levels are normal in patients with complete lipoprotein-lipase deficiency despite their massive hypertriglyceridaemia (Mitropoulos et al 1992), factor VII:Ag does not increase postprandially in healthy subjects (Table 8.1) and neither factor VII:Ag nor factor VIIa increases during postprandial lipaemia in patients with factor IX deficiency (Miller et al 1996). Thus, while the vitamin K-dependent clotting factors may associate with lipoproteins in vivo, such associations appear insufficient to influence factor VII turnover. Certainly any physical association of this type is broken during ultracentrifugation of plasma (Constantino et al 1977).

An alternative possibility might be that triglyceride-rich lipoproteins simply augment the expression of factor VIIa activity in the in vitro bioassay, but this seems unlikely for several reasons. Firstly, the addition of triglyceride-rich lipoproteins to plasma in vitro has no influence on the result of the factor VII:C bioassay (Constantino et al 1977, Miller et al 1985, Silveira et al 1994). Secondly, and as already noted, factor VII:C is not increased in the hypertriglyceridaemic state associated with familial lipoprotein-lipase deficiency (Mitropoulos et al 1992). Thirdly, factor VII:C does not increase postprandially in factor IX deficiency (Miller et al 1996). Thus the most likely explanation is that factor VIIa synthesis is increased after a fatty meal. How such activation of factor VII zymogen would occur is uncertain, but there are several pertinent observations to consider at this point.

Table 8.1 Mean (standard deviation) activated factor VII (VIIa, ng/ml) and factor VII zymogen (% standard)[*] in 14 adults in the baseline fasted state and 6.5 h after consumption of isocaloric high-fat and low-fat test meals

Factor	High fat meals		Low fat meals	
	Baseline	6.5 h	Baseline	6.5 h
VIIa	1.59(0.42)	2.17(0.67)[†]	1.53(0.45)	1.50(0.33)[NS]
VII zymogen	95(20)	98(17)[NS]	103(27)	95(30)[NS]

[*]Measured as factor VII antigen by ELISA (enzyme-linked immunosorbent assay).
In comparison with the baseline value (paired t-test): [†]$P = 5.88$, $t < 0.001$; NS, not statistically significant.

Lipids and the contact system of coagulation

The contact system of coagulation (factor XII–prekallikrein–high molecular weight kininogen) is activated in vitro when citrated plasma is incubated with a negatively charged surface such as presented by sulphatides (cerebroside sulphates). Such surfaces promote the autoactivation of factor XII (Tankersley & Finlayson 1984). Activated factor XII (XIIa) cleaves factor XI to factor XIa, which in turn activates factor IX to initiate the intrinsic pathway of coagulation. Both factor XIIa (Radcliffe et al 1977) and activated factor IX (IXa) (Seligsohn et al 1979b) activate factor VII zymogen in the absence of tissue factor (though these actions have not so far been demonstrated in vivo). Mitropoulos & Esnouf (1991) have shown that long-chain saturated fatty acids such as stearic acid serve as potent contact surfaces for the autoactivation of factor XII in vitro. Also, when triglyceride-rich plasma from patients with complete lipoprotein-lipase deficiency is incubated with lipoprotein-lipase, a prompt activation of factor XII is observed (Mitropoulos et al 1992). These in vitro findings suggested that in vivo lipolysis of lipoproteins may create a negatively charged surface, activating factor XII and thereby factor VII. As already men-

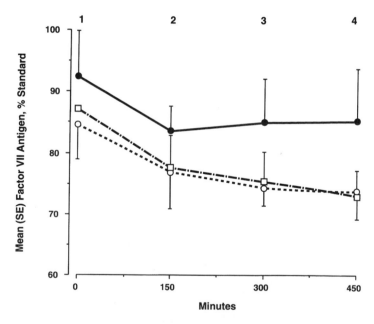

Fig. 8.1   Mean factor VII zymogen level (measured as factor VII antigen, VII:Ag) in five subjects at several times during the 28th day of three of isocaloric diets rich, respectively, in long-chain saturated fatty acids (●), polyunsaturated fatty acids (○) and carbohydrate (□). Measurements were made (1) fasting before breakfast, (2) late morning before lunch, (3) mid-afternoon after lunch, and (4) at late afternoon. Bars are standard errors about the means.

tioned, patients with familial lipoprotein-lipase deficiency have normal levels of factor VII:C and factor VII:Ag (Mitropoulos et al 1992). Furthermore, injection of a lipoprotein-lipase inhibitor in the rabbit causes a hyperlipidaemia that is not associated with any elevation in factor VII:C (Mitropoulos et al 1994a), suggesting that lipolysis is indeed required for activation of factor VII. However, an obligatory role for factor XII in this process would appear to be excluded by the demonstration of postprandial activation of factor VII in patients with homozygous factor XII deficiency (Miller et al 1993). Hence the details of the pathway linking postprandial lipolysis with factor VIIa generation remain to be elucidated.

FACTOR VII AND A HIGH-FAT DIET

Although factor VII:Ag concentration does not rise after a single high-fat meal, its fasting level does appear to increase when the habitual diet rather than the occasional meal is rich in fat. In a community survey of middle-aged men, Miller et al (1989) found those men consuming the most fat for their body size to have the highest levels of factor VII:C, a difference subsequently shown to be associated with an increased factor VII:Ag concentration (Miller et al 1995). These associations were independent of plasma triglyceride concentration. In another community survey of middle-aged men (Vaisanen et al 1995), fasting factor VII:C was found to be positively

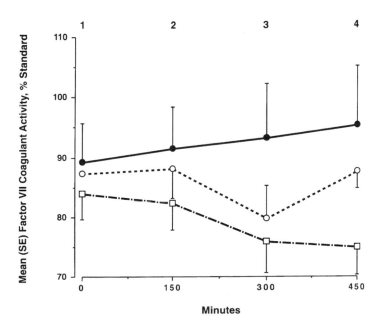

Fig. 8.2 Mean factor VII coagulant (VII:C) activity in five subjects at several times during the 28th day of three isocaloric diets. Symbols as in Figure 8.1.

associated with serum apolipoprotein B concentration (the major protein constituent of LDL and VLDL), serum triglyceride concentration and dietary fat intake. The association between factor VII:C and fat consumption was present only in the subgroup of men with apolipoprotein B levels below the upper tertile. Plasma factor VII:Ag and factor VIIa were not measured in this study.

The time required for factor VII to respond to a change in habitual fat intake appears to be variable. In two studies in which a reduced-fat diet was taken for 2 weeks (Marckmann et al 1994) and 20 weeks (Brace et al 1994) respectively, significant reductions in fasting factor VII:C were observed without any significant change in factor VII:Ag. By contrast, Marckmann et al (1990) reported significant decreases in fasting factor VII:C, factor VIIa and factor VII:Ag when a low-fat diet was consumed for 2 weeks, and the same group observed a significant decline in fasting factor VII:C (factor VII:Ag was not measured) after 4 weeks on a reduced-fat diet (Marckmann et al 1993a).

Mitropoulos et al (1994b) examined fasting and non-fasting levels of factor VII:C and factor VII:Ag in five adults on the final day of three diets of 4 weeks' duration: one rich in saturated fatty acids, another in polyunsaturated fatty acids, and the third in carbohydrate. The results are summarized in Figures 8.1 and 8.2. Neither fasting factor VII:C nor fasting factor VII:Ag differed on the polyunsaturated fatty acid and carbohydrate diets. However, both measures of factor VII were highest on the saturated fatty acid diet, the increase being statistically significant for factor VII:Ag in comparison with the polyunsaturated fatty acid diet ($P = 0.02$) and of borderline significance ($P = 0.07$) in comparison with the carbohydrate diet. Non-fasting factor VII:Ag levels declined similarly during the day irrespective of the composition of the meals consumed, but remained highest on the saturated fatty acid regimen.

Low-fat diets contain more fibre than high-fat diets. Marckmann et al (1993b) found no significant effect of fibre consumption on factor VII:C or factor VII:Ag over a period of 2 days, but in another study supplementation of the diet with 100 g/10 MJ of oat bran for 16 days produced significant reductions in factor VII:C and fasting triglyceride concentration after 16 days (Marckmann & Sandstrom 1995). Thus the low factor VII:C on a high-carbohydrate diet may be due not only to its low-fat content but also to the relatively high intake of fibre, both combining to lower triglyceride levels appreciably.

FACTOR VII AND DIETARY FAT COMPOSITION

Connor (1962) and Mitropoulos & Esnouf (1991) showed that factor XII was activated when incubated in whole plasma or in a purified system with long-chain saturated fatty acids, but not in the presence of unsaturated fatty acids. These in vitro findings raised the possibility that the postprandial responses of factor XII and factor VII in vivo may depend upon the composition of the fat consumed.

Dietary fat composition has been reported not to influence the responses of factor VII to a single meal (Salomaa et al 1993), a 7-day diet (Miller et al 1991) or a 2-week diet (Marckmann et al 1990). Two longer-term studies have observed significant effects of fat composition on factor VII, however, but are in apparent disagreement on the nature of these effects. Looking again at the study of Mitropoulos et al (1994b) summarized in Figures 8.1 and 8.2, a higher mean fasting factor VII:C and factor VII:Ag was observed after 4 weeks of a high-saturated fatty acid diet than after a high-polyunsaturated fatty acid diet, which was statistically significant for factor VII:Ag. In addition, the increase in non-fasting factor VII:C above the fasting level was marginally statistically significant on the saturated fatty acid regimen ($P = 0.06$), whereas non-fasting and fasting levels were similar on the polyunsaturated fatty acid diet. Stearic acid appeared primarily responsible for the effects of the high-saturated fatty acid diet on factor VII:C (Mitropoulos et al 1994b). Incidentally, the non-fasting differences in factor VII:C between the saturated and polyunsaturated fatty acid diets in this study were in contrast to the study of Salomaa et al (1993) discussed above, possibly because of differences in study design (4 weeks of dietary preparation in the former but none in the latter).

Tholstrup et al (1994) served three diets each of 3 weeks' duration. One diet supplied 36% of total energy in the form of shea butter (a Nigerian cooking fat very rich in stearic acid), while in the other two diets stearic acid was exchanged for palmitic acid and myristic plus lauric acids, respectively. Fasting factor VII:C was significantly reduced on the shea butter diet owing to a reduction in factor VII zymogen (Bladbjerg et al 1995). Why factor VII:Ag should have decreased in this study when the diet was rich in stearic acid, while it increased in the study of Mitropoulos et al (1994b), is unclear. However, shea butter also contains unidentified unsaponifiable substances and might therefore have had effects on factor VII unrelated to its stearic acid content. Stearic acid was supplied in ordinary dairy products and meat in the study of Mitropoulos et al (1994b).

Several studies have sought but failed to show any specific effects of fish oils (n-3 polyunsaturated fatty acids) on fasting levels of factor VII (Sanders et al 1981, Marckmann et al 1991). The effects of these oils on non-fasting levels have yet to be reported.

LIPIDS AND THE COFACTORS AND INHIBITORS OF FACTOR VII

The coagulation of blood begins when factor VIIa binds to its cofactor, tissue factor. The activity of the complex is regulated by tissue factor pathway inhibitor (TFPI), a protein which circulates in association with VLDL, LDL and high-density lipoproteins (HDL) (Novotny et al 1989). The first step in this regulation is the binding of TFPI to the active site of factor Xa (Xa), thereby inhibiting the proteolytic activity of factor Xa on factor VII zymogen. The second step is the inhibition of tissue factor–factor VIIa complexes by the formation of a quaternary complex of tissue factor–factor VIIa–factor Xa–TFPI (Gemmel et al 1990). Human apolipoprotein A-II, a major component of some classes of HDL particle, has been shown in vitro to inhibit human tissue factor in mixed brain lipids (Kondo & Kisiel 1987) and bovine tissue factor in phospholipid vesicles (Carson 1987). However, the pure apolipoprotein fails to inhibit tissue factor on the membranes of cultured fibroblasts (Gramzinski et al 1989). Thus the relevance of these findings for in vivo coagulation is not clear. The largest pool of TFPI in vivo is associated with the vascular endothelium, and the plasma concentration is not influenced by the concentration of the lipoproteins (Novotny et al 1991). Thus TFPI appears unlikely to play any prominent role in the hypercoagulability of hyperlipidaemic states.

Finally, there is some in vitro evidence for effects of plasma lipoproteins and dietary lipid on the expression of tissue factor activity by cells. Isolated triglyceride-rich lipoproteins are reported to enhance the expression of tissue factor activity on human peripheral blood mononuclear cells during incubation in vitro (Schwartz et al 1981). Increased concentrations of plasma HDL are also reported to promote the expression of tissue factor procoagulant activity in monocytes exposed to endotoxin in vitro (Crutchley et al 1989). The tissue factor expressed by adherent resting or endotoxin-exposed monocytes ex vivo has been found to be reduced by prolonged administration (3 months or more) of n-3 fatty acid ethyl ester at a dose of 3 g/day (Tremoli et al 1994).

LIPIDS AND FIBRINOGEN

Unlike factor VII, fibrinogen concentration, another major haemostatic marker of risk of CHD (Meade et al 1980, Yarnell et al 1991, Heinrich et al 1994), does not appear to be influenced by dietary fat content. Most studies have found fibrinogen concentration to be unaltered by enrichment of the diet with fish oils (Sanders et al 1981, Gans et al 1990) although a small number have reported a reduction (Berg-Schmidt et al 1990).

KEY POINTS FOR CLINICAL PRACTICE

• A high factor VII:C has been shown to be associated with an increased risk of fatal CHD in middle-aged men. In the Northwick Park Heart Study, the mean difference in factor VII:C between men who subsequently died of CHD and those who remained alive and well was 9.6% of standard after 16 years of follow-up. Increases in factor VII:C of 10%

of standard or more are frequently observed following large meals that are rich in fat, particularly long-chain saturated fatty acids. This postprandial rise in factor VII:C is due to a transient increase in the synthesis of factor VIIa, there being no related increase in factor VII:Ag concentration. Because of the short half-life of factor VIIa, basal concentrations are soon restored in the fasting state.

- The evanescent activation of factor VII zymogen after fatty meals seems to depend upon postprandial lipolytic activity, but the underlying mechanism is poorly understood. When the diet is habitually rich in fat, rather than occasional meals, plasma factor VII:Ag levels also tend to be increased.

- Few studies have so far examined the effects of dietary fat composition on factor VII, but one study of diets consisting of customary foods found that, when taken as part of a long-term diet of the same composition, single meals rich in long-chain saturated fatty acids were more potent as activators of factor VII than those rich in polyunsaturated fatty acids. More studies are needed on this topic.

- Plasma factor VII:C and factor VII:Ag levels are positively associated with the fasting triglyceride concentration, independent of their relationship with dietary fat. Plasma factor VII:C decreases when triglyceride levels are lowered by diet or drug therapy. The exception appears to be familial lipoprotein-lipase deficiency, in which both factor VII:C and factor VII:Ag levels are normal in the presence of massive hypertriglyceridaemia.

- Importantly, factor VII:C is not predictive of non-fatal CHD. This might indicate that a high factor VII:C does not accelerate atherosclerosis, but rather that it increases the thrombotic response to rupture of an atheromatous plaque and hence the attendant risk of fatality. The postprandial elevation in factor VII:C after fatty meals may temporarily increase such risk.

- Dietary fat content does not appear to influence fibrinogen concentration, but whether it affects clotting factors for which there is no established relation with risk of CHD is not known. Clinical hypertriglyceridaemia, however, is associated with increased levels of factors IX, X and prothrombin. The effects of a high-fat diet on factor VII add weight to recommendations to reduce the amount of fat in the 'Western' diet.

REFERENCES

Anitschkow N, Chatalow S 1913 Ueber experimentelle Cholesterinsteatose und ihre Bedeutung für die Entstehung einiger pathologischer Prozesse. Centralbl Allg Pathol 14: 1–9

ARIC Investigators 1989 The Atherosclerosis Risk in Communities (ARIC) Study: design and objectives. Am J Epidemiol 129: 687–702

Bainton D, Miller N E, Bolton C H et al 1992 Plasma triglyceride and high density lipoprotein cholesterol as predictors of ischaemic heart disease in British men. The Caerphilly and Speedwell Collaborative Heart Disease Studies. Br Heart J 68: 60–66

Baron J A, Mann J, Stukel T 1989 Effect of weight loss on coagulation factors VII and X. Am J Cardiol 64: 519–522

Barr D P, Russ E M, Eder H A 1951 Protein–lipid relationships in human plasma. II: In atherosclerosis and related conditions. Am J Med 11: 480–493

Berg-Schmidt E, Varming K, Ernst E et al 1990 Dose–response studies on the effect of n-3 polyunsaturated fatty acids on lipids and haemostasis. Thromb Haemost 63: 1–5

Bini A, Fenoglio J, Mesa-Tejada R et al 1989 Identification and distribution of fibrinogen, fibrin and fibrin(ogen) degradation products in atherosclerosis. Use of monoclonal antibodies. Arteriosclerosis 9: 109–121

Bladbjerg E M, Tholstrup T, Marckmann P et al 1995 Dietary changes in fasting levels of factor VII coagulant activity (FVIIC) are accompanied by changes in factor VII protein and other vitamin K-dependent proteins. Thromb Haemost 73: 239–242

Boas E P, Parets A D, Aldersberg D 1948 Hereditary disturbance of cholesterol metabolism: a factor in the genesis of atherosclerosis. Am Heart J 35: 611–622

Brace L D, Gittler-Buffa C, Miller G J et al 1994 Factor VII coagulant activity and cholesterol changes in premenopausal women consuming a long-term cholesterol-lowering diet. Arterioscler Thromb 14: 1284–1289

Bronte-Stewart B, Keys A, Brock J F 1955 Serum-cholesterol, diet, and coronary heart-disease. An inter-racial survey in the Cape Peninsula. Lancet ii: 1103–1108

Bruckert E, Carvalho de Sousa J, Giral P et al 1989 Interrelationship of plasma triglyceride and coagulant factor VII levels in normotriglyceridemic hypercholesterolemia. Atherosclerosis 75: 129–134

Carson S D 1987 Tissue factor (coagulation factor III) inhibition by apolipoprotein A-II. J Biol Chem 262: 718–721

Carvalho de Sousa J, Soria C, Ayrault-Jarrier M et al 1988 Association between plasma factors VII and X with triglyceride-rich lipoproteins. J Clin Pathol 41: 940–944

Carvalho de Sousa J, Bruckert E, Giral P et al 1989a Plasma factor VII, triglyceride concentration and fibrin degradation products in primary hyperlipidemia: a clinical and laboratory study. Haemostasis 19: 83–90

Carvalho de Sousa J, Bruckert E, Giral P et al 1989b Coagulation factor VII and plasma triglycerides. Decreased catabolism as a possible mechanism of factor VII hyperactivity. Haemostasis 19: 125–130

Chandler A B, Chapman I, Erhardt L R et al 1974 Coronary thrombosis in myocardial infarction. Report of a workshop on the role of coronary thrombosis in the pathogenesis of acute myocardial infarction. Am J Cardiol 34: 823–833

Connor W E 1962 The acceleration of thrombus formation by certain fatty acids. J Clin Invest 41: 1199–1205

Constantino M, Merskey C, Kudzma D J et al 1977 Increased activity of vitamin K-dependent clotting factors in human hyperlipoproteinaemia – association with cholesterol and triglyceride levels. Thromb Haemost 38: 465–474

Crutchley D J, McPhee G V, Terris M F, Canossa-Terris M A 1989 Levels of three hemostatic factors in relation to serum lipids. Monocyte procoagulant activity, tissue plasminogen activator, and type-1 plasminogen activator inhibitor. Arteriosclerosis 9: 934–939

De Wood M A, Spores J, Notske R et al 1980 Prevalence of total coronary occlusion during the early hours of transmural myocardial infarction. N Engl J Med 303: 897–902

Duncan G G, Waldron J M 1949 The effect of ingested fat on blood coagulation. Trans Assoc Am Physicians 62: 179–185

Elkeles R S, Chakrabarti R, Vickers M et al 1980 Effect of treatment of hyperlipidaemia on haemostatic variables. Br Med J 281: 973–974

Expert Panel 1988 Report of the National Cholesterol Education Program Expert Panel on detection, evaluation and treatment of high blood cholesterol in adults. Arch Intern Med 148: 36–69

Fair D S 1983 Quantitation of factor VII in the plasma of normal and warfarin-treated individuals by radioimmunoassay. Blood 62: 784–791

Fredrickson D S, Levy R I, Lees L S 1967 Fat transport in lipoproteins. An integrated approach to mechanisms and disorders. N Engl J Med 276: 94–103

Fuller J H, Keen H, Jarrett R J et al 1979 Haemostatic variables associated with diabetes and its complications. Br Med J 2: 964–966

Fullerton H W, Davie W J A, Anastasopoulos G 1953 Relationship of alimentary lipaemia to blood coagulability. Br Med J 2: 250–253

Gans R O B, Bilo H J G, Weersink E C G et al 1990 Fish oil supplementation in patients with stable claudication. Am J Surg 160: 490–495

Gemmel C H, Broze G J, Turitto V T et al 1990 Utilization of a continuous flow reactor to study the lipoprotein associated coagulation inhibitor that inhibits tissue factor. Blood 76: 2226–2271

Gofman J W, Lindgren F, Elliott H et al 1950 The role of lipids and lipoproteins in atherosclerosis. Science 111: 166–186

Graminski R A, Broze G J, Carson S D 1989 Human fibroblast tissue factor is inhibited by lipoprotein-associated coagulation inhibitor and placental anticoagulant protein but not by apolipoprotein A-II. Blood 73: 983–989

Hagen F S, Gray C L, O'Hara P et al 1986 Characterization of a cDNA coding for human factor VII. Proc Natl Acad Sci USA 83: 2412–2416

Hasselback R, Hjort P F 1960 Effect of heparin on in vivo turnover of clotting factors. J Appl Physiol 15: 945–948

Heinrich J, Balleisen L, Schulte H et al 1994 Fibrinogen and factor VII in the prediction of coronary risk. Arterioscler Thromb 14: 54–59

Hemker H C, Muller A D, Gonggrijp R 1976 The estimation of activated human blood coagulation factor VII. J Mol Med 1: 127–134

Hoffman C J, Miller R H, Hultin M B 1992 Correlation of factor VII activity and antigen with cholesterol and triglycerides in healthy young adults. Arterioscler Thromb 12: 267–270

Hubbard A R, Parr L J, Baines M G 1990 Pregnancy and factor VII. Br J Haematol 80: 265–266

Hulley S B, Avins A 1992 Asymptomatic hypertriglyceridaemia. Insufficient evidence to treat. Br Med J 304: 394–396

Kario K, Miyata T, Sakata T et al 1994 Fluorogenic assay for activated factor VII. Plasma factor VIIa levels in relation to arterial cardiovascular diseases in Japanese. Arterioscler Thromb 14: 265–274

Keys A 1952 The cholesterol problem. Voeding 13: 539–555

Kondo S, Kisiel W 1987 Evidence that plasma lipoproteins inhibit the factor VIIa–tissue factor complex by a different mechanism than extrinsic pathway inhibitor. Blood 70: 1947–1954

Law M R, Wald N J, Thompson S G 1994 By how much and how quickly does reduction in serum cholesterol concentration lower risk of ischaemic heart disease? Br Med J 308: 367–372

McMichael J 1979 Fats and atheroma: an inquest. Br Med J 1: 173–175

Manning P R, Walford R L 1954 Lack of effect of fat ingestion on blood coagulation. Am J Med Sci 228: 652–655

Marckmann P, Sandstrom B, Jespersen J 1990 Effects of total fat content and fatty acid composition in diet on factor VII coagulant activity and blood lipids. Atherosclerosis 80: 227–233

Marckmann P, Jespersen J, Leth T et al 1991 Effect of fish diet versus meat diet on blood lipids, coagulation and fibrinolysis in healthy young men. J Intern Med 229: 317–333

Marckmann P, Sandstrom B, Jespersen J 1993a Favorable long-term effect of a low-fat/high-fiber diet on human blood coagulation and fibrinolysis. Arterioscler Thromb 13: 505–511

Marckmann P, Sandstrom B, Jespersen J 1993b Dietary effects on circadian fluctuation in human blood coagulation factor VII and fibrinolysis. Atherosclerosis 101: 225–234

Marckmann P, Sandstrom B, Jespersen J 1994 Low-fat, high-fiber diet favorably affects several independent risk markers of ischemic heart disease: observations on blood lipids, coagulation, and fibrinolysis from a trial of middle-aged Danes. Am J Clin Nutr 59: 935–939

Marckmann P, Sandstrom B 1995 Personal communication.

Meade T W, Chakrabarti R 1972 Arterial-disease research: observation or intervention. Lancet ii: 913–916

Meade T W, North W R S, Chakrabarti R et al 1977 Population-based distributions of haemostatic variables. Br Med Bull 33: 283–288

Meade T W, North W R S, Chakrabarti R et al 1980 Haemostatic function and cardiovascular death: early results of a prospective study. Lancet i: 1050–1054

Messinger W J, Porosowska Y, Steele J M 1950 Effect of feeding egg yolk and cholesterol on serum cholesterol levels. Arch Intern Med 86: 189–195

Miller G J, Walter S J, Stirling Y et al 1985 Assay of factor VII activity by two techniques: evidence for increased conversion of VII to aVIIa in hyperlipidaemia, with possible implications for ischaemic heart disease. Br J Haematol 59: 249–258

Miller G J, Martin J C, Webster J et al 1986 Association between dietary fat intake and factor VII coagulant activity – a predictor of cardiovascular mortality. Atherosclerosis 60: 269–277

Miller G J, Cruickshank J K, Ellis L J et al 1989 Fat consumption and factor VII coagulant activity in middle-aged men. Atherosclerosis 78: 19–24

Miller G J, Martin J C, Mitropoulos K et al 1991 Plasma factor VII is activated by postprandial triglyceridaemia, irrespective of dietary fat composition. Atherosclerosis 86: 163–171

Miller G J, Martin J C, Mitropoulos K A et al 1993 Factor XII is not needed for factor VII activation by dietary fat. Circulation 88 (suppl): I-128

Miller G J, Stirling Y, Esnouf M P et al 1994 Factor VII-deficient substrate plasmas depleted of protein C raise the sensitivity of the factor VII bio-assay to activated factor VII: an international study. Thromb Haemost 71: 38–48

Miller G J, Martin J C, Mitropoulos K A et al 1996 Activation of factor VIII during alimentary lipemia occurs in healthy adults and patients with congenital factor XII or factor XI deficiency, but not in patients with factor IX deficiency. Blood (in press)

Miller G J, Stirling Y, Howarth D J et al 1995 Dietary fat intake and plasma factor VII antigen concentration. Thromb Haemost 73: 893

Mitropoulos K A, Esnouf M P 1991 The autoactivation of factor XII in the presence of long-chain saturated fatty acids. A comparison with the potency of sulphatides and dextran sulphate. Thromb Haemost 66: 446–452

Mitropoulos K A, Miller G J, Reeves B E A et al 1989 Factor VII coagulant activity is strongly associated with the plasma concentration of large lipoprotein particles in middle aged men. Atherosclerosis 76: 203–208

Mitropoulos K A, Miller G J, Watts G F et al 1992 Lipolysis of triglyceride-rich lipoproteins activates factor XII: a study in familial lipoprotein-lipase deficiency. Atherosclerosis 94: 119–125

Mitropoulos K A, Miller G J, Howarth D J et al 1994a The effects of intravenous Triton WR-1339 on factor VII coagulant activity and plasma lipoproteins in normocholesterolaemic and hypercholesterolaemic rabbits. Blood Coagulat Fibrinol 5: 583–591

Mitropoulos K A, Miller G J, Martin J C et al 1994b Dietary fat induces changes in factor VII coagulant activity through effects on plasma free stearic acid concentration. Arterioscler Thromb 14: 214–222

Morrissey J H, Macik B G, Neuenschwander P F et al 1993 Quantitation of activated factor VII levels in plasma using a tissue factor mutant selectively deficient in promoting factor VII activation. Blood 81: 734–744

Mustard J F 1957 Increased activity of the coagulation mechanism during alimentary lipaemia: its significance with regard to thrombosis and atherosclerosis. Can Med Assoc J 77: 308–314

Nemerson Y, Repke D 1985 Tissue factor accelerates the activation of coagulation factor VII: the role of a bifunctional coagulation cofactor. Thromb Res 40: 351–358

Neuenschwander P F, Morrissey J H 1992 Deletion of the membrane anchoring region of tissue factor abolishes autoactivation of factor VII but not cofactor function. J Biol Chem 267: 14477–14482

Novotny W F, Girard T J, Miletich J P et al 1989 Purification and characterization of the lipoprotein-associated coagulation inhibitor in human plasma. J Biol Chem 264: 18832–18837

Novotny W F, Brown S G, Miletich J P et al 1991 Plasma antigen levels of the lipoprotein-associated coagulation inhibitor in patient samples. Blood 78: 387–393

Olefsky J M, Crapo P, Reaven G M 1976 Postprandial plasma triglyceride and cholesterol responses to a low-fat meal. Am J Clin Nutr 29: 535–539

Oliver M F 1987 Dietary fat and coronary heart disease. Br Heart J 58: 423–428

Palareti G, Legnani C, Poggi M et al 1994 Prolonged very low calorie diet in obese subjects reduces factor VII and PAI but not fibrinogen levels. Fibrinolysis 8: 16–21

Papahadjopolous D, Hanahan D J 1964 Observations in the interaction of phospholipids and certain clotting factors in prothrombin activator formation. Biochim Biophys Acta 90: 436–439

Poggio M, Tripodi A, Mariani G et al 1991 Factor VII clotting assay: influence of different thromboplastins and factor VII-deficient plasmas. Thromb Haemost 65: 160–164

Radcliffe R, Bagdasarian A, Colman R W, Nemerson Y 1977 Activation of bovine factor VII by Hageman factor fragments. Blood 50: 611–617

Ruddock V, Meade T W 1994 Factor VII activity and ischaemic heart disease: fatal and non-fatal events. Q J Med 87: 403–406

Salomaa V, Rasi V, Pekkanen J et al 1993 The effects of saturated fat and n-6 polyunsaturated fat on postprandial lipemia and hemostatic activity. Atherosclerosis 103: 1–11

Sanders T A B, Vickers M, Haines A P 1981 Effects on blood lipids and haemostasis of a supplement of cod-liver oil rich in eicosapentaenoic and docosahexaenoic acids in healthy young men. Clin Sci 61: 317–324

Sanders T A B, Miller G J, de Grassi T et al 1996 Post-prandial activation of coagulant factor VII by long-chain dietary fatty acids. (in press)

Scandinavian Simvastatin Survival Study Group 1994 Randomised trial of cholesterol lowering in 4444 patients with coronary heart disease: the Scandinavian Simvastatin Survival Study (4S). Lancet 344: 1383–1389

Schwartz B S, Levy G A, Curtiss L K et al 1981 Plasma lipoprotein induction and suppression of the generation of cellular procoagulant activity in vitro. Two procoagulant activities are produced by peripheral blood mononuclear cells. J Clin Invest 67: 1650–1658

Seligsohn U, Osterud B, Rapaport S I 1978 Coupled amidolytic assay for factor VII: its use with a clotting assay to determine the activity state of factor VII. Blood 52: 978–988

Seligsohn U, Kasper C K, Osterud B et al 1979a Activated factor VII: presence in factor IX concentrates and persistence in the circulation after infusion. Blood 53: 828–837

Seligsohn U, Osterud B, Brown S F et al 1979b Activation of human factor VII in plasma and in purified systems. Roles of activated factor IX, kallikrein and activated factor XII. J Clin Invest 64: 1056–1065

Silveira A, Karpe F, Blomback M et al 1994 Activation of coagulation factor VII during alimentary lipemia. Arterioscler Thromb 14: 60–69

Simpson H C R, Mann J I, Meade T W et al 1983 Hypertriglyceridaemia and hypercoagulability. Lancet i: 786–790

Slabber M, Barnard H C, Kuyl J M et al 1992 Effect of a short-term very low calorie diet on plasma lipids, fibrinogen, and factor VII in obese subjects. Clin Biochem 25: 334–335

Stensvold I, Tverdal A, Urdal P et al 1993 Non-fasting serum triglyceride concentration and mortality from coronary heart disease and any cause in middle-aged Norwegian women. Br Med J 307: 1318–1322

Stirling Y, Woolf L, North W R S et al 1984 Haemostasis in normal pregnancy. Thromb Haemost 52: 176–182

Stuckey N W 1912 Ueber die Veranderungen der kaninchen Aorta bei der Futterung mit verschiedenen Fettsorten. Centralbl Allg Pathol 23: 910

Tankersley D L, Finlayson J S 1984 Kinetics of activation and autoactivation of human factor XII. Biochemistry 23: 273–279

Tholstrup T, Marckmann P, Jespersen J, Sandstrom B 1994 Fat high in stearic acid favorably affects blood lipids and factor VII coagulant activity in comparison with fats high in palmitic or high in myristic and lauric acids. Am J Clin Nutr 59: 371–377

Tremoli E, Elagini S, Colli S 1994 n-3 fatty acid ethyl ester administration to healthy subjects and to hypertriglyceridemic patients reduces tissue factor activity in adherent monocytes. Arterioscler Thromb 14: 1600–1608

Vaisanen S, Rankinen T, Penttila I, Rauramaa R 1995 Factor VII coagulant activity in relation to serum lipoproteins and dietary fat in middle-aged men. Thromb Haemost 73: 435–438

Van Amelsvoort J M M, van Stratum P, Kraal J H et al 1989 Effects of varying the carbohydrate: fat ratio in a hot lunch on postprandial variables in male volunteers. Br J Nutr 61: 267–283

Virchow R 1856 Endarteritis deformans und einfache Fettmetamorphose der Gefasswand. In: Gesammelte Abhandlungen zur wissenschaftlichen Medizin. von Meidinger, Sohn und Comp, Frankfurt-Main

Waxman E, Ross J B A, Lane T M et al 1992 Tissue factor and its extracellular soluble domain: the relationship between intermolecular association with factor VIIa and enzymatic activity of the complex. Biochemistry 31: 3998–4003

Weinhouse S, Hirsch E F 1940 Chemistry of atherosclerosis. Arch Pathol 29: 31–41

Wildgoose P, Nemerson Y, Hansen L L et al 1992 Measurement of basal levels of factor VIIa in haemophilia A and B patients. Blood 80: 25–28

Woolf N, Davies M J 1992 Interrelationship between atherosclerosis and thrombosis. In: Fuster V, Verstraete M (eds) Thrombosis in cardiovascular disorders. WB Saunders, Philadelphia

Wright D, Poller L, Thomson J M et al 1993 The inter-relationship of factor VII and its activity state with plasma lipids in healthy male adults. Br J Haematol 85: 348–351

Yamamoto M, Nakagaki T, Kisiel W 1992 Tissue factor-dependent autoactivation of human blood coagulation factor VII. J Biol Chem 267: 19089–19094

Yarnell J W G, Baker I A, Sweetnam P M et al 1991 Fibrinogen, viscosity, and white blood cell count are major risk factors for ischemic heart disease. The Caerphilly and Speedwell Collaborative Heart Disease Studies. Circulation 83: 836–844

9. Changing indications for warfarin therapy

C. Kearon   J. Hirsh

The anticoagulant effect of vitamin K antagonism was discovered in the 1930s when it was shown that hemorrhagic disease of cattle could be treated with vitamin K (Link 1959, Mueller & Scheidt 1994). Dicoumarol, a 4-hydroxy-coumarin compound formed in the spoilage process of sweet clover hay, was isolated as the responsible agent for this disease and became the first oral anticoagulant used in clinical practice. Warfarin (named after the Wisconsin Alumni Research Foundation and the terminal syllable of coumarin), which was initially developed as a rodenticide in the 1940s, subsequently became the oral anticoagulant of choice in Britain and North America because of its superior pharmacological profile, a position which it retains. However, based largely on the findings of randomized trials, the use of this familiar agent continues to be refined. Changes in the indications for long-term anticoagulants are continuously evolving, and the safety of warfarin therapy has been improved by the use of less intense levels of anticoagulation, which have been demonstrated to have similar antithrombotic efficacy but are associated with much less bleeding (Hull et al 1982b, Turpie et al 1988, Altman et al 1991). This development, coupled with recognition that low-dose aspirin therapy has equal antithrombotic efficacy but fewer bleeding complications than the higher doses of aspirin previously used (Hirsh et al 1992), has paved the way to combining these two medications in order to improve antithrombotic efficacy, particularly in the management of arterial thrombotic conditions.

In this chapter we will review current indications for oral anticoagulant therapy (Table 9.1), concentrating on changes that have occurred in the past decade, particularly with regard to the management of non-valvular atrial fibrillation (NVAF). We will also consider potential new therapeutic roles for warfarin that are currently under investigation.

The management of venous and arterial disease will be considered separately, and the results of randomized comparisons will be preferentially cited when considering specific indications for oral anticoagulants (Table 9.1). Although warfarin has not always been the oral anticoagulant evaluated in these studies – for example, nicoumalone, acenocoumarol and phenprocoumon are more commonly used in many parts of Europe – we will not distinguish between the different vitamin K antagonists; for the purposes of this review we will regard warfarin as synonymous with all types of coumarin anticoagulant.

ARTERIAL THROMBOSIS

Arterial indications for warfarin therapy can be divided into the prevention of (1) systemic embolism of cardiac origin and (2) myocardial ischaemia.

Prevention of systemic embolism

Until recently, the practice of anticoagulating patients to prevent systemic embolism was largely based on non-randomized comparisons (Levine et al 1992a, Stein et al 1992a), although a single randomized trial done in the early 1980s had demonstrated that warfarin was more effective than antiplatelet therapy at preventing thromboembolic complications in patients with mechanical heart valves (Mok et al 1985). Despite a lack of evidence from randomized trials to firmly establish the benefit of anticoagulation in patients with bioprosthetic heart valves, rheumatic mitral valve disease, or previous systemic embolism, it is widely accepted that anticoagulation is indicated in selected patients with these conditions (Levine et al 1992a, Stein et al 1992a).

Non-valvular atrial fibrillation (NVAF)

Six randomized controlled trials have established that oral anticoagulants prevent arterial embolism in patients with NVAF (Petersen et al 1989, Boston Area Anticoagulation Trial for Atrial Fibrillation Investigators 1990, Connolly et al 1991, Stroke Prevention in Atrial Fibrillation Investigators 1991, Ezekowitz et al 1992, European Atrial Fibrillation Trial Study Group 1993), overviews

Table 9.1   Indications for, and recommended intensity of, oral anticoagulation

Condition	Recommended INR
Prevention of central venous catheter thrombosis (warfarin 1 mg/day)	< 1.3
Prevention of VTE	2.0–3.0
Treatment of VTE	2.0–3.0
Atrial fibrillation	2.0–3.0
Systemic arterial embolism	2.0–3.0
Rheumatic mitral valve disease (right atrial diameter > 5.5 cm)	2.0–3.0
Prosthetic heart valves	
Bioprosthetic	
Uncomplicated (anticoagulate 3 months)	2.0–3.0
Complicated* (anticoagulate indefinitely)	2.0–3.0
Mechanical	2.5–3.5
Prevention of recurrent myocardial infarction	2.5–3.5

INR, international normalized ratio; VTE, venous thromboembolism.
*Atrial fibrillation, embolism.

demonstrating an approximately 65% risk reduction using intention-to-treat analyses (Atrial Fibrillation Investigators 1994, Barnett et al 1995). Given that the majority of patients in these trials who were randomized to receive warfarin and who had strokes were either markedly subtherapeutic (international normalized ratio (INR) <1.5) or had discontinued therapy when these events occurred (16/26 in the first five controlled trials) (Albers 1994, Atrial Fibrillation Investigators 1994), it is apparent that oral anticoagulation largely offsets the risk of thromboembolism associated with NVAF. Aspirin also reduces arterial embolism in patients with NVAF (Stroke Prevention in Atrial Fibrillation Investigators 1991, European Atrial Fibrillation Trial Study Group 1993), but is only associated with an approximately 22% risk reduction compared to controls (Barnett et al 1995). Oral anticoagulants, therefore, are much more effective than aspirin at preventing thromboembolic complications in association with NVAF, and have been shown to be associated with an additional 40% risk reduction in a meta-analysis (Barnett et al 1995) of trials which directly compared the two therapies (Petersen et al 1989, Stroke Prevention in Atrial Fibrillation Investigators 1991, European Atrial Fibrillation Trial Study Group 1993, Stroke Prevention in Atrial Fibrillation Investigators 1994). It is worthy of note that intermittent, as opposed to persistent, atrial fibrillation (Atrial Fibrillation Investigators 1994), gender (Atrial Fibrillation Investigators 1994) and duration of atrial fibrillation (European Atrial Fibrillation Trial Study Group 1993) have not been found to influence either the risk of thromboembolism or the response to anticoagulants. However, anticoagulation is associated with bleeding (Levine et al 1992b, Landefeld & Beyth 1993, Albers 1994, Atrial Fibrillation Investigators 1994), and this risk, coupled with the cost and inconvenience of therapy, has to be balanced against potential benefits in individual patients.

Because approximately 1500 control patients have been followed for a total of over 2000 patient-years in these randomized trials, it has been possible to identify clinical and echocardiographic risk factors for embolism in individual patients with NVAF. In the case of clinical risk factors, this process has been greatly facilitated by combining individual patient data from five of these trials (Petersen et al 1989, Boston Area Anticoagulation Trial for Atrial Fibrillation Investigators 1990, Stroke Prevention in Atrial Fibrillation Investigators 1991, Connolly et al 1991, Ezekowitz et al 1992) in a meta-analysis (Atrial Fibrillation Investigators 1994).

The presence of hypertension, diabetes mellitus, previous embolism and advancing age are independently associated with the risk of embolism in control patients (Atrial Fibrillation Investigators 1994) (Table 9.2). Although less convincingly demonstrated, there is also evidence that coronary artery disease (Petersen et al 1989, Boston Area Anticoagulation Trial for Atrial Fibrillation Investigators 1990, Ezekowitz et al 1992, Atrial Fibrillation Investigators 1994) and left ventricular dysfunction (Stroke Prevention in Atrial Fibrillation Investigators 1991, European Atrial Fibrillation Trial

Table 9.2   Risk of embolism in NVAF (control patients)

Patient characteristics			Risk of embolism	
Age (years)	Clinical risk factors	Echo risk factors	% per year	95% CI
Five trials				
<60	None*	N/S	0	0–2.3
60–69	None*	N/S	1.6	0.5–4.9
70–79	None*	N/S	2.1	0.8–5.9
≥ 80	None*	N/S	3.0	0.8–12.0
SPAF I				
N/S	None†	N/S	2.5	1.3–5.0
N/S	1†	N/S	7.2	4.8–10.8
N/S	≥2†	N/S	17.6	10.5–29.9
Five trials				
<65	≥1‡	N/S	4.9	3.0–8.1
65–75	≥1‡	N/S	5.7	3.9–8.3
>75	≥1‡	N/S	8.1	4.7–13.9
SPAF I	Clinical and/or echo			
N/S	1*		1.0	0.2–4.0
N/S	1–2*		6.0	4.1–8.8
N/S	≥3*		18.6	11.6–30.1
EAFT				
N/S	TIA/CVA	N/S	~13.2	~10.2–17.0

*Includes: previous stroke/TIA, history of hypertension or congestive heart failure, diabetes, angina, previous myocardial infarct.
†Includes: recent congestive heart failure, history of hypertension, previous arterial embolism.
‡Includes: previous stroke/TIA, history of hypertension, diabetes.
*Includes: recent congestive heart failure, history of hypertension, previous arterial embolism, global left ventricular dysfunction, enlarged left atrium.
95% CI, 95% confidence interval; N/S, not specified; TIA, transient ischemic attack; CVA, cerebrovascular accident; ~, approximated from the data reported.
Data sources: Five trials: Atrial Fibrillation Investigators 1994; SPAF I: Stroke Prevention in Atrial Fibrillation Investigators 1992a,b; EAFT: European Atrial Fibrillation Trial Study Group 1993.

Study Group 1993, Atrial Fibrillation Investigators 1994) are risk factors for embolism. In the absence of any risk factors, arterial embolism is exceedingly rare in patients with NVAF; no episode of arterial embolism occurred during follow-up in 112 control patients less than 60 years of age who had none of the previously noted risk factors (lone atrial fibrillation) (Atrial Fibrillation Investigators 1994) (Table 9.2). Conversely, the greater the number of risk factors, the greater the individual risk of systemic embolism. In the five-trial overview, the presence of one or more clinical risk factors increased the risk of thromboembolism in all age groups, ranging from 4.9% per year in patients younger than 65 years to 8.1% per year in those older than 75 years (Atrial Fibrillation Investigators 1994) (Table 9.2). This analysis did not further break down the risk of embolism according to different numbers of risk factors. This, however, was done in the SPAF I study which identified recent congestive heart failure, a history of hypertension and previous arterial embolism as clinical risk factors for thromboembolism in 568 patients assigned to placebo; the annual risk of embolism was 2.5% with none, 7.2% with one, and 17.6% with two or more of these factors (Stroke Prevention in Atrial Fibrillation Investigators 1991, 1992b) (Table 9.2).

SPAF I, which also evaluated the relationship of echocardiographic findings at randomization to thromboembolism, found that increased left atrial diameter and global left ventricular dysfunction were associated with subsequent embolism independently of clinical risk factors; the annual risk of embolism was 1.0% with none, 6.0% with one or two, and 18.6% with three or more of these combined clinical and echocardiographic risk factors (Stroke Prevention in Atrial Fibrillation Investigators 1992a) (Table 9.2). However, as has been shown with regard to the clinical prediction of embolism (Atrial Fibrillation Investigators 1994), individual studies tend to overestimate the strength of the association between specific risk factors and embolism, and consequently the strength of the association between echocardiographic features and subsequent embolism may be less than that reported in this single study. It should also be noted that, while the SPAF I study did not show an independent relationship between age and thromboembolism, and consequently did not include advanced age in the predictive model, there is convincing evidence that age is an independent risk factor for thromboembolism in patients with NVAF (Atrial Fibrillation Investigators 1994, Stroke Prevention in Atrial Fibrillation Investigators 1994) (Table 9.2). Unlike the first five randomized trials which included a minority (6%) of patients with previous embolism, the recently published EFAT study was confined to patients with atrial fibrillation and a previous transient ischemic attack or minor cerebral vascular accident (European Atrial Fibrillation Trial Study Group 1993). In keeping with the earlier observation that previous embolism is an independent risk factor for recurrence, the absolute rates of strokes in both control and anticoagulated arms were close to three times as high in this study than in earlier reports (e.g. 14% per year in controls, 4% per year in anticoagulated patients) (European Atrial Fibrillation Trial Study Group 1993).

Bleeding.   In the six randomized controlled trials of oral anticoagulants in patients with NVAF, the average rate of clinically important bleeding has been found to be low: approximately 1.6% per year in anticoagulated patients, compared to 0.8% per year in control patients (Atrial Fibrillation Investigators 1994, European Atrial Fibrillation Trial Study Group 1993) (Table 9.3). Of the 37 major bleeds which occurred in anticoagulated patients in these six trials, eight were fatal (four of these were intracranial) and there were two further non-fatal intracranial bleeds. As with the risk of embolism, the risk of bleeding is not the same for all patients. Previous randomized and non-randomized studies have established that the risk of bleeding on anticoagulants is influenced by anticoagulant (particularly the intensity of oral anticoagulation; Hull et al 1982b, Turpie et al 1988, Saour et al 1990, Altman et al 1991) and patient (advancing age, venous thromboembolism (VTE), cerebral vascular disease, concomitant antiplatelet therapy, peptic

Table 9.3   Risk of bleeding in NVAF

Therapy	Age (years)	Risk factors for embolism	Risk of bleeding	
			% per year	95% CI
Five trials				
No therapy	N/S	N/S	1.0	~0.6–1.6
Aspirin	N/S	N/S	1.0	~0.6–1.7
Warfarin (INR 1.5–4.5)	N/S	N/S	1.3	~0.8–2.0
EAFT				
No therapy	N/S	TIA/CVA	0.7	~0.2–1.5
Aspirin	N/S	TIA/CVA	0.9	~0.4–1.5
Warfarin (INR 2.5–4.0)	N/S	TIA/CVA	2.8	~1.6–4.7
SPAF II				
Aspirin	<75	N/S	0.9	~0.4–1.6
Warfarin (INR 2.0–4.5)	<75	N/S	1.7	~1.0–2.7
Aspirin	>75	N/S	1.6	~0.6–3.4
Warfarin (INR 2.0–4.5)	>75	N/S	4.2	~2.5–6.8

95% CI, 95% confidence interval; N/S, not specified; TIA, transient ischemic attack; CVA, cerebrovascular accident; ~, approximated from the data reported.
Data sources: Five trials: Atrial Fibrillation Investigators 1994; EAFT: European Atrial Fibrillation Trial Study Group 1993; SPAF II: Stroke Prevention in Atrial Fibrillation Investigators 1994.

ulcer disease, recent surgery or trauma; Levine et al 1992b, Landefeld & Beyth 1993) factors. Bleeding is also more likely to occur soon after anticoagulation is started (Landefeld & Beyth 1993). Evidence from randomized control trials performed in patients with NVAF support that bleeding, and more importantly intracranial hemorrhage, is associated with higher intensities of anticoagulation, and occurs more commonly in older patients (Albers 1994, Stroke Prevention in Atrial Fibrillation Investigators 1994). The combination of advanced age and higher intensity of anti-coagulation may be particularly dangerous (Albers 1994, Stroke Prevention in Atrial Fibrillation Investigators 1994). The SPAF II trial randomized patients, including a large proportion of older patients, to aspirin (325 mg/day) or warfarin (approximate target INR range 2.0–4.5). Although warfarin was more effective at preventing embolism (all ages, 1.9% versus 2.7%; <75 years, 1.3% versus 1.9%; ≥75 years 3.6% versus 4.8%), in patients over 75 years, stroke with residual deficit occurred as frequently with warfarin as it did with aspirin (4.6% and 4.3% per year, respectively), due to an increase in intracranial bleeding with the former (1.8% versus 0.8% per year) (Stroke Prevention in Atrial Fibrillation Investigators 1994).

Although less effective than warfarin, the risk of clinically important bleeding on low-dose aspirin (i.e. ≤325 mg/day, preferably enteric-coated) is minimally, if at all, increased compared to control patients in this population (European Atrial Fibrillation Trial Study Group 1993, Atrial Fibrillation Investigators 1994). SPAF II confirmed that advanced age, previous embolism, recent congestive cardiac failure and a history of hypertension were associated with an increased risk of thromboembolism, and a subgroup analysis suggested that the superior antithrombotic efficacy of warfarin was largely confined to patients (all ages) with these risk factors (Stroke Prevention in Atrial Fibrillation Investigators 1994).

A secondary analysis performed as part of the five-study overview suggested that the protective effect of aspirin may be greater in hypertensive patients (59% risk reduction for stroke) than for non-hypertensive patients (10% risk reduction) (Atrial Fibrillation Investigators 1994). This overview also suggested that higher blood pressure on study entry was a risk factor for intracranial bleeding, although this was not evident in SPAF II (Stroke Prevention in Atrial Fibrillation Investigators 1994). These interrelationships between hypertension, antithrombotic efficacy of aspirin and risk of intracranial bleeding may be chance observations, but, if confirmed, may support the preferential use of aspirin in patients with NVAF whose only risk factor is hypertension.

Because a large proportion of patients with NVAF were excluded from receiving anticoagulation in the above trials due to associated risk factors for bleeding, it is likely that the risk of anticoagulant-related bleeding in clinical practice will be higher than that reported above, unless the same patient selection criteria that were used in the trials are applied. However, a recent report suggests that the benefits of anticoagulation for patients with NVAF can be achieved in clinical practice without excessive bleeding (Gottlieb & Salem-Schatz 1994).

Recommendations.   Pending the findings of ongoing studies evaluating different intensities of anticoagulation, and combinations of oral anticoagulation and aspirin, we offer the following general guidelines for the selection of antithrombotic therapy in patients with NVAF. In the absence of contraindications, all patients with intermittent or persistent NVAF should be treated with aspirin (80–325 mg/day, preferably enteric-coated) or warfarin (INR 2.0–3.0). In patients less than 60 years without clinical or echocardiographic risk factors for embolism, oral anticoagulants are not justified. In patients more than 60 years of age without clinical or echocardiographic risk factors for embolism, it is not clear whether aspirin or warfarin are preferable; however, given that aspirin is easier to use and cheaper, we favor its selection in these patients. In patients of all ages with one or more clinical or echocardiographic risk factors for embolism, oral anticoagulants are indicated. In patients older than 75 years, a target INR of 1.5–2.5 may be preferable, in order to reduce the risk of intracranial hemorrhage associated with excessive anticoagulation (INR > 3.0).

In addition to considering a patient's individual risk of embolism, the decision to use aspirin or warfarin will be influenced by patient preference, individual risk of bleeding, accessibility to, and compliance with, laboratory monitoring, and stability of the INR response during long-term anticoagulation. If the individual risk of bleeding is very high (e.g. recurrent falls coupled with poor compliance), anticoagulation will not be feasible, even in patients with the highest risk of embolism. The possibility of converting the patient to sinus rhythm, thereby avoiding the need for long-term anticoagulation, should also be considered (Disch et al 1994).

Prosthetic heart valves

Patients with mechanical heart valves or bioprosthetic heart valve associated with a high risk of embolism (atrial fibrillation, previous embolism) should receive indefinite anticoagulation (Stein et al 1992a). Until recently, the recommended intensity of anticoagulation for patients with mechanical valves has been an INR of 3.0–4.5. However, on the basis of indirect evidence establishing that lower intensities of anticoagulation are effective and safer in patients with VTE (Hull et al 1982b) and prosthetic heart valves (Turpie et al 1988, Altman et al 1991), this recommendation has recently been modified to an INR of 2.5–3.5 (Stein et al 1992a). Current evidence suggests that these patients may also benefit from low-dose aspirin therapy (80–100 mg/day) (Stein et al 1992a, Turpie et al 1993) (see below). Anticoagulation with an INR of 2.0–3.0 is recommended for 3 months following insertion of a bioprosthetic heart valve, at which time, in the absence of risk factors for embolism, aspirin can be substituted.

Patients with severe left ventricular dysfunction or valvular heart disease (rheumatic or non-rheumatic) who have had a previous systemic embolus should receive anticoagulation (INR 2.0–3.0) for at least 3 months, and probably indefinitely (Clagett et al 1992b, Levine et al 1992a). Patients with rheumatic mitral stenosis who have an enlarged left atrium (diameter 5.5 cm) appear to be at a higher risk of systemic embolism, and current recommendations are that these patients should also be considered for indefinite anticoagulation (Levine et al 1992a). If anticoagulation is not undertaken in these groups of patients, aspirin should be considered. The arguments in favor of anticoagulating patients with rheumatic valvular disease or left ventricular dysfunction who do not have atrial fibrillation, have not had a previous episode of embolism, or do not have addition echocardiographic features known to be associated with systemic embolism (enlarged left atrium, mural thrombus) are not convincing (Tsevat et al 1989, Baker & Wright 1994). Following myocardial infarction, patients at high risk for arterial and/or venous embolism (large, generally anterior, myocardial infarcts; severe left ventricular dysfunction; prolonged immobility; mural thrombus) should be anticoagulated (INR 2.0–3.0) for approximately 3 months (Cairns et al 1992, 1994).

Prevention of myocardial ischaemia

The role of oral anticoagulants in the primary and secondary prevention of myocardial ischaemia is controversial due to a sparsity of evidence from randomized comparisons to guide these decisions. Aspirin has been shown to reduce clinical manifestations of myocardial ischaemia in diverse patient populations, achieving approximately a 21% risk reduction compared to placebo (Antiplatelet Trialists' Collaboration 1994). As low-dose aspirin is both cheap and safe, warfarin has to be shown to be superior to aspirin before it can be recommended as first-line therapy for primary or secondary prophylaxis of myocardial ischaemia. Warfarin (INR 1.5), with or without aspirin, is currently being evaluated for primary prophylaxis for coronary artery disease in high-risk men (Meade et al 1994, Meade & Miller 1995).

Secondary prevention of myocardial ischaemia

Post myocardial infarction.   A number of early randomized trials established that oral anticoagulants reduce the frequency of recurrent myocardial infarction and stroke (Chalmers et al 1977, Sixty Plus Reinfarction Study Research Group 1980, Smith et al 1990), findings which have recently been confirmed (Anticoagulants in the Secondary Prevention of Events in Coronary Thrombosis (ASPECT) Research Group 1994). However, these studies were performed before the widespread use of thrombolytic therapy and, more importantly, before long-term aspirin therapy was recommended following myocardial infarction. Few comparisons of aspirin and warfarin have been performed in postmyocardial infarction patients (Breddin et al 1980, EPSIM Research Group 1982, Meijer et al 1993), and patients were treated with thrombolytic therapy in only one of these studies (Meijer et al 1993). The results of these direct comparisons are inconclusive and it is therefore not clear whether aspirin or warfarin is superior in this setting, and, if warfarin is used for this purpose, what the optimal intensity of anticoagulation (INR) should be. Because the studies that have demonstrated that oral anticoagulants prevent recurrent myocardial infarction have used more intense anticoagulation (e.g. INR 2.8–4.5 in the ASPECT study), the Food and Drugs Administration 'of the USA has recently approved the use of warfarin, with an INR of 2.5–3.5, for this purpose. This position has been endorsed in the current antithrombotic recommendations of the American College of Chest Physicians (Cairns et al 1995).

Pending the results of further randomized comparisons of adequate size (such studies may also evaluate combinations of low-dose aspirin and warfarin; see below), current recommendations are that:

1. Aspirin should be given routinely for secondary prevention of coronary ischemia following myocardial infarction.
2. If aspirin is contraindicated, ticlopodine or warfarin (INR 2.5–3.5) should be substituted.
3. Warfarin should be administered for 3 months following myocardial infarction if the associated risk of venous or arterial embolism is high, in which case concomitant aspirin is not recommended unless

there are additional indications for its use (i.e. recurrent ischemia or systemic embolism despite adequate anticoagulation) (Cairns et al 1992, 1994); because oral anticoagulants are also responsible for prevention of recurrent myocardial infarction during this period, an INR of 2.5–3.5 is appropriate.

Other conditions.   Warfarin has not been adequately evaluated for the prevention of myocardial ischaemia in patients with stable or unstable angina; current recommendations are that aspirin is the antithrombotic agent of choice for patients with stable angina, and that aspirin in combination with heparin is used in patients with unstable angina (Cairns et al 1992, Hirsh & Fuster 1994a). Warfarin has not been found to be superior to aspirin at preserving graft patency following (1) coronary artery bypass surgery (Van der Meer et al 1993), or (2) peripheral artery reconstructions (Arfvidsson et al 1990, Clagett et al 1992b). Warfarin may be beneficial following complex peripheral artery reconstructions, or following thrombectomy of previous occluded peripheral arterial grafts, but this is also uncertain (Clagett et al 1992b). On the basis that mechanical heart valves are highly thrombogenic, that thrombosis is a common complication of intracoronary stenting, that heparin is believed to reduce thrombosis during coronary artery angioplasty (Stein et al 1992b) and that warfarin is an effective antithrombotic agent in other settings, warfarin – generally at a higher anticoagulant intensity (INR > 3.0) – is often used for 1–3 months following insertion of intracoronary stents. However, this practice has never been evaluated in randomized trials, and the need for routine anticoagulation of these patients has been questioned (Colombo et al 1995, Serruys & Di Mario 1995).

Combining aspirin and warfarin

Early studies found that combining aspirin (500–1000 mg/day) with warfarin (equivalent to an INR of approx. 3–5) resulted in increased bleeding and had an inconsistent effect on antithrombotic efficacy in patients with mechanical heart valves (Dale et al 1977, 1980, Chesebro et al 1983). As dipyridamole appeared to be at least as effective and less hemorrhagic in anticoagulated patients (Sullivan et al 1971, Chesebro et al 1983), the combination of aspirin and warfarin fell into disrepute. Subsequent demonstration that, similar to experience with lower intensities of oral anticoagulation, lowering the aspirin dose resulted in similar antithrombotic efficacy but reduced bleeding (Hirsh et al 1992), rekindled interest in combining aspirin and warfarin therapy. A recent randomized trial found that combining enteric-coated aspirin (100 mg/day) with warfarin (INR 3.0–4.5) resulted in a greater than 50% reduction in embolism and vascular deaths (including myocardial infarction) in patients with prosthetic heart valves (Turpie et al 1993). Consistent with previous reports, this study also found that the combination of aspirin and warfarin was associated with increased bleeding compared to warfarin alone, but most of these episodes were minor, and the magnitude of this effect was far outweighed by the benefits of therapy.

A further study randomized 214 patients with unstable angina or non-Q-wave myocardial infarction to aspirin (162.5 mg/day) or aspirin (same dose) plus anticoagulation (3–4 days of heparin followed by warfarin, INR 2.0–3.0) for 3 months (Cohen et al 1994). Combined therapy was associated with a statistically significant reduction in ischemic events at 14 days, but only a non-significant trend at 90 days. As the combination of aspirin and heparin appears to be superior to aspirin alone in the acute management of unstable coronary syndromes (Theroux et al 1988, The RISC Group 1990, Cohen et al 1994), it is not clear from this study whether combining warfarin with aspirin was of benefit; more ischemic events occurred between 2 and 14 weeks in patients on combined therapy than occurred in patients taking aspirin alone. Bleeding was also more frequent on combined therapy.

Preliminary safety data from the Thrombosis Prevention Trial, a placebo-controlled study evaluating aspirin alone (75 mg/day), warfarin alone (INR approx. 1.5), and aspirin and warfarin together, for the primary prevention of coronary artery disease in high-risk patients, indicates that, although this combination of aspirin and warfarin is associated with an increase of minor bleeding, the magnitude of this is very small (Meade et al 1994, Meade & Miller 1995). A pilot study evaluating the safety of combining 80 mg of aspirin with a fixed dose of warfarin (3 mg/day, reducing to 1 mg/day if the INR response is excessive) suggests that this approach may also be feasible, providing the INR is monitored in the initial stages to identify patients who require dose reduction or discontinuation of warfarin (Goodman et al 1994). A number of trials are in progress assessing different combinations of aspirin and warfarin (fixed and adjusted dose) for the primary and secondary prevention of myocardial ischaemia, and prevention of thromboembolic complications in patients with prosthetic heart valves, non-valvular atrial fibrillation, and following previous minor stroke or transient ischemic attack (Becker & Ansell 1995, Cairns & Markham 1995).

VENOUS THROMBOSIS

The efficacy of oral anticoagulants for the prevention and treatment of VTE has been established by a series of randomized controlled trials, many of which were performed in the late 1970s and early 1980s. Recent studies of oral anticoagulants in patients with acute VTE have focused on optimizing the intensity and duration of anticoagulation. In addition, recent studies have evaluated oral anticoagulants for the prophylaxis of VTE in populations other than postoperative and acute medical patients (e.g. metastatic breast cancer patients receiving chemotherapy, central venous catheters).

Prevention of VTE

The classic studies of Sevitt and Gallagher provided strong evidence that oral anticoagulants were effective at preventing DVT and pulmonary embolism in trauma and burn patients (Sevitt 1962). Subsequent randomized controlled trials have confirmed that oral anticoagulants, generally with an INR of 2.0–3.0, achieve a risk reduction of approximately 60% for DVT following orthopedic or major general surgery, when started either before surgery or on the first postoperative day (Clagett et al 1992a, Kearon & Hirsh 1995). The risk of clinically important bleeding with this relatively low-intensity regimen is small but, because warfarin prophylaxis is more complex than fixed low-dose heparin for patients at moderate risk of postoperative VTE and appears to be less effective than low-molecular-weight heparin for prophylaxis in very high-risk patients, its use is now generally confined to patients who have an additional indication for oral anticoagulation (e.g. atrial fibrillation) or who will require long-term prophylaxis (e.g. recurrent VTE, prolonged immobilization).

Very low-dose warfarin

A number of randomized controlled trials have established that very low-intensity anticoagulation (INR < 2.0) can prevent thromboembolic complications under a variety of circumstances. Warfarin 1 mg/day, started 2 weeks prior to surgery and continued postoperatively, reduced the incidence of leg scan detected DVT from 30% to 9% in patients undergoing gynecological surgery (Poller et al 1987). The prothrombin time was within the normal range at the time of surgery, and became prolonged by 2–4 s postoperatively. Similarly, warfarin 1 mg/day reduced central venous catheter thrombosis from 38% to 10% (Bern et al 1990). The prothrombin time generally remained within the normal range, although the occasional patient had an excessive anticoagulant response. Warfarin, initially 1 mg fixed dose daily adjusted after 6 weeks of treatment to an INR of 1.3–1.9, reduced VTE complication from 4.4% to 0.4% in women with metastatic breast cancer who were receiving combination chemotherapy (Levine et al 1994). In this study, warfarin was also estimated to reduce health-care costs by reducing the need to hospitalize and treat patients who developed symptomatic VTE (Rajan et al 1995). Very low-dose warfarin was not effective at preventing DVT following joint replacement (Dale et al 1991, Fordyce et al 1991).

Treatment of VTE

Three randomized trials provide evidence that oral anticoagulants are effective for the treatment of patients with acute VTE (Barritt & Jordan 1960, Hull et al 1979, Lagerstedt et al 1985). The first of these studies, by Barritt

& Jordan, established that a minimum of 14 days of the oral anticoagulant nicoumaolone (prothrombin time ratio 2.0–3.0), in combination with heparin, reduced symptomatic and fatal recurrent pulmonary embolism (Barritt & Jordan 1960). Subsequently, Hull and colleagues randomized patients with isolated calf or proximal DVT to either 5000 U of subcutaneous heparin every 12 h, or warfarin (INR 2.5–4.5), for 3 months, after an initial course of intravenous heparin (Hull et al 1979). Nine of the 19 patients (47%) with proximal DVT who were treated with subcutaneous heparin developed evidence of recurrence, whereas there were no recurrences in the 17 patients who were treated with warfarin – a highly significant difference. Regardless of treatment, none of the patients with isolated calf vein thrombosis (predominantly asymptomatic, postoperative clots detected by screening venography) experienced recurrence. In a subsequent study of patients with venographically confirmed symptomatic calf vein thrombosis who were randomly assigned to warfarin (INR 2.5–4.2) or placebo, with 5 days of initial heparin, none of the 23 warfarin patients experienced recurrence, whereas eight of the 28 (29%) control patients recurred during the first 3 months (one versus nine recurrences after 1 year) (Lagerstedt et al 1985).

The observation that bleeding was much more common in patients with DVT who were treated with warfarin (INR 2.5–4.5 approximately) compared to adjusted-dose heparin (Hull et al 1982a), and recognition that the intensity of therapeutic anticoagulation being used in North America in the late 1970s was higher than that used in Britain and parts of Europe (Hirsh et al 1989), led to a subsequent study designed to determine the optimal intensity of anticoagulation with warfarin for patients with VTE. Less intense anticoagulation (INR 2.0–2.5) was found to be as effective at preventing recurrent VTE as the traditional intensity of anticoagulation (INR 2.5–4.5), but was associated with a greatly reduced risk of bleeding (risk reduction of 81%) (Hull et al 1982b).

A number of small studies in the 1970s and 1980s evaluated the optimal duration of oral anticoagulant therapy for VTE, but their results were inconclusive (Hirsh & Fuster 1994b). Two recent larger studies have also addressed this question, comparing 4 weeks with 12 weeks of oral anticoagulation in patients with symptomatic VTE. The British Thoracic Society study randomized 712 patients with a clinical diagnosis of pulmonary embolism or DVT (confirmed by objective testing in 71%). Recurrence rate was higher in patients who were treated with anticoagulants for 4 weeks (7.8%) compared to those who were treated for 12 weeks (4.0%) (Research Committee of the British Thoracic Society 1992). Lack of blinding and infrequent use of objective tests to diagnose recurrent VTE undermines the conclusions which can be drawn from this study. A subsequent study randomized 220 patients with proximal DVT who had normal impedance plethysmography after 4 months of treatment to either 8 more weeks of warfarin or placebo (Levine et al 1995). In this double-blind study, recurrence was significantly less common during the 8 weeks on study medication in patients randomized to warfarin, but the difference in recurrence rates during the 11 months following randomization, a more clinically relevant period of follow-up, although less in patients treated with 3 months of therapy (11.2% versus 6.2%), was not statistically significant (Levine et al 1995). Subgroup analysis of these two studies strongly suggests that the risk of recurrence depends at least as much on patient characteristics as it does on the duration of anticoagulation. In both studies, the risk of recurrence was much higher if patients had continuing risk factors for thrombosis (including patients without any apparent risk factors, termed 'idiopathic') than if VTE occurred in association with a transient risk factor. Regardless of the duration of anticoagulation, of patients with a transient risk factor for thrombosis, only one of 116 patients in one study (Research Committee of the British Thoracic Society 1992), and two of 83 patients in the other (Levine et al 1995), developed recurrence during follow-up. These findings are supported by a prospective cohort study which found that 24% of patients with idiopathic DVT had a recurrence during 80 weeks of follow-up compared to 5% of patients with 'secondary' DVT, all patients receiving anticoagulation during the first 3 months (Prandoni et al 1992). Taken together these studies suggest that as little as 4 weeks of anticoagulation may be adequate for otherwise healthy patients with VTE whose risk factors for thrombosis resolve within that period. Conversely, patients with idiopathic VTE, or other continuing risk factors for thrombosis should be anticoagulated for a minimum of 3 months. Long-term anticoagulation should be considered for patients with active malignancy, recurrent thrombosis, or an hereditary hypercoagulable state, if VTE occurs without an additional transient risk factor.

PRIMARY PULMONARY HYPERTENSION

The role of thrombosis in primary pulmonary hypertension is controversial; thrombosis is commonly detected on lung biopsy, but its clinical significance is uncertain (Rubin 1993). Two non-randomized comparisons suggest that anticoagulation improves survival in patients with this condition (Fuster et al 1984, Rich et al 1992). However, non-randomized comparisons are likely to be biased in favor of anticoagulation. It is likely that some cases of pulmonary hypertension which were labelled as primary in early studies were due to major vessel chronic VTE, a condition which would benefit from long-term anticoagulation. It is also probable that the decision to use anticoagulants in these studies was influenced by the presence of clinical features suggestive of associated VTE, and that these patients may have a better prognosis, particularly when anticoagulated. Consistent with this, it was noted in one of the above studies that patients were more likely to have been treated with anticoagulants if they had patchy perfusion scans

(Rich et al 1992). Although supporting evidence is limited, indefinite anticoagulation is currently recommended by many authorities for patients with primary pulmonary hypertension (Rubin 1993, Rich 1994). A recently reported observation that patients with primary pulmonary hypertension may develop in situ thrombosis of major pulmonary arteries provides further anecdotal support for this practice (Moser et al 1995).

CONCLUSION

Randomized studies continue to refine the optimal use of, and indications for, warfarin therapy. Such studies also provide evidence that warfarin is both safe and cost-effective in a number of settings. Although the demands of oral anticoagulation are often considered onerous, this burden may have been overstated. In the case of atrial fibrillation, a recent study found that, in the absence of previous bleeding, long-term warfarin therapy did not decrease quality of life; the peace of mind associated with protection from thromboembolism at least compensated for the inconvenience of therapy (Lancaster et al 1991). Therefore, it appears likely that the number of patients on long-term warfarin will continue to expand.

KEY POINTS FOR CLINICAL PRACTICE

- The recommended intensity of anticoagulation corresponds to an INR of 2.0–3.0 for most indications.

- The risk of bleeding increases approximately threefold with an INR of 3.0–4.5, compared to an INR of 2.0–3.0.

- Warfarin is at least twice as effective as aspirin at preventing systemic embolism in patients with NVAF. However, warfarin is also associated with approximately twice as much bleeding as aspirin, and the relative risk:benefit ratio needs to be assessed in individual patients.

- Advanced age, diabetes, hypertension, previous embolism, impaired left ventricular function, and left atrial enlargement are risk factors for embolism in patients with NVAF. In general, anticoagulation is not indicated in patients less than 60 years old without risk factors, and is indicated in patients of all ages who have one or more risk factors. Embolic risk increases with the number of risk factors.

- Three months of warfarin is indicated for prevention of venous and arterial embolism in selected patients following myocardial infarction (e.g. anterior myocardial infarct, mural thrombus, left ventricular failure, previous embolism), during which time concomitant aspirin is not recommended.

- The addition of low-dose aspirin (80–100 mg/day) to warfarin (INR 2.5–3.5) is indicated in patients with mechanical heart valves, despite a small increase in associated bleeding. The antithrombotic efficacy and safety of different combinations of low-dose aspirin and warfarin are currently being evaluated in other patient populations.

- Very low-dose warfarin (INR <2.0) may provide effective prophylaxis in selected patients without established thrombosis (e.g. central venous catheters, metastatic breast cancer on chemotherapy, moderate risk surgery).

- Three months of warfarin is generally recommended following a first episode of VTE, provided there are no continuing risk factors for thrombosis. Four weeks may be adequate in otherwise healthy patients who develop VTE following surgery.

Note

Since preparation of this manuscript a large study has demonstrated that 6 months of anticoagulation is superior to 6 weeks of anticoagulation in patients with a first episode of VTE (Schulman et al 1995 N Engl J Med 332: 1661–1665). The report of the Fourth American College of Chest Physicians Consensus Conference on Antithrombotic Therapy has also been published (1995 Chest 108: 2255–5225).

REFERENCES

Anticoagulants in the Secondary Prevention of Events in Coronary Thrombosis (ASPECT) Research Group 1994 Effect of long-term oral anticoagulant treatment on mortality and cardiovascular morbidity after myocardial infarction. Lancet 343: 499–503

Albers G W 1994 Atrial fibrillation and stroke three new studies, three remaining questions. Arch Intern Med 154: 1443–1448

Altman P, Rouvier J, Gurfinkel E et al 1991 Comparison of two levels of anticoagulant therapy in patients with substitute heart valves. J Thorac Cardiovasc Surg 101: 427–431

Antiplatelet Trialists' Collaboration 1994 Collaborative overview of randomised trials of antiplatelet therapy-I: Prevention of death, myocardial infarction, and stroke by prolonged antiplatelet therapy in various categories of patients. Br Med J 308: 81–106

Arfvidsson B, Lundgren F, Drott C 1990 Influence of coumarin treatment on patency and limb salvage after peripheral arterial reconstructive surgery. Am J Surg 159: 556–560

Atrial Fibrillation Investigators 1994 Risk factors for stroke and efficacy of antithrombotic therapy in atrial fibrillation. Analysis of pooled data from five randomized trials. Arch Intern Med 154: 1449–1457

Baker D W, Wright R F 1994 Management of heart failure IV. Anticoagulation for patients with heart failure due to left ventricular systolic dysfunction. JAMA 272: 1614–1618

Barnett H J M, Eliasziw M, Meldrum H E 1995 Drugs and surgery in the prevention of ischemic stroke. N Engl J Med 332: 238–248

Barritt D W, Jordan S C 1960 Anticoagulant drugs in the treatment of pulmonary embolism: a controlled trial. Lancet i: 1309–1312

Becker R C, Ansell J 1995 Antithrombotic therapy, an abbreviated reference for clinicians. Arch Intern Med 155: 149–161

Bern M M, Lokich J J, Wallach S R et al 1990 Very low doses of warfarin can prevent thrombosis in central venous catheters. Ann Intern Med 112(6): 423–428

Boston Area Anticoagulation Trial for Atrial Fibrillation Investigators 1990 The effect of low-dose warfarin on the risk of stroke in patients with nonrheumatic atrial fibrillation. N Engl J Med 323(22): 1505–1511

Breddin K, Loew D, Lechner K et al 1980 The German–Austrian Aspirin Trial: A comparison of acetylsalicylic acid, placebo and phenprocoumon in secondary prevention of myocardial infarction. Circulation 62(suppl V): 63–72

Cairns J A, Markham B A 1995 Economics and efficacy in choosing oral anticoagulants or aspirin after myocardial infarction. JAMA 273: 965–967

Cairns J A, Hirsh J, Lewis H D Jr et al 1992 Antithrombotic agents in coronary artery disease. Chest 102: 456S–481S

Cairns J, Armstrong P, Belenkie I et al 1994 Canadian consensus conference on coronary thrombolysis – 1994 recommendations. Can J Cardiol 10: 522–529

Cairns J A, Lewis D, Meade T W, Sutton G C, Théroux P. 1995 Antithrombotic agents in coronary artery disease Chest 108: 3805–4005

Chalmers T C, Matta R J, Smith H Jr, Kunzler A 1977 Evidence favoring the use of anticoagulants in the hospital phase of acute myocardial infarction. N Engl J Med 297: 1091–1096

Chesebro J H, Fuster V, Elveback L R et al 1983 Trial of combined warfarin plus dipyridamole or aspirin therapy in prosthetic heart valve replacement: danger of aspirin compared with dipyridamole. Am J Cardiol 51: 1537–1541

Clagett G P, Anderson F A, Levine M N et al 1992a Prevention of venous thromboembolism. Chest 102: 391S–407S

Clagett G P, Graor R A, Salzman E W 1992b Antithrombotic therapy in peripheral arterial occlusive disease. Chest 102: 516S–528S

Cohen M, Adams P C, Parry G et al 1994 Combination antithrombotic therapy in unstable rest angina and non-Q-wave infarction in nonprior aspirin users. Primary end points analysis from the ATACS trial. Circulation 89: 81–88

Colombo A, Hall P, Nakamura S et al 1995 Intracoronary stenting without anticoagulation accomplished with intravascular ultrasound guidance. Circulation 91: 1676–1688

Connolly S J, Laupacis A, Gent M et al 1991 Canadian Atrial Fibrillation Anticoagulation (CAFA) Study. J Am Coll Cardiol 18: 349–355

Dale J, Myhre E, Storstein O et al 1977 Prevention of arterial thromboembolism with acetylsalicylic acid. Am Heart J 94: 101–111

Dale J, Myhre E, Loew D 1980 Bleeding during acetylsalicylic acid and anticoagulant therapy in patients with reduced platelet reactivity after aortic valve replacement. Am Heart J 99: 746–752

Dale C, Gallus A, Sycherley A et al 1991 Prevention of venous thrombosis with minidose warfarin after joint replacement. Br Med J 303: 224

Disch D L, Greenberg M L, Holzberger P T et al 1994 Managing chronic atrial fibrillation: a markov decision analysis comparing warfarin, quinidine, and low-dose amiodarone. Ann Intern Med 120: 449–457

EPSIM Research Group 1982 A controlled comparison of aspirin and oral anticoagulants in prevention of death after myocardial infarction. N Engl J Med 307: 701–708

European Atrial Fibrillation Trial Study Group 1993 Secondary prevention in non-rheumatic atrial fibrillation after transient ischaemic attack or minor stroke. Lancet 342: 1255–1262

Ezekowitz M D, Bridgers S L, James K E et al 1992 Warfarin in the prevention of stroke associated with nonrheumatic atrial fibrillation. N Engl J Med 327: 1406–1412

Fordyce M J F, Baker A S, Staddon G E 1991 Efficacy of fixed minidose warfarin prophylaxis in total hip replacement. Br Med J 303: 219–220

Fuster V, Steele P M, Edwards W D et al 1984 Primary pulmonary hypertension: natural history and the importance of thrombosis. Circulation 70(4): 580–587

Goodman S, Langer A, Durica S S et al 1994 Safety and anticoagulation effect of a low-dose combination of warfarin and aspirin in clinically stable coronary artery disease. Am J Cardiol 74: 657–661

Gottlieb L K, Salem-Schatz S 1994 Anticoagulation in atrial fibrillation. Does efficacy in clinical trials translate into effectiveness in practice? Arch Intern Med 154: 1945–1953

Hirsh J, Fuster V 1994a Guide to anticoagulant therapy. Part 1: Heparin. Circulation 89: 1449–1468

Hirsh J, Fuster V 1994b Guide to anticoagulant therapy. Part 2: Oral anticoagulants. Circulation 89: 1469–1480

Hirsh J, Poller L, Deykin D et al 1989 Optimal therapeutic range for oral anticoagulants. Chest 95 (suppl): 5S–11S

Hirsh J, Dalen J E, Fuster V et al 1992 Aspirin and other platelet-active drugs; the relationship between dose, effectiveness and side effects. Chest 102: S327–S336

Hull R D, Delmore T J, Genton E et al 1979 Warfarin sodium versus low dose heparin in the long-term treatment of venous thrombosis. N Engl J Med 301: 855–858

Hull R, Delmore T, Carter C et al 1982a Adjusted subcutaneous heparin versus warfarin sodium in the long-term treatment of venous thrombosis. N Engl J Med 306: 189–194

Hull R, Hirsh J, Jay R et al 1982b Different intensities of oral anticoagulant therapy in the treatment of proximal-vein thrombosis. N Engl J Med 307: 1676–1681

Kearon C, Hirsh J 1995 Starting prophylaxis for venous thromboembolism postoperatively. Arch Intern Med 155: 366–372

Lagerstedt C I, Olsson C G, Fagher B O et al 1985 Need for long-term anticoagulant treatment in symptomatic calf-vein thrombosis. Lancet ii: 515–518

Lancaster T R, Singer D E, Sheehan M A et al 1991 The impact of long-term warfarin therapy on quality of life. Arch Intern Med 151: 1944–1949

Landefeld C S, Beyth R J 1993 Anticoagulant-related bleeding: clinical epidemiology, prediction, and prevention. Am J Med 95: 315–328

Levine H J, Pauker S G, Salzman E W, Eckman M H 1992a Antithrombotic therapy in valvular heart disease. Chest 102: 434S–444S

Levine M N, Hirsh J, Landefelt S, Raskob G 1992b Hemorrhagic complications of anticoagulant therapy. Chest 102: 352S–363S

Levine M N, Hirsh J, Gent M et al 1995 Optimal duration of oral anticoagulant therapy: a randomized trial comparing four weeks with three months of warfarin in patients with proximal deep vein thrombosis. Thromb Haemost 74: 606–611

Levine M, Hirsh J, Gent M et al 1994 Double-blind randomised trial of very-low-dose warfarin for prevention of thromboembolism in stage IV breast cancer. Lancet 343: 886–889

Link K P 1959 The discovery of dicoumarol and its sequels. Circulation 19: 97–107

Meade T W, Miller G J 1995 Combined use of aspirin and warfarin in primary prevention of ischemic heart disease in men at high risk. Am J Cardiol 75: 23B–26B

Meade T W, Howarth D J, Brennan P J 1994 Effects of low intensity antithrombotic regimes on the haemoglobin level. Thromb Haemost 71: 284–285

Meijer A, Verheugt F W A, Werter C J P J et al 1993 Aspirin versus coumadin in the prevention of reocclusion and recurrent ischemia after successful thrombolysis: a prospective placebo-controlled angiographic study results of the APRICOT study. Circulation 87: 1524–1530

Mok C K, Boey J, Wang R et al 1985 Warfarin versus dipyridamole–aspirin and pentoxifylline–aspirin for the prevention of prosthetic heart valve thromboembolism: a prospective randomized clinical trial. Circulation 72: 1059–1063

Moser K M, Fedullo P F, Finkbeiner W E, Golden J 1995 Do patients with primary pulmonary hypertension develop extensive central thrombi? Circulation 91: 741–745

Mueller R L, Scheidt S 1994 History of drugs for thrombotic disease: discovery, development, and directions for the future. Circulation 89: 432–449

Petersen P, Godtfredsen J, Boysen G et al 1989 Placebo-controlled, randomised trial of warfarin and aspirin for prevention of thromboembolic complications in chronic atrial fibrillation; the Copenhagen AFASAK study. Lancet 8631: 175–179

Poller L, McKernan A, Thomson J M et al 1987 Fixed minidose warfarin: a new approach to prophylaxis against venous thrombosis after major surgery. Br Med J 295: 1309–1312

Prandoni P, Lensing A W A, Buller H R et al 1992 Deep-vein thrombosis and the incidence of subsequent symptomatic cancer. N Engl J Med 327: 1128–1133

Rajan R, Gafni A, Levine M et al 1995 Very low-dose warfarin prophylaxis to prevent thromboembolism in women with metastatic breast cancer receiving chemotherapy: an economic evaluation. J Clin Oncol 13: 42–46

Research Committee of the British Thoracic Society 1992 Optimum duration of anticoagulation for deep-vein thrombosis and pulmonary embolism. Lancet 340: 873–876

Rich S, Kaufmann E, Levy P S 1992 The effect of high doses of calcium-channel blockers on survival in primary pulmonary hypertension. N Engl J Med 327: 76–81

Rich S 1994 The medical treatment of primary pulmonary hypertension: proven and promising strategies. Chest 105(2): 17S–20S

Rubin L J 1993 Primary pulmonary hypertension. Chest 104: 236–250

Saour J N, Sieck J O, Mamo L A R, Gallus A S 1990 Trial of different intensities of anticoagulation in patients with prosthetic heart valves. N Engl J Med 322: 428–432

Serruys P W, Di Mario C 1995 Who was thrombogenic: the stent or the doctor? Circulation 91: 1891–1893

Sevitt S 1962 Venous thrombosis and pulmonary embolism: their prevention by oral anticoagulants. Am J Med 33: 703

Sixty Plus Reinfarction Study Research Group 1980 A double-blind trial to assess long-term oral anticoagulant therapy in elderly patients after myocardial infarction. Lancet ii: 989–994

Smith P, Arnesen H, Holme I 1990 The effect of warfarin on mortality and reinfarction after myocardial infarction. N Engl J Med 323: 147–151

Stein P D, Alpert J S, Copeland J et al 1992a Antithrombotic therapy in patients with mechanical and biological prosthetic heart valves. Chest 102: 445S–455S

Stein P D, Dalen J E, Goldman S et al 1992b Antithrombotic therapy in patients with saphenous vein and internal mammary artery bypass grafts following percutaneous transluminal coronary angioplasty. Chest 102: 508S–515S

Stroke Prevention in Atrial Fibrillation Investigators 1991 Stroke prevention in atrial fibrillation study. Final results. Circulation 84: 527–539

Stroke Prevention in Atrial Fibrillation Investigators 1992a Predictors of thromboembolism in atrial fibrillation: I. Clinical features of patients at risk. Ann Intern Med 116: 1–5

Stroke Prevention in Atrial Fibrillation Investigators 1992b Predictors of thromboembolism in atrial fibrillation: II. Echocardiographic features of patients at risk. Ann Intern Med 116: 6–12

Stroke Prevention in Atrial Fibrillation Investigators 1994 Warfarin versus aspirin for prevention of thromboembolism in atrial fibrillation: stroke prevention in atrial fibrillation II study. Lancet 343: 687–691

Sullivan J M, Harken D E, Gorlin R 1971 Pharmacologic control of thromboembolic complications of cardiac-valve replacement. N Engl J Med 284: 1391–1394

The RISC Group 1990 Risk of myocardial infarction and death during treatment with low dose aspirin and intravenous heparin in men with unstable coronary artery disease. Lancet 336: 827–830

Theroux P, Ouimet N, McCans J et al 1988 Aspirin, heparin or both to treat unstable angina. N Engl J Med 319: 1105–1111

Tsevat J, Eckman M H, McNutt R A, Pauker S G 1989 Warfarin for dilated cardiomyopathy: a bloody pill to swallow? Med Decis Making 9: 162–169

Turpie A G G, Gunstensen J, Hirsh J et al 1988 Randomised comparison of two intensities of oral anticoagulant therapy after tissue heart valve replacement. Lancet i: 1242–1245

Turpie A G G, Gent M, Laupacis A et al 1993 A comparison of aspirin with placebo in patients treated with warfarin after heart-valve replacement. N Engl J Med 329: 524–529

Van der Meer J, Hillege H L, Kootstra G J et al 1993 Prevention of one-year vein-graft occlusion after aortocoronary-bypass surgery: a comparison of low-dose aspirin, low-dose aspirin plus dipyridamole, and oral anticoagulants. Lancet 342: 257–264

10. Progress in clinical fibrinolysis

E. J. P. Brommer   J. J. Emeis   J. H. Verheijen
P. Brakman

Fibrinolysis seems to have attained a firm place in clinical medicine, and has transcended mere scientific curiosity. Equipment for routine fibrinolytic assays is no longer restricted to the clinical laboratory of academic hospitals only. As a consequence, important contributions to our knowledge are being made not only by renowned research institutes, but also by a growing number of non-academic hospitals. Furthermore, in this brief review of advances in clinical fibrinolysis over the last 2 years, quite a few publications could be included from countries that were formerly mere bystanders, or at most formed the rearguard. This survey omits progress reported in previous editions of this series, which the reader is recommended to consult (Brommer et al 1993).

FIBRIN(OGEN)

A remarkable observation regarding the breakdown of fibrin clots has been published by Beer et al (1994). The authors highlight the uniqueness of the individual, not because of his physionomy, cellular antigens or acquired antibody constitution, but because of the – presumably genetically determined – molecular specificity of his enzymes and their substrates. In a simple, elegant experiment, Beer and coworkers demonstrated that whole blood clots dissolve more easily in autologous plasma than in heterologous plasma. Although the differences were relatively small, the principle is of great importance in showing at least two things. First, not only does the big fibrin(ogen) molecule, with its large domains and its frequent, often 'silent', mutations, display individual variation, but also the enzyme(s) involved in fibrin breakdown – variations not noticed before, let alone identified, by the customary biochemical analyses. Second, lysis experiments which involve the use of a single (individual) source for enzyme or substrate may give erroneous results in the analysis of an individual patient sample.

Another new insight into the interpretation of laboratory results regarding fibrin metabolism has been presented by Nieuwenhuizen (1994). The parallel plasma disappearance curves of fibrinogen-related molecules of very different sizes, such as fibrinogen degradation products (FgDP) and fibrin degradation products (FbDP) such as D-dimers, have been difficult to explain. A new hypothesis, proposing the existence of circulating complexes composed of fibrinogen, fibrin and various partially degraded and/or crosslinked fibrin(ogen) molecules, explains the laboratory data. If FgDP and FbDP (and D-dimer) circulate in one and the same complex, they will be detected by any 'specific' antibody! The clinical implication of the model is that the inferences derived from different assays would still yield information on the relative rates of fibrin formation (inclusive crosslinking) and degradation, i.e. the haemostatic balance. A novel approach is the detection of small fragments of the Aα-chain of fibrinogen, using a monoclonal antibody. According to Sobel et al (1994), Aα-FDPs are very early markers of intravascular fibrinolysis, detectable within 15 min of the initiation of thrombolytic treatment.

PLASMIN

Plasmin is the main fibrinolytic enzyme active in the degradation of fibrin. Inside a thrombus, plasmin is generated from plasminogen by any plasminogen activator that is able to penetrate the thrombus structure. During thrombolysis, plasminogen binds to the outer layer of the thrombus, presumably to new epitopes exposed by plasmin-mediated proteolysis (Sakharov & Rijken 1994). Permeation, hence clot lysis, can moreover be furthered greatly by pressure (Wu et al 1994) and ultrasound (Francis et al 1992, Lauer et al 1992). Local application of ultrasound may – in combination with thrombolytic enzyme infusion – become a novel approach to thrombolytic therapy (see for example Kashyap et al 1994).

In the last few years, an unexpected property of the apparently well-known enzyme plasmin has been revealed. As a consequence, the old problem of the pathogenesis of hypotension following streptokinase infusion has been solved. Mashina & Bashkov (1994) discovered that plasmin could potently induce endothelium-dependent, nitric oxide mediated, vasodilatation. This suggests that plasmin formation during thrombolytic treatment might result in local vasodilatation, promoting restoration of blood flow through a partly occluded vessel. Another consequence could be hypotension, known to be associated with thrombolytic therapy. The vasorelaxing effect could be blocked by pretreatment with the synthetic fibrinolytic inhibitor ε-aminocaproic acid.

PLASMINOGEN ACTIVATORS

Since its first detection in the blood in the late 1970s, the occurrence of urokinase-type plasminogen activator (uPA) in plasma has for a long time received relatively little attention. Until recently, tissue-type plasminogen activator (tPA) was presumed to play the leading role in blood fibrinolysis, uPA being preferentially involved in tissue proteolysis. Views have changed, though, and uPA promises to become an important blood activator in the body's defence against thrombosis as well, and perhaps even against arteriosclerotic occlusion.

The sensitive and reliable detection methods, developed by Dooijewaard and coworkers, allowed the separate appraisal of the plasma levels of 'plasmin-activatable' single-chain uPA (scuPA, or pro-urokinase), active two-chain uPA (tcuPA, or urokinase), and total plasma uPA antigen (uPA:Ag), the latter including uPA circulating in complex with an inhibitor. The application of the methods to plasma samples of several groups of patients under a variety of circumstances has given insight in many clinical problems (see Brommer et al 1993). In addition to the data published earlier, we now found that, during the postovulatory period of the menstrual cycle, the plasma scuPA level is lower than during the preovulatory period, and also lower than the mean level in a mixed population including men (Dörr et al 1993). This finding seems relevant for the interpretation of individual scuPA levels, especially in women.

The commercial production of scuPA for thrombolysis has greatly favoured the apprehension of the potential efficacy of this zymogen, not yet activated to tcuPA. From its thrombolytic effect it has been inferred that self-activation of scuPA takes place at the fibrin surface. In vitro, the enzymatic properties of scuPA had been overlooked by most investigators, probably due to the chelation of metal ions, during the chelation of calcium. Zinc ions have now been shown to play an essential role in scuPA activation (Husain 1993). In our experience, scuPA is a potent thrombolytic agent, dissolving pathological human thrombi, in vitro, as fast or even faster than streptokinase, anisoylated plasminogen streptokinase activator complex (APSAC), tPA or tcuPA (Brommer & Van Bockel 1992). It has furthermore been demonstrated that scuPA is a powerful inhibitor of platelet aggregation (Romanova et al 1994). Thrombolytic treatment with scuPA, however, results in defibrination and α_2-antiplasmin consumption similar to other thrombolytic agents. Optimal use of this plasminogen activator requires another way of administration, presumably continuously and at a low rate (Dooijewaard 1993). Since scuPA is a naturally occurring, non-antigenic substance which is not immediately captured by inhibitors, it could be an ideal prophylactic anticoagulant. For this prophylactic application, a scuPA blood concentration of 1% of the usual thrombolytic blood level of, for instance, tPA should be sufficient. Low-dose scuPA infusion into volunteers does not cause detectable fibrinogen breakdown, as De Boer et al (1993a) have shown, though α_2-antiplasmin consumption indicated conversion of plasminogen to plasmin. Large-scale clinical investigations to demonstrate the efficacy of prophylactic administration of low-dose scuPA are underway.

Endogenous tPA is, in contrast to scuPA, neutralized in the blood by PAI-1 (plasminogen activator inhibitor 1). It will reach an effective concentration especially after it has been released in high concentrations during stressful conditions, such as physical, mental or emotional strain. In addition to receptors (for thrombin and bradykinin, for instance) described previously, muscarinic (Bashkov et al 1993, Jern et al 1994b) and adrenergic (Chandler et al 1992, 1995) receptors have been found to mediate acute release of tPA. tPA, whether released locally or presented systemically, can be regarded as a protector against fibrin formation within blood vessels. High concentrations might even prevent coagulation: by its incorporation into the clotting fibrin, tPA contributes to the due removal of intra- and extravascular fibrin deposits. This theoretical role is difficult to ascertain in vivo, clinically or experimentally. In this regard, the approach of Tromholt et al (1993), who injected radiolabelled anti-tPA antibodies into six patients, 1 day before resection of their aortic aneurysm, is of interest. The radiolabel accumulated in the wall of the aneurysm, indicating an active fibrinolytic process generating FbDPs and mimicking a 'lytic state'.

Conclusions about the patient's tendency to thrombosis by evaluation of the 'fibrinolytic capacity', as deduced from the baseline concentration of tPA (activity or antigen) only, are bound to be false. The value of stimulation tests (desmopressin infusion, exercise testing or venous occlusion) has still not yet been established (Emeis 1996), although it can function as a measure of the tPA-neutralizing capacity of plasma. The increase in the uPA concentration, along with tPA, during exercise suggests that the scuPA level also is subject to physiological adaptation. scuPA has a higher fibrin specificity than tcuPA, which is even enhanced by oxidative injury: oxidized fibrin stimulates the activation of scuPA more rapidly than non-oxidized fibrin, and also promotes the conversion of scuPA to active tcuPA by plasmin (Stief 1993).

α_2-Antiplasmin prevents the conversion of scuPA into tcuPA outside the clot. Exhaustion of α_2-antiplasmin during thrombolytic therapy will thus allow the systemic conversion of scuPA to tcuPA; in this way it causes loss of the fibrin specificity of scuPA (Declerk et al 1991).

A new, and exciting, approach towards elucidating the role of plasminogen activators in fibrinolysis was initiated by Carmeliet and coworkers (Carmeliet et al 1994, review by Carmeliet & Collen 1994), who created transgenic mice in which either the tPA gene, or the uPA gene, or both, had been functionally disrupted ('knock-out' mice). In the uPA-deficient mice, minor fibrin deposits were seen in the liver, skin and intestines. These mice developed no spontaneous thrombotic phenotype, but were more susceptible to endotoxin-induced venous thrombosis. Spontaneous lysis of plasma clots embolized to the lungs was normal in the uPA-deficient mice. In contrast, 'tPA knock-out' mice, that consequently do not have tPA circulating in their blood, lysed these pulmonary emboli at a significantly reduced rate, compared with control mice, and showed in general an increased thrombogenic tendency. In the 'double knock-out' mice (neither uPA nor tPA present), the abnormalities found were similar in kind, but much more severe, than in the 'single knock-out' animals (Carmeliet et al 1994). Although the interpretation in clinical terms of these data is still being discussed, 'knock-out' mice will probably in the future greatly contribute to our understanding of the physiological role of plasminogen activators.

INHIBITORS

There is ample evidence for the involvement, besides α_2-antiplasmin, of other plasma protease inhibitors in the inhibition of plasmin. However, the relevance of this for clinical management of a patient with intravascular coagulation and fibrinogenolysis, or for the control of thrombolytic therapy, is not clear. Levi et al (1993) tried to address this topic by measuring, in various disease states, circulating complexes of plasmin with a variety of potential plasmin inhibitors. They concluded that antitrypsin and C_1-inhibitor were involved in disseminated intravascular coagulation, whereas α_2-macroglobulin and antithrombin neutralized plasmin during thrombolytic therapy, apart from α_2-antiplasmin. In septic disease α_2-macroglobulin formed complexes with thrombin, elastase and cathepsin-G, and also with plasmin (De Boer et al 1993b).

Histidine-rich glycoprotein (HRG) has been considered as an inhibitor of the plasminogen–plasmin system, elevated levels being sometimes present in thrombophilia. A congenital HRG deficiency was, however, detected in a patient with sinus thrombosis during contraceptive pill usage (Shigekiyo et al 1993). The association of elevated HRG levels and thrombosis remains unclear, as recently discussed in detail by Hennis (1995).

An induction of high PAI-1 levels by the infusion of angiotensin II has been observed by Ridker et al (1993a). Is this an allusion to a link between the renin–angiotensin system in hypertension and thrombotic risk? It is not yet clear whether the decrease in tPA antigen and of PAI-1 activity (the decrease of the former presumably being a consequence of the decrease of the latter) after the administration of angiotensin converting enzyme (ACE) inhibitors (Wright et al 1994) should be regarded from the same point of view. Whatever the mechanism, the possibility of reducing thrombotic complications (e.g. after myocardial infarction) by the administration of ACE inhibitors is intriguing.

The belief in the thrombogenic effect of high PAI-1 activity levels has been strengthened by the results of a study performed by Rosenfeld et al (1993). This group set up a clinical trial to compare the effects of either general anaesthesia, or regional (epidural) anaesthesia, on the development of postoperative arterial thrombosis. Two otherwise comparable groups of patients who underwent lower extremity vascular surgery were studied. Rosenfeld et al measured, at 24 h postoperatively, an increase in PAI activity level only in the general anaesthesia group, and not in the epidural anaesthesia group. Of those patients in whom thrombosis developed, the majority had received general anaesthesia (77%). This outcome may persuade others to change their mind on the risk/benefit ratio of regional anaesthesia (Gelman 1993). For those interested in the mechanism of thrombosis, it points to a (causal ?) relationship between high inhibitor levels and arterial thrombosis. Of note too was the description, by Lang et al (1994), of high PAI-1 levels in chronic pulmonary thromboemboli.

GENETIC ASPECTS OF FIBRINOLYSIS

During the last few years, various papers have appeared describing the effect of genetic factors in fibrinolysis (see also Green & Humphries 1994). As regards tPA, only one paper has appeared thus far, describing a poly-morphism in a non-coding sequence of the tPA gene (Ludwig et al 1992). No functional correlate of this polymorphism has yet been reported.

In the PAI-1 gene, three polymorphisms have been found: a *HindIII* re-striction fragment length polymorphism downstream of the 3'-end of the gene (Klinger et al 1987, Dawson et al 1991), a $(CA)_n$ dinucleotide repeat polymorphism in the intron between exons 3 and 4 (Dawson et al 1991), and a 4G/5G polymorphism in the promotor region (Dawson et al 1993). All three polymorphisms are of great practical interest, because they influ-ence plasma PAI-1 levels. The *HindIII* allele 1 was associated with higher PAI-1 levels, as were the shorter alleles of the dinucleotide repeat poly-morphism (Dawson et al 1991). Interestingly, the genotype also determined the correlation with serum triglycerides: PAI-1 levels increased at a greater rate with increasing very low-density lipoprotein in the *HindIII* 1/1 geno-type than in the 1/2 or 2/2 genotype (Dawson et al 1991). A similar effect was seen for the 4G/5G polymorphism in non-insulin-dependent diabetes mellitus (NIDDM) patients: only in patients carrying the 4G/4G genotype did PAI-1 levels correlate with triglycerides (Panahloo et al 1995). In a cultured hepatic cell line, the 4G allele proved much more responsive to interleukin-1 (IL-1) than the 5G allele, resulting in a 5-fold greater in-crease in PAI-1 mRNA levels after IL-1 stimulation (Dawson et al 1993).

Allelic frequencies for the *HindIII* polymorphism and for the dinucleotide repeat polymorphism did not differ between type 1 or type 2 diabetics and controls (Mansfield et al 1994, Panahloo et al 1995).

The greater prevalence of the 4G allele in patients with myocardial infarction before the age of 45 years, associated with a higher plasma PAI-1 level (Eriksson et al 1995), is highly interesting. This finding pro-vides the first direct evidence of an independent, etiological role of PAI-1 in coronary heart disease.

Various mutations resulting in a complete (functional) absence of PAI-1 have been described, as recently reviewed in detail by Fearns et al (1995).

FIBRINOLYSIS AND PLATELETS

The influence of platelets on thrombolysis remains enigmatic. Unfortu-nately, most 'thrombolysis' experiments are performed with artificial clots, loosely called 'thrombi'. Theoretically, large numbers of platelets within a thrombus would hamper thrombolysis since platelets contain a rather high concentration of PAI-1, though this PAI-1 is largely inactive. The report of Fay et al (1994), describing the lysis of clots prepared from platelet-rich plasma of a patient completely lacking PAI-1 expression, suggests that inhibitory mechanisms other than PAI-1 may be present in platelets as well. Still, human arterial thrombi with a layered structure (indicating a large platelet component), even pathological ones, lysed with an amazing speed in all the thrombolytic agents tested, including tPA (Brommer & Van Bockel 1992).

Serizawa et al (1993) showed that at least a certain amount of platelet PAI-1 is activated during platelet aggregation and effectively inhibits fibrinolysis. Bremer (1994) measured a significant decrease in PAI-1 activity during low-dose aspirin prophylaxis for toxaemia in pregnancy. He suggests that the reduction in PAI-1 activity is the consequence of an aspirin-induced reduction in platelet activation. Although this observation is in agreement with the work of Serizawa et al (1993), changes in PAI activity under the influence of aspirin have not been found by others in non-pregnant subjects. The problem would be solved if pregnancy brings about changes in platelet behaviour, but this has not yet been demonstrated.

The efficacy of aprotinin in reducing blood loss during cardiopulmonary bypass surgery (CPB) has been attributed by some authors to its action on platelets. A recent report challenges this idea. Orchard et al (1993) concluded from platelet aggregometry, and determinations of platelet counts, β-thromboglobulin, glycocalicin and D-dimer levels during CPB, that the reduction in blood loss correlated with inhibition of plasmin-mediated fibrinolysis, but was independent of platelet integrity or platelet function. The increase in fibrinolytic activity during CPB has been shown to be factor XII dependent (Chung et al 1994).

Platelets display an affinity for scuPA, and presumably incorporate it, thus prolonging its half-life in the circulation, and enhancing the therapeutic efficacy of scuPA (Gurewich et al 1993). It is not known whether this platelet-conveyed scuPA also affects other processes, such as platelet adhesion and aggregation, which both involve fibrinogen-mediated platelet bridging. We have already mentioned that scuPA is a powerful inhibitor of platelet aggregation (Romanova et al 1994). Platelet-bound prekallikrein seems to promote fibrinolysis induced by scuPA as well (Loza et al 1994).

BIOLOGICAL REGULATION OF FIBRINOLYSIS

Interest in the exact mechanism of the release of plasminogen activators under the influence of physiological or artificial stimuli remains vivid. Notwithstanding excellent work in the past, new discoveries on old themes have come to light. Bashkov et al (1993) demonstrated the release of tPA in anaesthetized cats upon the electric stimulation of a transected isolated sympathetic nerve chain, in spite of α-adrenergic blockade. Both vasorelaxation and release of tPA, stimulated by electric impulses or by intra-arterial infusion of acetylcholine, were blocked by atropine. The authors propose the presence of a neurogenic pathway to vascular muscarinic cholinergic receptors. Recently, muscarine-type cholinergic receptor-mediated release of tPA has been confirmed in human subjects. Jern et al (1994b) infused metacholine for 5 min into a forearm artery of healthy men and found a more than 10-fold increase in net tPA antigen release, and a 25-fold increase in net tPA activity release, over the forearm vascular bed. Sodium nitroprusside infusion caused vasodilatation, but had little influence on tPA release. This latter observation negates hypotheses about a direct relation between vasorelaxation and acute tPA release. No PAI-1 antigen release was observed in the studies of Jern et al (1994a,b). The discussion about the role of α- versus β-adrenergic activation in tPA release gained new impetus by the demonstration (Chandler et al 1995) that tPA release from endothelial cells was β-adrenergically mediated. The effect of α-adrenergic activation was to increase plasma tPA levels by decreasing liver blood flow, and hence to decrease the clearance of tPA by the liver.

Lifestyle

If, by modifying our lifestyle – including eating habits, physical training, smoking, drinking alcoholic beverages, etc. – we could modify either the constitutive production of plasminogen activators, or the potential to release tPA and scuPA, or else the baseline level of PAI-1, we could possibly enhance our protection against thrombosis and arterial occlusive disease without having recourse to drugs. The last years have seen an upsurge of interest in the investigation of the effects of lifestyle factors on fibrinolysis. Unfortunately, only a few investigators have included the measurement of scuPA levels in their studies. Conclusions, therefore, have to be provisional.

An optimistic indication as to the protective effect of moderate alcohol consumption at dinner was given by the study of Hendriks et al (1994): although tPA and PAI-1 levels increase a few hours after the consumption of alcohol (Veenstra et al 1993), in the early morning hours of the day after – the peak hours of myocardial infarction – PA activity was higher than in controls. Also, Ridker et al (1994) and Lee et al (1995) found a positive correlation between self-reported alcohol consumption and plasma tPA antigen levels. However, neither tPA nor PAI-1 activity was measured in these studies.

A diet rich in fish-oil did not affect fibrinolytic parameters in the study of Hellsten et al (1993). Dietary supplementation with ω3-polyunsaturated fatty acids (MaxEPA) reduced triglycerides, but increased PAI-1, as had been reported before, in healthy young men (Fumeron et al 1991), in NIDDM patients (Boberg et al 1992), and in moderately hyper-triglyceridemic patients undergoing coronary artery bypass (Eritsland et al

1994). The fish-oil effect on PAI-1 was not obliterated by co-administration of pyridixine and folic acid (Haglund et al 1993). Others found an increase in plasma PAI activity the morning after a high dose of ω3-polyunsaturated fatty acids given as a supplement to the evening meal (Møller et al 1992).

A low-fat, high-fibre diet increased fibrinolytic parameters (Marckmann et al 1992, 1993, 1994, review in Marckman & Jespersen 1994), as did high-fibre diets (Sundell & Rånby 1993, Guzic et al 1994). Drastic measures, such as jejunoileal bypass surgery for morbid obesity also have an effect: the mean PAI activity and tPA antigen concentrations were, 14–20 years after surgery, lower in operated subjects compared to non-operated obese controls (Sylvan et al 1992). Weight loss also proved effective in decreasing PAI-1 in moderately overweight adults (Folsom et al 1993), though tPA antigen also decreased to some extent.

Exercise

The association between physical exertion and myocardial infarction was observed as early as 1910, and has been repeatedly confirmed (Willich et al 1993). Whereas clotting activity and fibrinolytic activity increase concomitantly during exercise, partly through a decrease in PAI activity (de Geus et al 1992), factor VIII levels and APTT (activated partial thromboplastin time) remain elevated in the recovery phase, while fibrinolytic activity rapidly diminishes (Van den Burg 1994). A hypercoagulable state after physical exertion, unbalanced by hyperfibrinolysis, may confront untrained people with a short-lasting elevation of the risk of thrombosis. Van den Burg et al (1994) followed haemostatic parameters after exercise testing, before and after 6 and 12 weeks of physical training. During the training period a gradual rise in both coagulation and fibrinolysis response to exercise testing was observed, but the haemostatic balance did not change. However, after the training period the hypercoagulable state was enhanced during recovery from submaximal exercise. In a later paper the same investigators described a gradual increase in peak scuPA levels during exercise testing after the training period (Huisveld et al 1994). The conclusion is that regular physical training should be beneficial: firstly, because it elevates the threshold of submaximal exercise: the same physical work can be performed with less exertion, without risking a hypercoagulable state; secondly, because of the rise of the postexercise scuPA level, which might have a prophylactic effect. Interestingly, mechanisms regulating postexercise increases in tPA and uPA seem to be different (Van den Burg et al 1994).

A favourable reduction of coagulation, and an increase in fibrinolytic potential, were reported by Suzuki et al (1992) during physical training after myocardial infarction. Long-term, heavy excercise improved the fibrinolytic risk factor profile in the study of Boman et al (1994).

INFLAMMATION

The role of fibrinolytic enzymes in inflammation is beyond doubt. Nevertheless, the subject has received relatively little attention. The inflammatory mediator tumour necrosis factor-α (TNF-α) has been shown to induce increased levels of tPA and uPA. TNF-α also plays a pivotal role in the mediation of fibrinolytic activation during the acute inflammatory response to endotoxin exposure in primates: anti-TNF antibodies largely suppressed fibrinolysis in chimpanzees, but left coagulation undisturbed (Van der Poll et al 1994b). In contrast, IL-6 neutralizing antibodies did not affect fibrinolysis, but fully inhibited coagulation activation (Van der Poll et al 1994a). In a similar study, this group demonstrated that the activation of coagulation was mediated through the extrinsic, tissue factor dependent pathway, while the concomitant fibrinolytic response to endotoxin was independent of the generation of thrombin (Levi et al 1994, Biemond et al 1995).

The low fibrinolytic activity, and the poor response to stimulation by desmopressin, in children with haemolytic uraemic syndrome were attributed by Menzel et al (1994) to high plasma levels of PAI-1. We discovered, however, a high percentage of poor responders among patients with glomerulonephritis with regard to tPA antigen, uPA antigen and von Willebrand factor antigen, totally unrelated to PAI-1 levels (Brommer et al 1993). In both reports a gradual normalization of responses was described during follow-up of the patients, the uPA response lagging behind in Menzel's patients.

The similarity of tumour infiltration to invasive growth of inflammatory tissue has led to the investigation of fibrinolytic enzymes and inhibitors in synovial tissue of rheumatic joints. Plasmin formation (Kummer et al 1992), possibly uPA-mediated (Brommer et al 1992, Saxne et al 1993) was found in synovial fluid. Recent (our unpublished) studies confirmed that invading cells used plasminogen activators for the degradation of extracellular matrix components. A closer investigation of the role of the plasminogen/plasmin system in joint destruction in rheumatoid arthritis looks promising.

INSULIN RESISTANCE, DIABETES MELLITUS, AND FIBRINOLYTIC IMPAIRMENT

Elevated PAI-1 levels are now regarded as part of the insulin resistance syndrome (Syndrome X) (Juhan-Vague et al 1993b, Reaven 1994). The mechanisms involved are still being debated, though, and the factor(s) responsible (insulin, insulin precursors, insulin resistance) have not yet been identified. PAI-1 synthesis by a cultured liver cell line is enhanced by insulin precursors (Nordt et al 1994), as is synthesis in endothelial cells (Schneider et al 1992). An enhancing effect of insulin itself has been re-

ported for liver cells, but not for endothelial cells. Glucose increased
PAI-1 in arterial endothelial cell cultures (Nordt et al 1993). In survivors
of myocardial infarction, Gray et al (1995) found a good correlation, in
multiple regression analysis, between proinsulin, des-31,32-proinsulin, and
triglyceride levels on the one hand, and the PAI-1 level on the other. Jain
et al (1993) described a decrease in PAI activity during insulin treatment,
in close correlation with the concentration of intact proinsulin, but not with
split products or C-peptide. Nagi & Yudkin (1993) reported that metformin
concomitantly decreased insulin resistance and PAI-1, without any changes
in insulin itself. During an oral glucose load, PAI-1 levels decreased with
a concomitant increase in tPA activity (Seljeflot et al 1994).

According to Gough et al (1993), elevated PAI-1 levels in NIDDM are
not the result of obesity or coexistent arteriosclerosis. However, peripheral
arteriosclerosis is associated with increased PAI-1 levels (Cortellaro et al
1994), possibly due to endothelial damage by smoking as well (Smith et al
1993). An elevated PAI-1 level appeared to be an independent characteristic of intermittent claudication (Johansson et al 1993). In young adults
with early-onset arteriosclerosis, Oudenhoven et al (1994) found a significant difference in PAI-1 and triglyceride levels between smokers and
non-smokers, suggesting a causal relationship between some parameters
commonly associated with hyperinsulinism and smoking. A positive correlation of PAI-1 levels with insulin and C-peptide levels was confirmed by
their study.

What is most interesting is the recent study by Panahloo et al (1995),
who demonstrated in NIDDM patients a much stronger correlation between triglycerides and PAI-1 in patients with the PAI-1 genotype 4G/4G
(compare the section on genetic aspects of fibrinolysis), than in patients
with the PAI-1 genotypes 4G/5G or 5G/5G. Upon multiple regression
analysis, insulin sensitivity and the interaction between the PAI-1 G4/5
genotype and triglyceride proved the strongest determinants of PAI-1 activity. This would be in agreement with Potter van Loon et al (1993), who
also concluded that insulin resistance was a major determinant. Mykkänem
et al (1994) found, however, no independent effect of insulin sensitivity on
plasma PAI-1 activity. In patients with hypertension and obesity, also an
unfavourable combination, Urano et al (1993) found high PAI-1 levels,
especially in the case of habitual alcohol drinking or smoking.

Wieczorek et al (1993) confirmed in a detailed study that insulin-
dependent diabetics have an increased baseline fibrinolytic activity, but
that the response to stimulation (venous occlusion, or insulin-induced
hypoglycaemia) is reduced.

The negative correlation between plasma testosterone levels and PAI-1
levels, previously reported by Caron et al (1989), was confirmed by Glueck
et al (1993). Johansson et al (1994) found increased PAI-1 levels in growth
hormone deficient adults.

CANCER

The role of fibrinolytic enzymes in cancer has been studied extensively. These enzymes are thought to be involved in proteolytic degradation of the extracellular matrix, one of the steps involved in invasion and metastasis. The list of cancer types with increased levels of urokinase grows steadily. Recently such observations have been reported for cancer of the oesophagus, stomach, endometrium, brain, prostate and for skin and eye melanoma (Achbarou et al 1994, Delbaldo et al 1994, deVries et al 1994, 1995, Gleeson et al 1993a,b, Landau et al 1994, Rao et al 1993, Sier et al 1993, Yamamoto et al 1994a,b). The remarkable finding of a concomitant increase of both urokinase and its inhibitor PAI-1, originally observed in colon and breast tumours, appears to be a general phenomenon, since it has also been found in endometrium, brain and melanoma (DeVries 1994, Gleeson et al 1993a,b, Landau et al 1994, Yamamoto et al 1994b). PAI-1 is believed to act as a regulator of the local proteolytic activity in the vicinity of the tumour cells.

In addition to an increase of urokinase and PAI-1, in a number of cancers an increased level of urokinase receptor (uPAR) also was shown (Bianchi et al 1994, DeVries et al 1994, Yamamoto et al 1994c). More interestingly, the levels of uPA appear to increase with the tumour progression, as has been found for cancers of the prostate and colon and in melanoma. (Achbarou et al 1994, De Vries et al 1994, Mulcahy et al 1994). At least in some cases a similar increase with progression has been discovered for PAI-1 (De Vries et al 1994). Very high levels of this inhibitor have been found in liver metastases originating from colon tumours. This suggests a direct involvement in the process of metastasis formation (Sier et al 1994). In colon and melanoma the urokinase receptor too increases in more advanced stages of cancer (Bianchi et al 1994, De Vries et al 1994).

A very important new development is the use of fibrinolytic components as prognostic factors for tumour relapse and survival. It has now been established by several studies that urokinase and, in some cases also PAI-1, is a strong independent prognostic marker in breast cancer (Bouchet et al 1994, Duffy et al 1994, Foekens et al 1992, 1994, Grøndahl-Hansen et al 1993, Jänicke et al 1993). It has become clear that this is not limited to breast cancer but might be a more general phenomenon, since it has been described for cancer of the stomach, colon, bladder, lung and cervix (Ganesh et al 1994b, Hasui et al 1994, Kobayashi et al 1994, Nekarda et al 1994a,b, Mulcahy et al 1994, Pedersen et al 1994a,b).

In a few cases also the other plasminogen activator inhibitor PAI-2 appears to be of prognostic significance (Bouchet et al 1994, Ganesh et al 1994a). The use of fibrinolytic components for prognostic purposes might be of great importance for the adaptation of therapy to the relative risk for each individual patient. The strong correlation between a more active local proteolysis on the one hand, and tumour progression and survival of patients on the other, moreover suggests a causal relationship between urokinase-mediated pericellular proteolysis and the invasive and metastatic behaviour of tumour cells, which might lead to novel therapeutic possibilities. Especially interference with the binding of urokinase to its receptor is a new target for therapeutic intervention, since *in vitro* experiments in this direction show very promising results (Weidle et al 1994).

RENAL DISEASE

The relationship between disturbances of fibrinolysis and renal disease is not firmly established. Nevertheless, quite a few observations even point to the possibility of a causal relationship. On the other hand, disturbance of the normal anatomy or function of the kidney may have repercussions for fibrinolytic parameters in blood and urine. We have found that the release of tPA or uPA into the blood in response to desmopressin is impaired in about 50% of patients with glomerulonephritis (Brommer et al 1993). We have not seen any other group of patients with a similar high percentage of poor responders.

Urokinase – the name was coined after the biological fluid in which it was first detected – is not only secreted by the kidney into the urine, but also into the blood (Hong & Yang 1993). Brown et al (1994) localized the synthesis of urokinase to glomerular epithelial cells. No synthesis was detected in the mesangial cells.

It has been suggested that elevated tPA levels in urine may lead to the diagnosis of renal disease (Heussen-Schemmer et al 1993). The relevance of this finding has not yet been established, but the assay is simple, and does not impose a burden upon the patient. Urinary levels of fibrinopeptide A and FDP appear to allow discrimination between diabetic subjects with and without nephropathy (Kaizu et al 1993).

Glomerular plasmin – antiplasmin (PAP) complexes were studied in glomerulopathy by Suzuki et al (1993). They found these complexes in the mesangium, and along capillary loops, in patients with various forms of glomerulopathy. Deposition of PAP complexes correlated with the decrease in glomerular filtration rate, phenolphthalein excretion and haematuria. The authors conclude that deposition of PAP complexes in the glomerulus could play a role in the progression of renal damage in various forms of glomerulopathy.

SKIN DISEASE

Fibrin cuffs around capillaries beneath venous ulcers might reduce exchange of nutrients and other essentials and hamper healing. Mulder et al (1993) showed that the application of hydrocolloid bandages with fibrinolytic properties resulted in a reduction of fibrin cuff thickness in a significant greater percentage of patients than after treatment with fibrinolytically inert bandages. Gertner & Lie (1994) treated patients with non-healing cutaneous ulcers with tPA plus heparin, and reported resolution of the ulcers. These promising data suggest that these conditions merit more attention than they have received thus far. Recent reports (Veraart et al 1994, Ibbotson et al 1994) suggest that increased levels of PAI-1 may be present in patients with chronic leg ulcers, though this is not invariably found (Vanscheidt et al 1992).

FIBRINOLYTIC FACTORS AND CARDIOVASCULAR DISEASE

The role of the fibrinolytic system in cardiovascular disease ('athero-thrombosis') is receiving increasing attention, as evidenced by the number of recent reviews of the subject (Hamsten 1995, Hamsten & Eriksson 1994, Hamsten et al 1994, Juhan-Vague & Alessi 1993, Juhan-Vague et al 1993a, Rabbani & Loscalzo 1994, Ridker 1992, Wilcox 1994, Zysow & Lawn 1993). Especially high PAI-1 levels might be one of the factors promoting not only venous thrombosis but also arterial disease. The Angina Pectoris Group of the ECAT (European Concerted Action on Thrombosis and Disabilities) study have presented their data. A positive correlation of the PAI-1 level and of the fibrinogen concentration with coronary events was reported (Haverkate et al 1992, Juhan-Vague et al 1993b, Thompson et al 1995), underscoring the presumed effect of fibrinolytic inhibition on arterial thrombotic events. Probably, the results published by Jansson et al (1993) and by Ridker et al (1993b) point to the same issue: the concentration of tPA antigen (usually correlating with PAI-1 levels) was a significant risk factor related to mortality.

CONCLUDING REMARKS

During the last 2 years some interesting achievements have been reported in the field of clinical fibrinolysis. However, the number of scientific reports by clinicians is not proportional to the dissemination of the analytical techniques involved over the hospitals. There are quite a few disorders (rheumatoid arthitis, Raynaud's disease, vasculitis, Crohn's disease and ulcerative colitis, postoperative thrombosis, microembolism syndrome, to name only a few) where clinical contributions could promote insight into the role of fibrinolysis/plasminogen activation in disease mechanisms, and might suggest potential treatment modalities. This applies as well to studies with regard to lifestyle and other non-pharmacological means of prevention.

KEY POINTS FOR CLINICAL PRACTICE

- Despite considerable progress in our understanding of basic aspects of the fibrinolytic/thrombolytic system in the years covered by this review, clinical progress has been painstakingly slow.

- A major development though was the renewed realization that increased plasma levels of PAI-1 (and fibrinogen) are major risk factors for cardio-vascular disease.

- In particular, the results of the large European Concerted Action on Thombosis and Disabilities (ECAT) angina pectoris study (Thompson et al 1995) showed that PAI-1 is not only a risk factor for venous, but also for arterial thrombosis (see also Rosenfeld et al 1993).

- PAI-1 reduction may therefore become an attractive goal for intervention. Promising approaches are life-style interventions such as high fibre diets, and exercise training. Elevated PAI-1 levels are now also regarded as part of the insulin resistance syndrome (syndrome X; Reaven, 1994), and may, in these patients, prove susceptible to pharmacological intervention (for example, Nagi & Yudkin, 1993).

- The regulation of PAI-1 metabolism may become one the major areas of clinical research in fibrinolysis over the next years.

REFERENCES

Achbarou A, Kaiser S, Tremblay G et al 1994 Urokinase overproduction results in increased skeletal metastasis by prostate cancer cells in vivo. Cancer Res 54: 2372–2377

Bashkov G V, Sergeev I Y, Medvedeva N A 1993 Role of sympathetic cholinergic pathway in the neurogenous control of tissue-type plasminogen activator release into the blood. Blood Coagulat Fibrinol 4: 993–998

Beer J H, Kläy H-P, Herren T et al 1994 Whole blood clot lysis: enhanced by exposure to autologous but not homologous plasma. Thromb Haemost 71: 622–626

Bianchi E, Cohen R L, Thor A T et al 1994 The urokinase receptor is expressed in invasive breast cancer but not in normal breast tissue. Cancer Res 54: 861–866

Biemond B J, Levi M, ten Cate H et al 1995 Complete inhibition of endotoxin-induced coagulation activation in chimpanzees with a monoclonal Fab fragment against factor VII/VIIa. Thromb Haemost 73: 223–230

Boberg M, Pollare T, Siegbahn A, Vessby B 1992 Supplementation with n-3 fatty acids reduces triglycerides but increases PAI-1 in non-insulin-dependent diabetes mellitus. Eur J Clin Invest 22: 645–650

Boman K, Hellsten G, Bruce Å et al 1994 Endurance physical activity, diet and fibrinolysis. Atherosclerosis 106: 65–74

Bouchet C, Spyratos F, Martin P M et al 1994 Prognostic value of urokinase-type plasminogen activator (uPA) and plasminogen activator inhibitors PAI-1 and PAI-2 in breast carcinomas. Br J Cancer 69: 398–405

Bremer H A 1994 Aspirin in pregnancy: clinical and biochemical studies. Thesis, Rotterdam

Brommer E J P, van Bockel J H 1992 Composition and susceptibility to thrombolysis of human arterial thrombi and the influence of their age. Blood Coagulat Fibrinol 3: 717–725

Brommer E J P, Dooijewaard, G, Dijkmans B A C, Breedveld F C 1992 Plasminogen activators in synovial fluid and plasma from patients with arthritis. Ann Rheum Dis 51: 965–968

Brommer E J P, Dooijewaard G, Rijken D C, Kluft C, Emeiss J J, Brakman P 1993 Progress in clinical fibrinoloysis. In Poller L (ed) Recent Advances in Blood Coagulation. Churchill Livingstone, Edinburgh, Volume 6, pp 1–15

Brommer E J P, van den Wall Bake A W L, Dooijewaard G et al 1994 Blood fibrinolysis and the response to desmopressin in glomerulonephritis. Thromb Haemost 71: 19–25

Brown P A, Wilson H M, Reid F J et al 1994 Urokinase-plasminogen activator is synthesized in vitro by human glomerular epithelial cells but not by mesangial cells. Kidney Int 45: 43–47

Carmeliet P, Collen D 1994 Evaluation of the plasminogen/plasmin system in transgenic mice. Fibrinolysis 8 (suppl 1): 269–276

Carmeliet P, Schoonjans L, Kieckens L et al 1994 Physiological consequences of loss of plasminogen activator gene function in mice. Nature 368: 419–424

Caron P, Bennet A, Camare R et al 1989 Plasminogen activator inhibitor in plasma is related to testosterone in men. Metabolism 38: 1010–1015

Chandler W L, Veith R C, Fellingham G W et al 1992 Fibrinolytic response during exercise and epinephrine infusion in the same subjects. J Am Coll Cardiol 19: 1412–1420

Chandler W L, Levy W C, Stratton J R 1995 The circulatory regulation of tPA and uPA during exercise and alpha- and beta-adrenergic agonist infusions. Circulation 92: 2904–2994

Chung H I, Burman J F, Balogun B A et al 1994 Elevated fibrinolysis in cardiopulmonary bypass is factor XII dependent. Fibrinolysis 8 (suppl 2): 84–88

Cortellaro M, Cofrancesco E, Boschetti C et al 1994 Association of increased fibrin turnover and defective fibrinolytic capacity with leg atherosclerosis. Thromb Haemost 72: 292–296

Dawson S, Hamsten A, Wiman B et al 1991 Genetic variation at the plasminogen activator inhibitor-1 locus is associated with altered levels of plasma plasminogen activator inhibitor-1 activity. Arterioscler Thromb 11: 183–190

Dawson S J, Wiman B, Hamsten A et al 1993 The two allele sequences of a common polymorphism in the promotor of the plasminogen activator inhibitor-1 (PAI-1) gene respond differently to interleukin-1 in HepG2 cells. J Biol Chem 268: 10739–10745

De Boer A, Kluft C, Gerloff J et al 1993a Pharmacokinetics of saruplase, a recombinant unglycosylated human single-chain urokinase-type plasminogen activator and its effects on fibrinolytic and haemostatic parameters in healthy male subjects. Thromb Haemost 70: 320–325

De Boer J P, Creasey A A, Chang A et al 1993b Alpha-2-macroglobulin functions as an inhibitor of fibrinolytic, clotting, and neutrophilic proteinases in sepsis: studies using a baboon model. Infect Immun 61: 5035–5043

Declerk P J, Lijnen H R, Verstrecken M, Collen D 1991 Role of α_2-antiplasmin in fibrin-specific clot lysis with single-chain urokinase-type plasminogen activator in human plasma. Thromb Haemost 65: 394–398

De Geus E J, Kluft C, de Bart A C, van Doornen L J 1992 Effects of exercise training on plasminogen activator inhibitor activity. Med Sci Sports Exerc 24: 1210–1219

Delbaldo C, Masouye I, Saurat J H et al 1994 Plasminogen activation in melanocytic neoplasia. Cancer Res 54: 4547–4552

De Vries T J, Quax P H A, Denijn M et al 1994 Plasminogen activators, their inhibitors, and urokinase receptor emerge in late stages of melanocytic tumor progression. Am J Pathol 144: 70–81

De Vries T J, Mooy C M, Vanbalken M R et al 1995 Components of the plasminogen activation system in uveal melanoma – a clinico-pathological study. J Pathol 175: 59–67

Dooijewaard G 1993 The post-thrombolytic era: is it possible to prevent thrombosis by stimulating indigenous fibrinolysis. Fibrinolysis 7 (suppl 1): 42–43

Dörr P J, Brommer E J P, Dooijewaard G, Vemer H M 1993 Parameters of fibrinolysis in peritoneal fluid and plasma in different stages of the menstrual cycle. Thromb Haemost 70: 873–875

Duffy M J, Reilly D, Mcdermott E et al 1994 Urokinase plasminogen activator as a prognostic marker in different subgroups of patients with breast cancer. Cancer 74: 2276–2280

Emeis J J 1996 Normal and abnormal endothelial release of tissue-type plasminogen activator. In: Glas-Greenwalt P (ed) Fibrinolysis in disease. CRC Press, Boca Raton, pp 54–63

Eriksson P, Kallin B, van't Hooft F M et al 1995 Allele-specific increase in basal PAI-1 transcription associated with myocardial infarction. Proc Natl Acad Sci USA 92:

1851–1855

Eritsland J, Seljeflot I, Abdelmoor M, Arnesen H 1994 Long-term influence of omega-3 fatty acids on fibrinolysis, fibrinogen, and serum lipids. Fibrinolysis 8: 120–125

Fay W P, Eitzman D T, Shapiro A D et al 1994 Platelets inhibit fibrinolysis in vitro by both plasminogen activator inhibitor-1-dependent and -independent mechanisms. Blood 83: 351–356

Fearns C, Samad F, Loskutoff D J 1996 Synthesis and localization of PAI-1 in the vessel wall. In: Van Hinsbergh V W M (ed) Vascular control of haemostasis. Gordon and Breach, Australia (in press)

Foekens J A, Schmitt M, van Putten W L J et al 1992 Prognostic value of urokinase-type plasminogen activator in 671 primary breast cancer patients. Cancer Res 52: 6101–6105

Foekens J A, Schmitt M, van Putten W L J et al 1994 Plasminogen activator inhibitor-1 and prognosis in primary breast cancer. J Clin Oncol 12: 1648–1658

Folsom A R, Qamhieh H T, Wing R R et al 1993 Impact of weight loss on plasminogen activator inhibitor (PAI-1), factor VII, and other hemostatic risk factors in moderately overweight adults. Arterioscler Thromb 13: 162–169

Francis C W, Önundarson P T, Carstensen E L et al 1992 Enhancement of fibrinolysis in vitro by ultrasound. J Clin Invest 90: 2063–2068

Fumeron F, Brigant L, Ollivier V et al 1991 n-3 polyunsaturated fatty acids raise low-density lipoproteins, high-density lipoprotein 2, and plasminogen activator inhibitor in healthy young men. Am J Clin Nutr 54: 118–122

Ganesh S, Sier C F, Griffioen G et al 1994a Prognostic relevance of plasminogen activators and their inhibitors in colorectal cancer. Cancer Res 54: 4065–4071

Ganesh S, Sier C F M, Heerding M M et al 1994b Urokinase receptor and colorectal cancer survival. Lancet 344: 401–402

Gelman S 1993 General versus regional anesthesia for peripheral vascular surgery. Is the problem solved? Anesthesiology 79: 415–418

Gertner E, Lie J T 1994 Systemic therapy with fibrinolytic agents and heparin for recalcitrant nonhealing cutaneous ulcer in the antiphospholipid syndrome. J Rheumatol 21: 2159–2161

Gleeson N C, Buggy F, Sheppard B L, Bonnar J 1993a The effect of tranexamic acid on measured menstrual loss and endometrial fibrinolytic enzymes in dysfunctional uterine bleeding. Eur J Gynaecol Oncol 14: 369–373

Gleeson N C, Gonsalves R, Bonnar J 1993b Plasminogen activator inhibitors in endometrial adenocarcinoma. Cancer 72: 1670–1672

Glueck C J, Glueck H I, Stroop J et al 1993 Endogenous testosterone, fibrinolysis, and coronary heart disease risk in hyperlipidemic men. J Lab Clin Med 122: 412–420

Gough S C, Rice P J, McCormack L et al 1993 The relationship between plasminogen activator inhibitor-1 and insulin resistance in newly diagnosed type-2 diabetes mellitus. Diabet Med 10: 638–642

Gray R P, Mohamed-Ali V, Patterson D L H, Yudkin J S 1995 Determinants of plasminogen activator inhibitor-1 activity in survivors of myocardial infarction. Thromb Haemost 73: 261–267

Green F, Humphries S 1994 Genetic determinants of arterial thrombosis. Baillières Clin Haematol 7: 675–692

Grøndahl-Hansen J, Christensen I J, Rosenquist C et al 1993 High levels of urokinase-type plasminogen activator and its inhibitor PAI-1 in cytosolic extracts of breast carcinomas are associated with poor prognosis. Cancer Res 53: 2513–2521

Gurewich V, Johnstone M, Loza J P, Pannell R 1993 Pro-urokinase and prekallikrein are both associated with platelets. Implications for the intrinsic pathway of fibrinolysis and for therapeutic thrombolysis. FEBS Lett 318: 317–321

Guzic B, Sundell I B, Keber I, Keber D 1994 The effect of oat husk supplementation in diet on plasminogen activator inhibitor type-1 in diabetic survivors of myocardial infarction. Fibrinolysis 8 (suppl 2): 44–46

Haglund O, Hamfelt A, Hambraeus L, Saldeen T 1993 Effects of fish oil supplemented with pyridoxine and folic acid on homocysteine, atherogenic index, fibrinogen and plasminogen activator inhibitor-1 in man. Nutr Res 13: 1351–1365

Hamsten A 1995 Haemostatic function and coronary artery disease. N Engl J Med 332: 677–678

Hamsten A, Eriksson P 1994 Fibrinolysis and atherosclerosis: an update. Fibrinolysis 8 (suppl 1): 253–262

Hamsten A, Eriksson P, Karpe F, Silveira A 1994 Relationships of thrombosis and fibrinolysis to atherosclerosis. Curr Opin Lipidol 5: 382–389

Hasui Y, Marutsuka K, Nishi S et al 1994 The content of urokinase-type plasminogen activator and tumor recurrence in superficial bladder cancer. J Urol 151: 16–19

Haverkate F, Thompson S G, van de Loo J C 1992 The relationship between hemostatic tests and cardiovascular risk factors in patients with angina pectoris. Ann Epidemiol 2: 521–524

Hellsten G, Boman K, Saarem K et al 1993 Effects on fibrinolytic activity of corn oil and a fish oil preparation enriched with omega-3-polyunsaturated fatty acids in a long-term study. Curr Med Res Opin 13: 133–139

Hendriks H F, Veenstra J, Velthuis-te Wierik E J et al 1994 Effect of moderate dose of alcohol with evening meal on fibrinolytic factors. Br Med J 308: 1003–1006

Hennis B C 1995 Histidine-rich glycoprotein and thrombosis. Thesis, Leiden

Heussen-Schemmer C, Barron J R, Swanepoel C R, Dowdle E B 1993 Urinary tissue plasminogen activator in renal disease. Nephron 64: 42–44

Hong S Y, Yang D H 1993 Fibrinolytic activity in end-stage renal disease. Nephron 63: 188–192

Huisveld I A, van den Burg P J M, van Vliet M et al 1994 The urokinase-type, rather than the tissue-type plasminogen system is influenced by regular physical training. Fibrinolysis 8 (suppl 1): 13 (abstract)

Husain S S 1993 Fibrin affinity of urokinase-type plasminogen activator. Evidence that Zn^{2+} mediates strong and specific interaction of single-chain urokinase with fibrin. J Biol Chem 268: 8574–8579

Ibbotson S H, Layton A M, Davies J A, Goodfield M J D 1994 Plasminogen activator inhibitor-1 (PAI-1) levels in patients with chronic venous leg ulceration (letter). Br J Dermatol 131: 738

Jain S K, Nagi D K, Slavin B M et al 1993 Insulin therapy in type-2 diabetic subjects suppresses plasminogen activator inhibitor (PAI-1) activity and proinsulin-like molecules independently of glycaemic control. Diabet Med 10: 27–32

Janicke F, Schmitt M, Pache L et al 1993 Urokinase (uPA) and its inhibitor PAI-1 are strong and independent prognostic factors in node-negative breast cancer. Breast Cancer Res Treat 24: 195–208

Jansson J H, Olofsson B O, Nilsson T K 1993 Predictive value of tissue plasminogen activator mass concentration on long-term mortality in patients with coronary artery disease. A 7-year follow-up. Circulation 88: 2030–2034

Jern C, Selin L, Jern S 1994a In vivo release of tissue-type plasminogen activator across the human forearm during mental stress. Thromb Haemost 72: 285–291

Jern S, Selin L, Bergbrant A, Jern C 1994b Release of tissue-type plasminogen activator in response to muscarinic receptor stimulation in human forearm. Thromb Haemost 72: 588–594

Johansson J, Egberg N, Johnsson H, Carlson L A 1993 Serum lipoproteins and hemostatic function in intermittent claudication. Arterioscler Thromb 13: 1441–1448

Johansson J-O, Landin K, Tengborn L et al 1994 High fibrinogen and plasminogen activator inhibitor activity in growth hormone-deficient adults. Arterioscler Thromb 14: 434–437

Juhan-Vague I, Alessi M C 1993 Plasminogen activator inhibitor 1 and atherothrombosis. Thromb Haemost 70: 138–143

Juhan-Vague I, Alessi M C, Nalbone G 1993a Fibrinolysis and atherothrombosis. Curr Opin Lipidol 4: 477–483

Juhan-Vague I, Thompson S G, Jespersen J 1993b Involvement of the hemostatic system in the insulin resistance syndrome. A study of 1500 patients with angina pectoris. Arterioscler Thromb 13: 1865–1873

Kaizu K, Uriu K, Eto S 1993 Role of intrarenal coagulation and anticoagulant therapy in the progression of diabetic nephropathy. Nippon Jinzo Gakkai Shi 35: 35–42

Kashyap A, Blinc A, Marder V J et al 1994 Acceleration of fibrinolysis by ultrasound in a rabbit ear model of small vessel injury. Thromb Res 76: 475–485

Klinger K, Winqvist R, Riccio A et al 1987 Plasminogen activator inhibitor type 1 gene is located at region q21.3–q22 of chromosome 7 and genetically linked with cystic fibrosis. Proc Natl Acad Sci USA 84: 8548–8552

Kobayashi H, Fujishiro S, Terao T 1994 Impact of urokinase-type plasminogen activator and its inhibitor type 1 on prognosis in cervical cancer of the uterus. Cancer Res 54: 6539–6548

Kummer J A, Abbink J J, de Boer J P et al 1992 Analysis of intraarticular fibrinolytic pathways in patients with inflammatory and noninflammatory joint diseases. Arthritis Rheum 35: 884–893

Landau B J, Kwaan H C, Verrusio E N, Brem S S 1994 Elevated levels of urokinase-type plasminogen activator and plasminogen activator inhibitor type 1 in malignant human brain tumors. Cancer Res 54: 1105–1108

Lang I M, Marsh J J, Olman M A et al 1994 Expression of type 1 plasminogen activator inhibitor in chronic pulmonary thromboemboli. Circulation 89: 2715–2721

Lauer C G, Burge R, Tang D B et al 1992 Effect of ultrasound on tissue-type plasminogen activator-induced thrombolysis. Circulation 86: 1257–1264

Lee A J, Flanagan P A, Rumley A et al 1995 Relationship between alcohol intake and tissue plasminogen activator antigen and other haemostatic factors in the general population. Fibrinolysis 8: 49–54

Levi M, Roem D, Kamp A M et al 1993 Assessment of the relative contribution of different protease inhibitors to the inhibition of plasmin in vivo. Thromb Haemost 69: 141–146

Levi M, ten Cate H, Bauer K A et al 1994 Inhibition of endotoxin-induced activation of coagulation and fibrinolysis by pentoxifylline or by a monoclonal anti-tissue factor antibody in chimpanzees. J Clin Invest 93: 114–120

Loza J P, Gurewich V, Johnstone M, Pannell R 1994 Platelet-bound prekallikrein promotes pro-urokinase-induced clot lysis: a mechanism for targeting the factor XII dependent intrinsic pathway of fibrinolysis. Thromb Haemost 71: 347–352

Ludwig M, Wohn K-D, Schleuning W-D, Olek K 1992 Allelic dimorphism in the human tissue-type plasminogen activator (TPA) gene as a result of an Alu insertion/deletion event. Hum Genet 88: 388–392

Mansfield M W, Stickland M H, Carter A M, Grant P J 1994 Polymorphisms of the plasminogen activator inhibitor-1 gene in type 1 and type 2 diabetes, and in patients with diabetic retinopathy. Thromb Haemost 71: 731–736

Marckman P, Jespersen J 1994 Introduction to diet and endogenous fibrinolysis. Fibrinolysis 8 (suppl 2): 37–40

Marckmann P, Sandström B, Jespersen J 1992 Fasting blood coagulation and fibrinolysis of young adults unchanged by reduction in dietary fat content. Arterioscler Thromb 12: 201–205

Marckmann P, Sandström B, Jespersen J 1993 Favorable long-term effect of a low-fat/high-fiber diet on human blood coagulation and fibrinolysis. Arterioscler Thromb 13: 505–511

Marckmann P, Sandström B, Jespersen J 1994 Low-fat, high-fiber diet favorably affects several independent risk markers of ischemic heart disease: observations on blood lipids, coagulation, and fibrinolysis from a trial of middle-aged Danes. Am J Clin Nutr 59: 935–939

Mashina S Y, Bashkov G V 1994 Plasmin-induced endothelium-dependent vasodilatation versus fibrinolysis – two pathways of blood flow restoration in the thrombotically occluded vessels? Fibrinolysis 8 (suppl 2): 113–115

Menzel D, Levi M, Dooijewaard G et al 1994 Impaired fibrinolysis in the hemolytic-uremic syndrome of childhood. Ann Hematol 68: 43–48

Møller J M, Svaneborg N, Lervang H H et al 1992 The acute effect of a single very high dose of n-3 fatty acids on coagulation and fibrinolysis. Thromb Res 67: 569–577

Mulcahy H E, Duffy M J, Gibbons D et al 1994 Urokinase-type plasminogen activator and outcome in Dukes' B colorectal cancer. Lancet 344: 583–584

Mulder G, Jones R, Cederholm-Williams S et al 1993 Fibrin cuff lysis in chronic venous ulcers treated with a hydrocolloid dressing. Int J Dermatol 32: 304–306

Mykkänen L, Rönnemaa T, Marniemi J et al 1994 Insulin sensitivity is not an independent determinant of plasma plasminogen activator inhibitor-1 activity. Arterioscler Thromb 14: 1264–1271

Nagi D K, Yudkin J S 1993 Effects of metformin on insulin resistance, risk factors for cardiovascular disease, and plasminogen activator inhibitor in NIDDM subjects. Diabetes Care 16: 621–629

Nekarda H, Schmitt M, Ulm K et al 1994a Prognostic impact of urokinase-type plasminogen activator and its inhibitor PAI-1 in completely resected gastric cancer. Cancer Res 54: 2900–2907

Nekarda H, Siewert J R, Schmitt M, Ulm K 1994b Tumour-associated proteolytic factor-uPA and factor-PAI-1 and survival in totally resected gastric cancer. Lancet 343: 117

Nieuwenhuizen W 1994 Personal communication

Nordt T K, Klassen K J, Schneider D J, Sobel B E 1993 Augmentation of synthesis of plasminogen activator inhibitor type 1 in arterial endothelial cells by glucose and its implications for local fibrinolysis. Arterioscler Thromb 13: 1822–1828

Nordt T K, Schneider D J, Sobel B E 1994 Augmentation of the synthesis of plasminogen activator inhibitor type 1 by precursors of insulin. A potential risk factor for vascular disease. Circulation 89: 321–330

Orchard M A, Goodchild C S, Prentice C R M et al 1993 Aprotinin reduces cardiopulmonary bypass-induced blood loss and inhibits fibrinolysis without influencing platelets. Br J Haematol 85: 533–541

Oudenhoven L F I J, Brommer E J P, Aronson D C et al 1994 Impaired fibrinolysis in young adults with arterial occlusive disease: the relationship with hyperinsulinism and smoking. Fibrinolysis 8: 263–269

Panahloo A, Mohamed-Ali V, Lane A et al 1995 Determinants of plasminogen activator inhibitor 1 activity in treated NIDDM and its relation to a polymorphism in the plasminogen activator inhibitor 1 gene. Diabetes 44: 37–42

Pedersen H, Brunner N, Francis D et al 1994a Prognostic impact of urokinase, urokinase receptor, and type 1 plasminogen activator inhibitor in squamous and large cell lung cancer tissue. Cancer Res 54: 4671–4675

Pedersen H, Grøndahl-Hansen J, Francis D et al 1994b Urokinase and plasminogen activator inhibitor type 1 in pulmonary adenocarcinoma. Cancer Res 54: 120–123

Potter van Loon B J, Kluft C, Radder J K et al 1993 The cardiovascular risk factor plasminogen activator inhibitor type 1 is related to insulin resistance. Metabolism 42: 945–949

Rabbani L E, Loscalzo J 1994 Recent observations on the role of hemostatic determinants in the development of the atherothrombotic plaque. Atherosclerosis 105: 1–7

Rao J S, Rayford A, Morantz R A et al 1993 Increased levels of plasminogen activator inhibitor-1 (PAI-1) in human brain tumors. J Neurooncol 17: 215–221

Reaven G M 1994 Syndrome X: 6 years later. J Intern Med 236 (suppl 736): 13–22

Ridker P M 1992 An epidemiological assessment of thrombotic risk factors for cardiovascular disease. Curr Opin Lipidol 3: 285–290

Ridker P M, Gaboury C L, Conlin P R et al 1993a Stimulation of plasminogen activator inhibitor in vivo by infusion of angiotensin II. Evidence of a potential interaction between the renin–angiotensin system and fibrinolytic function. Circulation 87: 1969–1973

Ridker P M, Vaughan D E, Stampfer M J et al 1993b Endogenous tissue-type plasminogen activator and risk of myocardial infarction. Lancet 341: 1165–1168

Ridker P M, Vaughan D E, Stampfer M J et al 1994 Association of moderate alcohol consumption and plasma concentration of endogenous tissue-type plasminogen activator. J Am Med Assoc 272: 929–933

Romanova E P, Gorbunova N A, Jitkova J V, Bashkov G V 1994 Anti-aggregatory activity of recombinant single-chain urokinase-type plasminogen activator. Fibrinolysis 8 (suppl 2): 111–112

Rosenfeld B A, Beattie C, Christopherson R et al 1993 The effects of different anesthetic regimens on fibrinolysis and the development of postoperative arterial thrombosis. Anesthesiology 79: 435–443

Sakharov D V, Rijken D C 1994 Superficial accumulation of plasminogen during clot lysis. Fibrinolysis 8 (suppl 1): 83 (abstract)

Saxne T, Lecander I, Geborek P 1993 Plasminogen activators and plasminogen activator inhibitors in synovial fluid. Difference between inflammatory joint disorders and osteoarthritis. J Rheumatol 20: 91–96

Schneider D J, Nordt T K, Sobel B E 1992 Stimulation by proinsulin of expression of plasminogen activator inhibitor type 1 in endothelial cells. Diabetes 41: 890–895

Seljeflot I, Eritsland J, Torjesen P, Arnesen H 1994 Insulin and PAI-1 levels during oral glucose tolerance test in patients with coronary heart disease. Scand J Clin Lab Invest 54: 241–246

Serizawa K, Urano T, Kozima Y et al 1993 The potential role of platelet PAI-1 in t-PA mediated clot lysis of platelet rich plasma. Thromb Res 71: 289–300

Shigekiyo T, Ohshima T, Oka H et al 1993 Congenital histidine-rich glycoprotein deficiency. Thromb Haemost 70: 263–265

Sier C F M, Verspaget H W, Griffioen G et al 1993 Plasminogen activators in normal tissue and carcinomas of the human oesophagus and stomach. Gut 34: 80–85

Sier C F M, Vloedgraven H J M, Ganesh S et al 1994 Inactive urokinase and increased levels of its inhibitor type 1 in colorectal cancer liver metastasis. Gastroenterology 107: 1449–1456

Smith F B, Lowe G D, Fowkes F G et al 1993 Smoking, haemostatic factors and lipid peroxides in a population case control study of peripheral arterial disease. Atherosclerosis 102: 155–162

Sobel J H, Wu H Q, Canfield R E 1994 The development of assays for the detection of fibrin(ogen)olysis based on COOH-terminal A alpha chain epitopes. Blood 84: 535–546

Stief T W 1993 Oxidized fibrin stimulates the activation of pro-urokinase and is the preferential substrate of human plasmin. Blood Coagulat Fibrinol 4: 117–121

Sundell I B, Rånby M 1993 Oat husk fiber decreases plasminogen activator inhibitor type 1 activity. Haemostasis 23: 45–50

Suzuki S, Sato H, Shimada H et al 1993 Significance of glomerular deposition of plasmin–alpha 2-plasmin inhibitor complexes in various glomerulopathies. Clin Nephrol 40: 270–276

Suzuki T, Yamauchi K, Yamada Y et al 1992 Blood coagulability and fibrinolytic activity before and after physical training during the recovery phase of acute myocardial infarction. Clin Cardiol 15: 358–364

Sylvan A, Rutegard J N, Janunger K G et al 1992 Normal plasminogen activator inhibitor levels at long-term follow-up after jejuno-ileal bypass surgery in morbidly obese individuals. Metabolism 41: 1370–1372

Thompson S G, Kienast J, Pyke S D M et al 1995 Hemostatic factors and the risk of myocardial infarction and sudden death in patients with angina pectoris. N Engl J Med 332: 635–641

Tromholt N, Jorgensen S J, Hesse B, Hansen M S 1993 In vivo demonstration of focal fibrinolytic activity in abdominal aortic aneurysms. Eur Vasc Surg 7: 675–679

Urano T, Kojima Y, Takahashi M et al 1993 Impaired fibrinolysis in hypertension and obesity due to high plasminogen activator inhibitor-1 level in plasma. Jpn J Physiol 43: 221–228

Van den Burg P J 1994 The effects of physical exercise and training on blood coagulation and fibrinolysis. Thesis, Utrecht

Van den Burg P J, Dooijewaard G, van Vliet M et al 1994 Differences in u-PA and t-PA increase during acute exercise; relation with exercise parameters. Thromb Haemost 71: 236–239

Van der Poll T, Levi M, Hack C E et al 1994a Elimination of interleukin 6 attenuates coagulation activation in experimental endotoxemia in chimpanzees. J Exp Med 179: 1253–1259

Van der Poll T, Levi M, van Deventer S J 1994b Differential effects of anti-tumor necrosis factor monoclonal antibodies on systemic inflammatory responses in experimental endotoxemia in chimpanzees. Blood 83: 446–451

Vanscheidt W, Kresse O, Hach-Wunderle V et al 1992 Leg ulcer patients: no decreased fibrinolytic response but white cell trapping after venous occlusion of the upper limb. Phlebology 7: 92–96

Veenstra J, Kluft C, van de Pol H et al 1993 Acute effects of moderate alcohol consumption on fibrinolytic factors in healthy middle-aged men. Fibrinolysis 7: 177–182

Veraart J C J M, Hamalyuk K, Neumann H A M, Engelen J 1994 Increased plasma activity of plasminogen activator inhibitor 1 (PAI-1) in two patients with Klinefelter's syndrome complicated by leg ulcers. Br J Dermatol 130: 641–644

Weidle U H, Wollisch E, Ronne E et al 1994 Studies on functional and structural role of urokinase receptor and other components of the plasminogen activation system in malignancy. Ann Biol Clin 52: 775–782

Wieczorek I, Pell A C H, McIver B et al 1993 Coagulation and fibrinolytic systems in type 1 diabetes: effects of venous occlusion and insulin-induced hypoglycaemia. Clin Sci 84: 79–86

Wilcox J N 1994 Thrombotic mechanisms in atherosclerosis. Coronary Artery Dis 5: 223–229

Willich S N, Lewis M, Löwel H 1993 Physical exertion as a trigger of acute myocardial infarction. N Engl J Med 329: 1684–1690

Wright R A, Flapan A D, Alberti K G et al 1994 Effects of captopril therapy on endogenous fibrinolysis in men with recent, uncomplicated myocardial infarction. J Am Coll Cardiol 24: 67–73

Wu J-H, Siddiqui K, Diamond S L 1994 Transport phenomena and clot dissolving therapy: an experimental investigation of diffusion-controlled and permeation-enhanced fibrinolysis. Thromb Haemost 72: 105–112

Yamamoto M, Sawaya R, Mohanam S et al 1994a Expression and cellular localization of messenger RNA for plasminogen activator inhibitor type 1 in human astrocytomas in vivo. Cancer Res 54: 3329–3332

Yamamoto M, Sawaya R, Mohanam S et al 1994b Expression and localization of urokinase-type plasminogen activator in human astrocytomas in vivo. Cancer Res 54: 3656–3661

Yamamoto M, Sawaya R, Mohanam S et al 1994c Expression and localization of urokinase-type plasminogen activator receptor in human gliomas. Cancer Res 54: 5016–5020

Zysow B R, Lawn R M 1993 The relationship of lipoprotein (a) to hemostasis. Curr Opin Lipidol 4: 484–489

11. New antithrombotic agents

H. ten Cate   J. W. ten Cate

Investigation of the complex mechanism of the blood coagulation system has enabled the development of more specific agents for inhibiting selected pathways leading to fibrin formation. Enhanced specificity could have the theoretical advantage of fewer undesired interactions and side-effects which are at present associated with antithrombotic treatment. While current antithrombotic agents interact with different proteases of the coagulation mechanism (heparin), or inhibit the synthesis of all vitamin K-dependent proteins (coumarin), or inhibit platelet functions (aspirin), new generations of antithrombotic drugs are being designed with the aim of inhibiting a single target function. First, we will briefly review a few key elements of the coagulation system, in relation to therapeutic interventions.

The currently proposed mechanism of thrombosis involves interactions between platelets, coagulation proteins and the vessel wall (Colman et al 1994, Fig. 11.1). Other potential participants (i.e. lipids, inflammatory components, complement factors and acute phase proteins) and cells (mononuclear leucocytes) are likely to play an important role in coagulation, but will not be considered in the context of this chapter. In the formation of thrombus, platelets adhere to the subendothelium through interaction of the glycoprotein (GP) Ib/IX complex with adhesive proteins such as von Willebrand factor (vWF) and integrin receptors. Platelet aggregation is facilitated through platelet activation by compounds such as thrombin, and mediated through interaction of the GPIIb/IIIa complex with fibrinogen and other proteins. The thrombus plug is formed by the assembly of aggregated platelets and polymerized fibrin (Fig. 11.1). This process is markedly enhanced by activated platelets, which provide a surface for enzymatic complex formation (such as the tenase and prothrombinase complexes), stimulating the formation of factor Xa and thrombin (Harker & Mann 1992). The process of fibrin formation is initiated by the assembly of the factor VIIa–tissue factor (TF) complex at cell surfaces (Davie et al 1991, Broze 1992). This complex rapidly activates factors IX and X, leading to thrombin generation. The amount of thrombin may determine the rate of coagulation propagation, because thrombin is crucial as a procoagulant feedback catalyst. Furthermore, thrombin induces fibrinogen conversion and is probably the most important activator of platelets in vivo.

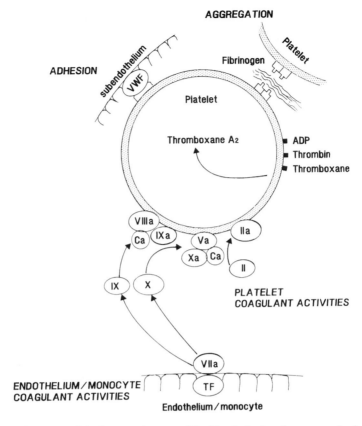

Fig. 11.1 Summary of the hemostatic system. The blood platelet plays a central role, interacting with the (sub)endothelium and with other platelets, as well as providing surface receptors for specific substances that mediate platelet or procoagulant functions. Part of the 'plasmatic' coagulation system is indicated at the lower part of the platelet, illustrating that the platelet provides an important surface for catalyzing procoagulant reactions. The hemostatic process is driven by the endothelial cell or monocyte bound factor VIIa–tissue factor complex. TF, tissue factor; VWF, von Willebrand factor.

These procoagulant actions are counteracted by the thrombin-induced activation of the protein C mechanism, through interaction of thrombin with the endothelial cell bound protein thrombomodulin (Esmon 1987). Thus, in the formation of thrombus, platelet interactions with the vessel wall and with fibrinogen, the formation of the factor VIIa–TF complex, and the enzymes factor Xa and particularly thrombin play pivotal roles. It should be noted that there are apparent differences in the etiology of venous and arterial thrombosis; however, the major difference may consist of a principal role of platelets in the developing arterial thrombus, while derangements of the coagulation system are more relevant to venous thrombosis. This differentiation in contribution of the key elements to the formation of thrombus seems to be supported by major clinical studies showing therapeutic inhibition of platelet function to be particularly effective in preventing arterial occlusion, while anticoagulants remain the cornerstone therapy for the prevention and treatment of venous thromboembolism.

The insight gained into the pathways leading to fibrin formation has led to the extensive experimental and clinical evaluation of new compounds that interfere with specific steps in the coagulation mechanism. In this chapter we will discuss new developments in the agents that inhibit platelet function or specific steps in the coagulation cascade.

PLATELET INHIBITORS

In spite of extensive research aimed at improving antiplatelet therapy, aspirin is still the preferred agent for clinical use (Roth & Calverley 1994). Its clinical efficacy, particularly in preventing arterial thrombosis, the lack of major side-effects and low costs make it the 'gold standard' drug against which new agents are being compared (Antiplatelet Trialists' Collaboration 1994). During the past decades only a few compounds have emerged as potential alternatives: for example, ticlopidine, which is a suitable alternative for aspirin especially in stroke prevention in spite of potential significant side-effects (particularly granulocytopenia) (Rothrock & Hart 1994), and prostacyclin, which is not suitable for long-term administration, however, because of its short half-life, high cost and side-effects (Szczeklik et al 1978).

Inhibition of platelet thrombogenicity may be effected by:

1. Inhibition of platelet adhesion to the subendothelium.
2. Inhibition of platelet–platelet interaction through adhesive proteins (particularly fibrinogen).
3. Inhibition of the platelet thromboxane pathway.
4. Inhibition of specific platelet receptors such as those for thromboxane and thrombin (Harker et al 1994).

Several novel agents have been studied in animal models with regard to their potency to block platelet adhesion with the subendothelium, mostly through inhibition of the interaction with vWF. These substances include monoclonal antibodies and peptides. These studies have demonstrated that antithrombotic effects may be obtained in models of arterial thrombosis, which are, however, sometimes associated with thrombocytopenia and/or prolonged bleeding times. The fact that multiple adhesive proteins and receptors are involved makes it less likely that effective inhibition of platelet adhesion can be easily obtained pharmacologically (Bellinger et al 1987, Miller et al 1991, Krupski et al 1992, Harker et al 1994).

Of greater clinical importance are substances that interfere with platelet interaction with adhesive proteins (e.g. fibrinogen) which facilitate platelet aggregation. Currently at least four such agents are being tested in phase II and phase III clinical trials: c7E3 (monoclonal antibody Fab fragment),

Integrelin (cyclic heptapeptide), MK-383 and Ro-44 (both peptidomimetics) (Topol 1995). These drugs act through interfering with the platelet GPIIb/IIIa receptor interaction with fibrinogen. Most agents are not fully specific and may also interact with other integrins with structural similarity (e.g. the vitronectin receptor) (Harker et al 1994).

The monoclonal antibody c7E3 has been extensively studied in patients with coronary disease. In a randomized double-blind study in 2099 patients scheduled to undergo coronary angioplasty or atherectomy, c7E3 was given either as a single bolus injection or as a bolus plus continuous infusion for 12 h. In addition, all patients received conventional treatment with aspirin and heparin. Compared with placebo, a 35% reduction (12.8% versus 8.3%; $P = 0.008$) was observed in the primary end-point during the first 30 days in patients treated with c7E3 bolus plus infusion, whereas this reduction was 10% in those treated with a bolus only ($P = 0.43$) (Boehrer et al 1994). In this study, the primary end-point was a composite, including death from any cause, non-fatal myocardial infarction, or one of several interventions. In particular, there were far fewer indications for emergency PTCA (percutaneous transluminal coronary angioplasty) in those treated with bolus monoclonal antibody plus infusion. Major bleeding complications requiring blood transfusion occurred more often in those receiving c7E3 (14% in bolus plus infusion, 11% in bolus only, 7% in placebo; $P = 0.001$ for the comparison of treated versus placebo patients), but were mostly confined to puncture sites. The significant advantage of bolus plus infusion treatment persisted at 6 months with 35.1% of place-bo-treated patients having had a major ischemic event or elective revascularization, versus 27.0% in the group treated with bolus plus infusion of c7E3 (23% reduction; $P = 0.001$) (Topol et al 1994a). The subgroup requiring emergency surgery had comparable high rates of perioperative bleeding (72% placebo, 100% c7E3 bolus, 76% bolus plus infusion).

The peptide Integrelin has been investigated in the IMPACT study, including 150 patients scheduled to undergo routine coronary angioplasty being randomized to placebo, a 4-h infusion, or a 12-h infusion with Integrelin (Tcheng et al 1993). Active treatment reduced the composite end-point (death, myocardial infarction, emergency procedures) from 11.9% to 5.6%.

The GPIIb/IIIa inhibitors are also being studied for other indications. In a placebo-controlled study in 60 patients with refractory myocardial ischemia, administration of c7E3 led to a reduction in clinical events from 20% to 3% (Simoons et al 1994). In a similar population the non-peptide inhibitor MK-383 reduced the incidence of refractory angina compared to intravenous heparin from 13% to 1% (Theroux et al 1994). In this particular study most patients (83%) also received aspirin.

The potential of these agents as adjuncts to thrombolysis is being evaluated. Future studies may address the potential efficacy of recently developed orally active GPIIb/IIIa inhibitors such as SC-54684A, a prodrug from a non-peptide mimetic of RGDF (Nicholson et al 1995). Finally, a combination of a fibrinogen receptor antagonist with a direct thrombin inhibitor has shown considerable potential compared to either agent alone as adjunct therapy to thrombolysis in a dog model of intracoronary thrombosis (Nicolini et al 1994). The combination of a continuous infusion of relatively low doses of Integrelin plus recombinant hirudin produced complete restoration of blood flow for 92 min and reduced the reocclusion rate after tissue plasminogen activator (tPA)-induced clot lysis, whereas each compound alone was not effective.

From the other classes of newly developed platelet inhibitors a few appear to have interesting additional properties. The observation that aspirin not only reduces thromboxane formation in platelets but also inhibits prostacyclin formation in endothelial cells has led to the development of selective inhibitors of the thromboxane pathway. In addition to inhibiting thromboxane formation, these inhibitors enhanced prostacyclin formation in some studies, while having no effect in others (FitzGerald & Oates 1984, Reilly & FitzGerald 1987, Morio et al 1993). One major clinical study has been published to date, in which the effect of Ridogrel – a combined thromboxane A_2 synthase inhibitor and weak thromboxane A_2 receptor antagonist – on vessel patency after thrombolysis with streptokinase for myocardial infarction was compared with aspirin (The RAPT Investigators 1993). Vessel patency was similar in the two groups (72.2% for Ridogrel and 75.5% for aspirin) while there was no increase in bleeding complications. Animal experiments suggest that agents that specifically block thromboxane A_2 receptors may be more effective than aspirin in models of arterial (and venous) thrombosis (Schumacher et al 1993).

In addition, a new series of serotonin receptor antagonists is being developed which may improve the mild antithrombotic effect obtained by the non-selective serotonin inhibitor ketanserin in arterial disease, particularly intermittent claudication. Three such compounds (MCI-9042, LY 53857, SR 46349) showed antithrombotic efficacy in animal models of arterial thrombosis and extracorporeal shunt occlusion (Hara et al 1991, Wilson et al 1991, Herbert et al 1993). Clinical trials must be awaited to evaluate their antithrombotic potential.

Another emerging inhibitor of (primarily ADP-induced) platelet aggregation is Clopidogrel (a ticlopidine analogue) (Gachet et al 1990), which may also have the interesting potential to inhibit TF expression in endothelial cells (Savi et al 1994). Its antithrombotic potency has been determined in different animal models (Maffrand et al 1988) and the compound is currently being investigated in a multicenter clinical trial (CAPRIE study) as to its efficacy to reduce mortality in patients with cardiovascular disease.

An evolving strategy is the inhibition of the thrombin receptor on platelets. Since it is generally thought that thrombin is an important physiological agonist of platelet activation, effective inhibition of its interaction with platelets may be relevant (Harker et al 1994). In vitro studies have confirmed that thrombin activation of platelets is dependent on ligand–receptor interaction (Hung et al 1992). There are no published data from animal experiments with this drug.

In conclusion, it appears that specific inhibitors of platelet aggregation may significantly improve antithrombotic treatment in specific arterial disorders. It is noteworthy that even short-term blockade of the GPIIb/IIIa receptor of platelets, in addition to conventional treatment with aspirin (and heparin), appears to improve clinical outcome in patients requiring angioplasty. This indicates that the combination of differently acting platelet inhibitors, and probably also in combination with specific anticoagulants, may enhance efficacy of antithrombotic treatment. The main challenge will be to carefully ascertain the safety of these combinations.

THROMBIN INHIBITORS

The best known and most extensively studied thrombin inhibitor is hirudin (Markwardt 1994). Originally derived from the leech (*Hirudo medicinalis*), the structure of the anticoagulant molecule hirudin has been determined. The native molecule is a polypeptide of 65 amino acids with a relative molecular mass of approximately 7000. It specifically and reversibly binds thrombin (in 1:1 molar complexes) with a very low dissociation constant of approximately 20×10^{-9}, and neutralizes its enzymatic activity. Recombinant hirudin has been produced by various methods, and is virtually identical to the native molecule except for a missing sulfate group at tyrosine 63. The affinity of recombinant hirudin (further referred to as hirudin) for thrombin is 10-fold lower than that of the native molecule. Based on the structure of hirudin, synthetic peptides have been designed and tested for their anticoagulant potential; one such compound, Hirulog (a 20 amino acid molecule) (Maraganore et al 1990), has been evaluated clinically.

Hirudin has an immediate anticoagulant effect after intravenous injection, which is measured as a prolongation of the APTT (activated partial thromboplastin time) or thrombin clotting time. After intravenous injection the anticoagulant effect parallels the clearance of hirudin from the circulation (Marbet et al 1993). It is predominantly cleared by the renal route in unmetabolized form; its elimination half-life is between 60 and 100 min and is directly influenced by renal clearance. The half-life can be markedly prolonged by conjugating hirudin to a high molecular weight molecule such as polyethylene glycol (PEG). PEG–hirudin has a half-life of between 5 and 9 h. Hirulog has a shorter half-life (about 36 min) and its clearance is dependent on metabolism by the liver (Fox et al 1993).

Several factors have contributed to the development of hirudin and analogues for clinical studies (Markwardt 1994):

1. Hirudin acts directly on thrombin, i.e. without interaction with cofactors.
2. It appears to be a weak immunogen.

3. It is not neutralized by any of the physiological inhibitors.
4. It inhibits clot-bound thrombin.

As far as these aspects are involved, hirudin differs from heparin (and most of the low molecular weight heparins, LMWH), because heparin needs the presence of the cofactor antithrombin, it can act as an immunogen after complexing with platelet factor 4, which also neutralizes its anticoagulant action, and it is not a potent inhibitor of clot-bound thrombin. Specific disadvantages of hirudin are the fact that it is a strong inhibitor of thrombin and thus potentially predisposes to bleeding, because of the ability to inhibit thrombin-induced platelet activation. A practical disadvantage is the lack of an antidote. In preclinical animal testing hirudin was a strong antithrombotic agent and more potent than heparin, particularly in models of arterial thrombosis (and angioplasty) and disseminated intravascular coagulation (DIC) (Markwardt 1994).

The principal clinical trials with hirudin have focused on PTCA, myocardial infarction and venous thromboembolism. The application of hirudin (20 mg bolus prior to PTCA, followed by continuous infusion of 0.16 mg/kg for 24 h) versus heparin in patients undergoing PTCA resulted in a significant reduction in primary outcome (sum of myocardial infarction and emergency bypass procedures) from 10.3% in those patients receiving heparin to 1.4% in hirudin-treated patients (Van den Bos et al 1993). Bleeding was confined to puncture sites and occurred in four patients on hirudin. In a dose-finding study, hirudin was compared with heparin as an adjunct to front-loaded tPA for treatment of acute myocardial infarction (Cannon et al 1994). All four doses of hirudin tested (bolus of 0.1–0.6 mg/kg, continuous infusion of between 0.05 and 0.2 mg/kg/h for up to 5 days) had a comparable efficacy, and improved outcome compared to heparin with respect to TIMI grade 2–3 flow after 18–36 h upon repeat angiogram, reocclusion of patent arteries, and late perfusion of occluded arteries. The clinical end-point of death or reinfarction was significantly lower in hirudin-treated patients (6.8% versus 16.7% for heparin, $P = 0.02$). Major spontaneous hemorrhage in-hospital occurred in 4.7% of heparin-treated patients and 1.2% of hirudin-treated individuals. For total major hemorrhage these were 23.3% and 17.5%, respectively (NS). There was one intracranial hemorrhage in the heparin group and none in the hirudin groups.

In patients with unstable angina a similar range of hirudin doses (bolus plus continuous infusion) was compared against heparin at two target intensities given for 3–5 days as to the effect on change in the average cross-sectional area of the culprit lesion on angiography (Topol et al 1994b). Slight but not significant outcome improvements were seen in the 116 hirudin-treated patients compared to the 50 heparin-treated patients. No deaths occurred in-hospital and the number of myocardial infarctions was lower among the hirudin-treated patients (2.6% versus 8.0% on heparin, NS). No intracranial or other major spontaneous bleeds occurred in any patient.

Based on these dose-finding studies, phase III studies were initiated in patients with coronary disease. Three major trials were terminated before completion, however, because of excess bleeding in the hirudin-treated patients (Antman 1994, The GUSTO Investigators 1994, Neuhaus et al 1994). The results are summarized in Table 11.1. Thus, the chosen hirudin regimens tended to be less safe than the heparin doses selected in terms of bleeding complications. In GUSTO II the APTT was longer in patients with hemorrhagic stroke compared to those without (The GUSTO Investigators 1994). Also, the average age of those suffering a hemorrhagic stroke was higher than in those without stroke (71.8 versus 63.8 years, NS). Similar findings regarding the importance of APTT prolongation and bleeding in relation to hirudin, and also to heparin, were made in the other two studies. Therefore, subsequent trials have been designed to study the efficacy of hirudin versus heparin at lower doses adjusted by the APTT.

The use of the synthetic thrombin inhibitor hirulog was also investigated in coronary patients. In a pilot study of 45 patients, hirulog was given as adjunct to streptokinase treatment for acute myocardial infarction; this resulted in better flow characteristics than with heparin, at comparable bleeding rates (Lidon et al 1994). Further large trials with this compound are needed to evaluate the bleeding risks appropriately.

Small-scale studies have reported on the efficacy of hirudin for the treatment of venous thromboembolism, administered either as continuous intravenous infusion at much lower doses than given in the arterial studies (e.g. 0.07 mg/kg bolus plus 0.05 mg/kg/h for 5 days) (Parent et al 1993),

Table 11.1   Summary of safety data from three phase III trials with recombinant hirudin in patients with acute coronary syndromes

Study Drug	GUSTO Heparin	GUSTO Hirudin	HIT3 Heparin	HIT3 Hirudin	TIMI Heparin	TIMI Hirudin
Total patients	1291	1273	154	148	368	345
Dose	5000 U + 1000–1300 U/h	0.6 mg/kg + 0.2 mg/kg/h	70 U/kg + 15 U/kg/h	0.4 mg/kg + 0.15 mg/kg/h	5000 U + 1000 –1300 U/h	0.6 mg/kg + 0.2 mg/kg/h
HS: tPA	4 (0.9)	8 (1.7)	0	4 (2.7)	nd	nd
HS: SK	5 (2.7)	6 (3.2)	–	–	nd	nd
Total HS	9 (1.5)	14 (2.2)	0	4 (2.7)	7 (1.9)	6 (1.7)
Major bleeds*	nd	nd	3 (1.9)	5 (3.4)	11 (3.0)	24 (7.0)
Cardiac rupture and EMD	nd	nd	1 (0.6)	3 (2.0)	3 (0.8)	6 (1.7)
Cardiac death	nd	nd	5 (3.2)	9 (6.1)	nd	nd

*Major bleeds other than stroke.
EMD, electromechanical dissociation; HS, intracranial hemorrhages; nd, not determined (or not specified in the published investigation); SK, streptokinase; tPA, tissue plasminogen activator.
Numbers in brackets = % of total number of patients in study group.

or by twice-daily subcutaneous injection (Schiele et al 1994). Both routes appeared safe, but efficacy studies have not yet been published.

Assuming that a direct thrombin inhibitor would also be of advantage over heparin or LMWH for the prevention of DVT (deep venous thrombosis) postoperatively, a fairly large-scale, uncontrolled phase II trial with hirulog was undertaken in patients undergoing major hip or knee surgery (Ginsberg et al 1994). The drug was commenced 12–24 h after surgery. The highest dose regimen (1.0 mg/kg every 8 h) was most effective, with an impressive low rate of proximal DVT of 2% (one out of 46 patients). Overall, three patients suffered a major bleeding, one occurring in the highest dose group.

On the basis of these data it appears that hirudin, and the hirudin-derived synthetic peptide hirulog, can induce antithrombotic effects in diverse patient groups; however, substantial bleeding complications can still occur in conjunction with thrombolytic treatment, and careful dose adjustment will thus be required. So far, the claim that hirudin is more efficacious than heparin, because of its potential to block fibrin-bound thrombin, has not been convincingly substantiated. Two ways of improving hirudin's safety profile are:

1. Fibrin-specific targeting through coupling of hirudin to a fibrinspecific monoclonal antibody (Bode et al 1994).
2. Local application of high concentrations of hirudin through catheters, which can be suitable for preventing local thrombus formation such as after angioplasty (Meyer et al 1994).

Several other classes of naturally occurring or synthetic thrombin inhibitors, some of which may act by the oral route, have been investigated in vitro and in animal models (Harker et al 1994, Topol 1995). So far, it appears that the potential of strong inhibition of thrombin may facilitate much higher antithrombotic efficacy, particularly in models of arterial thrombosis, however at the cost of inhibition of hemostasis. The recent clinical studies with hirudin demonstrate that bleeding may easily occur in spite of pilot studies suggesting safety. This observation will hamper the clinical application of direct thrombin inhibitors.

GLYCOSAMINOGLYCANS

The therapeutic effect of heparin is through its enhancement of the action of antithrombin to inactivate coagulant proteases. In the past decade heterogeneous heparin has been further fractionated on molecular weight and/or affinity for antithrombin, and the various fractions have been further investigated. It appeared that heparin fractions of lower than average molecular weight (LMWH) still contained antithrombotic potency in animal models, while their associated bleeding inducing effect was reduced compared with unfractionated heparin (UFH) (Hirsh & Levine 1992). It was also shown that with lowering molecular weight (MW) the overall antico-agulant effect (measured by APTT) diminished, while the specific action of LMWH against factor Xa persisted, which was characterized as the 'anti-Xa' activity of LMWH (mediated by antithrombin) (Andersson et al 1979). Since then a number of LMWH preparations have been commercially produced and are currently available in most countries. The LMWH com-pounds have an average MW of between 4000 and 6500 (unfractionated heparin is about 15 000), and consist of molecules of different chain length and thus different inhibitory activity against the various clotting proteases (Hirsh & Levine 1992).

A large number of clinical studies have been carried out and have been reviewed recently. For details the reader is referred to those summaries of clinical data (Hirsh & Levine 1992, Leizorovicz et al 1992, Nurmohamed et al 1992, Jorgensen et al 1993) that allow for the following conclusions to be drawn:

1. LMWH have a greater bioavailability at low doses, longer half-life (approximately 2–3 times UFH) and more predictable response when administered at fixed doses than UFH.

2. LMWH provide an antithrombotic efficacy in the prevention of post-operative DVT and pulmonary embolism (PE) at least as good as UFH in general surgery. This effect may be obtained with a once-daily injection for some preparations. In the meta-analyses by Nurmohamed et al (1992) and Leizorovicz et al (1992), the calculated relative risks of DVT in general surgery were 0.79 (95% CI (confidence intervals) 0.65–0.95) and 0.86 (95% CI 0.72–1.04), respectively, for LMWH versus UFH (a value < 1 repre-senting an advantage of LMWH over UFH). The relative risks (RR) of PE in these meta-analyses were 0.44 and 0.62, respectively, for LMWH versus UFH, while the risk of hemorrhage was identical (RR 1.01 and 1.02, respectively).

3. In orthopedic surgery LMWH is superior to UFH as prophylaxis for postoperative DVT in terms of efficacy without increasing the bleeding risk. This observation is based on the same meta-analyses from Nurmohamed et al (1992) and Leizorovicz et al (1992), and supported by the results from the meta-analysis of Jorgensen et al (1993). The analyses by Nurmohamed et al (1992) and Leizorovicz et al (1992) showed an overall reduction in the relative risk of DVT (RR 0.68, 95% CI 0.54–0.86; RR 0.83, 95% CI 0.68–1.02) and a more impressive 50% reduction in non-fatal PE after ortho-pedic surgery (RR 0.43, 95% CI 0.22–0.82; RR 0.53, 95% CI 0.27–1.03). Again, there was no increase in blood loss compared to UFH. According to the analysis by Jorgensen et al (1993), the reduction in PE by LMWH compared to UFH was comparable for elective and fractured hip surgery (which constitutes the majority of orthopedic procedures in the studies with LMWH).

4. Subcutaneous LMWH may be superior to UFH (intravenous or sub-

cutaneous) for the initial treatment of DVT (Leizorovicz et al 1994). In their meta-analysis Leizorovicz et al demonstrated that treatment with LMWH (mostly by the subcutaneous route) significantly reduced thrombus extension compared to UFH (odds ratio 0.51 (95% CI 0.32–0.83), $P = 0.006$) and also showed a trend towards fewer recurrent thromboembolic events (odds ratio 0.66 (95% CI 0.41–1.07), $P = 0.09$), while the risk of bleeding was not significantly reduced in those receiving LMWH versus UFH (odds ratio 0.65 (95% CI 0.36–1.16), $P = 0.15$). Further management studies will need to demonstrate whether this will also allow for home treatment of DVT and PE, which may substantially lower the costs.

5. LMWH are effective as anticoagulants in chronic hemodialysis, given as a single predialysis bolus injection; no other clear advantages over UFH have been observed (Nurmohamed et al 1991).

6. LMWH treatment may be associated with a lower incidence of thrombocytopenia, and fewer cases of 'heparin-induced thrombocytopenia' (HIT) and thrombosis, although it is not clear whether this is true for each LMWH (Hirsh & Levine 1992). No comparative data on the incidence of HIT associated with each of the LMWH are available yet.

Initial small studies investigated the potential of a LMW heparinoid in patients at high risk for, or actively, bleeding since animal studies showed this compound to be much safer than UFH in terms of blood loss (ten Cate et al 1988). Although these initial studies were successful in selected patients, where the heparinoid Org 10172 (a mixture of different glycosaminoglycans of LMW) was used to provide therapeutic anticoagulation, later studies showed that this compound produced a dose-dependent increase in postoperative blood loss at prophylactic doses (ten Cate et al 1987), which, although lower than with UFH, made it less likely that this compound would be substantially safer than UFH in clinical practice. Org 10172 may, however, be a suitable compound to replace UFH or LMWH in case of a HIT developing. The cumulative evidence indicates that in most cases antithrombotic treatment can be safely carried out, with recovery of the platelet count, after replacement with Org 10172 (Magnani 1993).

Currently, clinical studies are being carried out to assess the suitability of LMWH in neurosurgery, trauma surgery and stroke, and in specific arterial indications such as PTCA. In the latter condition, the use of UFH or LMWH is being studied also because of the possible inhibitory actions against smooth muscle cell proliferation (Buchwald et al 1992).

More recent developments include experimental studies with dermatan sulfate, heparan sulfate, low-affinity heparin, and a synthetic pentasaccharide. Dermatan sulfate is a glycosaminoglycan that acts as anticoagulant by potentiating the inhibitory action of heparin cofactor II against thrombin, and should therefore be considered an antithrombin drug. Animal studies showed that dermatan sulfate possesses antithrombotic activity at relatively high doses, but only minimally influences experimental bleeding (Fernandez et al 1986, Hoppensteadt et al 1990). Clinical studies (Agnelli et al 1992, Prandoni et al 1992) have shown that dermatan sulfate can be used for thrombosis prevention in high-risk patients; however, significant advantages over LMWH have not so far been demonstrated. Preliminary evidence suggests that the combination of a LMWH and dermatan sulfate may give additive antithrombotic activity in an animal model (Cosmi et al 1993).

Heparan sulfate and low-affinity (for antithrombin) heparin (LAH) have also been shown to possess significant antithrombotic activity in animal models. Heparan sulfate is currently being tested as an orally active preparation; however, its efficacy in man is not known. LAH inhibits thrombus formation, by antithrombin-independent pathways, most likely also through heparin cofactor II. Its efficacy in man is unknown.

For the near future, the clinical testing of the new synthetically prepared pentasaccharide and derivatives will be of interest. The pentasaccharide represents the minimal sequence required for heparin binding to antithrombin and for accelerating the inhibition of factor Xa (Olson et al 1992). The potential advantages are that it is chemically synthesized – and therefore of well-defined structure and in vitro potency – and will probably be much less immunogenic than UFH and LMWH. In animal models it has antithrombotic potency, which also demonstrates that the absence of antithrombin activity (because the pentasaccharide is too small to enhance inhibition of thrombin by antithrombin, lacking the thrombin-binding sequence) does not impair the antithrombotic activity (Walenga et al 1987, Carrie et al 1994). Factors that may be responsible for the antithrombotic mechanism of the pentasaccharide may include the factor Xa-mediated antiprothrombinase activity, and the unexplained reduced fibrin clot thrombogenicity (Vogel et al 1993).

AGENTS INHIBITING THE FACTOR VIIa–TF COMPLEX

In the present models of hemostasis and thrombosis, the factor VIIa–TF complex is the source of fibrin formation. From this point of view, interference in the factor VIIa–TF system represents a therapeutic possibility. The main problems with this strategy may be the lack of understanding of the in vivo distribution of TF under normal and pathological conditions and, more importantly, the physiological role of TF in vivo, in addition to its cofactor function in coagulation. The TF structure has strong similarity with a family of cytokine receptors and it is therefore possible that TF may be involved in immunologic responses of unknown nature (Edgington et al 1992). Certain organs such as the brain contain substantial amounts of TF, and it is possible that inhibition of its activity may result in excess bleeding. As far as its role in coagulation is concerned, a number of animal experiments, also in non-human primates, indicate that inhibition of the factor VIIa–TF complex effectively inhibits coagulation activation, or even DIC, in models of sepsis (Creasey et al 1993, Taylor 1993, Levi et al 1994, Biemond et al 1995). These studies were done with intact monoclonal antibodies, or Fab fragments, or the recombinant physiological inhibitor of the extrinsic system, tissue factor pathway inhibitor (TFPI). In animal models of DIC due to sepsis, or thrombosis, TFPI has been shown to be a potent anticoagulant (Wun 1992, Creasey et al 1993). Interestingly, its action is markedly accelerated by the presence of glycosaminoglycans; in fact, heparin or LMWH may act in part through endogenous TFPI (Haskel et al 1991). In view of the uncertainties about the physiological roles of TF, clinical trials with factor VIIa–TF inhibitors may be delayed. In certain life-threatening conditions such as sepsis, however, clinical testing of a substance like TFPI may be justified, given the substantial improvement observed in septic baboons treated with TFPI.

KEY POINTS FOR CLINICAL PRACTICE

- Current development of drugs aimed at specific sites within the coagulation cascade appears to gradually improve the antithrombotic potency of existing agents like heparin and aspirin. However, the therapeutic margins are small, and bleeding may unexpectedly occur at dose levels considered safe on the basis of preliminary clinical studies. Thus, improvement is expected to take place by only small increments in future.

- Selective platelet inhibitors such as GpIIb/IIIa blocking agents enhance the platelet inhibitory activity of aspirin in conditions with a high risk of thrombotic occlusion such as after PTCA.

- Thrombin inhibitors, such as hirudin, are potent anticoagulants in conditions associated with arterial and venous thrombosis (after hip surgery), however, optimal dose ranges still have to be established.

- Low molecular weight heparins offer enhanced protection against DVT and PE in high thrombotic risk situations such as hip surgery; they may also increase the efficacy of treatment for DVT/PE as compared to unfractionated heparin. The heparinoid Org 10172 is a good replacement drug for the treatment of heparin induced thrombocytopenia.

- Inhibition of the factor VII/TF mechanism may become an effective strategy for limiting DIC in sepsis.

REFERENCES

Agnelli G, Cosmi B, Di Filippo P et al 1992 A randomized, double blind, placebo-controlled trial of dermatan sulphate for prevention of deep vein thrombosis in hip fracture. Thromb Haemost 67: 203–208
Andersson L O, Barrowcliffe T W, Holmer E et al 1979 Molecular weight dependency of

the heparin potentiated inhibition of thrombin and activated factor X. Effect of heparin neutralization in plasma. Thromb Res 15: 531–541

Antiplatelet Trialists' Collaboration 1994 Collaborative overview of randomised trials of antiplatelet therapy–I: prevention of death, myocardial infarction, and stroke by prolonged antiplatelet therapy in various categories of patients. Br Med J 308: 81–106

Antman E M for the TIMI 9A Investigators 1994 Hirudin in acute myocardial infarction. Circulation 90: 1624–1630

Bellinger D A, Nichols T C, Read M S et al 1987 Prevention of occlusive coronary artery thrombosis by a murine monoclonal antibody to porcine vWF 1987 Proc Natl Acad Sci USA 84: 8100–8104

Biemond B J, Levi M, ten Cate H et al 1995 Complete inhibition of endotoxin-induced coagulation activation in chimpanzees with a monoclonal Fab fragment against factor VII/VIIa. Thromb Haemost 73: 223–230

Bode C, Hudelmayer M, Mehwald P et al 1994 Fibrin-targeted recombinant hirudin inhibits fibrin deposition on experimental clots more efficiently than recombinant hirudin. Circulation 90: 1956–1963

Boehrer J D, Kereiakes D J, Navetta F I et al for the EPIC Investigators 1994 Effects of profound platelet inhibition with c7E3 before coronary angioplasty on complications of coronary bypass surgery. Am J Cardiol 74: 1166–1170

Broze G J Jr 1992 The role of tissue factor pathway inhibitor in a revised coagulation cascade. Semin Hematol 29: 159–169

Buchwald A B, Unterberg C, Nebendahl K et al 1992 Low-molecular weight heparin reduces neointimal proliferation after coronary stent implantation in hypercholesterolemic minipigs. Circulation 86: 531–537

Cannon C P, McCabe C H, Henry T D et al 1994 A pilot trial of recombinant desulfatohirudin compared with heparin in conjunction with tissue-type plasminogen activator and aspirin for acute myocardial infarction: results of the thrombolysis in myocardial infarction (TIMI) 5 trial. J Am Coll Cardiol 23: 993–1003

Carrie D, Caranobe C, Saivin S et al 1994 Pharmacokinetic and antithrombotic properties of two pentasaccharides with high affinity to antithrombin III in the rabbit: comparison with CY 216. Blood 84: 2571–2577

Colman R W, Marder V J, Salzman E W, Hirsh J 1994 Overview of hemostasis. In: Colman R W, Hirsh J, Marder V J, Salzman E W (eds) Hemostasis and thrombosis: basic principles and clinical practice, 3rd edn. JB Lippincott, Philadelphia, pp 3–17

Cosmi B, Agnelli G, Young E et al 1993 The additive effect of low molecular weight heparins on thrombin inhibition by dermatan sulfate. Thromb Haemost 70: 443–447

Creasey A A, Chang A C K, Feigen L et al 1993 Tissue factor pathway inhibitor reduces moratlity from Escherichia coli septic shock. J Clin Invest 91: 2850–2860

Davie E W, Fujikawa K, Kisiel W 1991 The coagulation cascade: initiation, maintenance, and regulation. Biochemistry 30: 10363–10370

Edgington T S, Mackman N, Fan S T, Ruf W 1992 Cellular immune and cytokine pathways resulting in tissue factor expression and relevance to septic shock. Nouv Rev Fr Hematol 34: S15–S27

Esmon C T 1987 The regulation of natural anticoagulant pathways. Science 235: 1348–1352

Fernandez F, van Rijn J, Ofosu F A et al 1986 The haemorrhagic and antithrombotic effects of dermatan sulphate. Br J Haematol 64: 309–317

FitzGerald G A, Oates J A 1984 Selective and nonselective inhibition of thromboxane formation. Clin Pharmacol Ther 35: 633–640

Fox I, Dawson A, Loynds P et al 1993 Anticoagulant activity of Hirulog, a direct thrombin inhibitor, in humans. Thromb Haemost 69: 157–163

Gachet C, Stierle A, Cazenave J-P et al 1990 The thienopyridine PCR 4099 selectively inhibits ADP-induced platelet aggregation and fibrinogen binding without modifying the membrane glycoprotein IIb–IIIa complex in rat and in man. Biochem Pharmacol 40: 229–238

Ginsberg J S, Nurmohamed M, Gent M et al 1994 Use of hirulog in the prevention of venous thrombosis after major hip or knee surgery. Circulation 90: 2385–2389

Hara H, Kitajima A, Shimada H, Tamao Y 1991 Antithrombotic effect of MCI-9042, a new antiplatelet agent on experimental thrombosis models. Thromb Haemost 66: 484–488

Harker L A, Mann K G 1992 Thrombosis and fibrinolysis. In: Fuster V, Verstraete M (eds) Thrombosis in cardiovascular disorders. W B Saunders, Philadelphia

Harker L A, Maraganore J M, Hirsh J 1994 Novel antithrombotic agents. In: Colman R W, Hirsh J, Marder V M, Salzman E W (eds) Hemostasis and thrombosis: basic principles and clinical practice, 3rd edn. J B Lippincott, Philadelphia, pp 1638–1660

Haskel E J, Torr S R, Day K C et al 1991 Prevention of arterial reocclusion after thrombolysis with recombinant lipoprotein-associated coagulation inhibitor. Circulation 84: 821–827

Herbert J M, Bernat A, Barthelemy G et al 1993 Antithrombotic activity of SR 46349, a novel, potent and selective 5-HT2 receptor antagonist. Thromb Haemost 69: 262–267

Hirsh J, Levine M N 1992 Low molecular weight heparin. Blood 79: 1–17

Hoppensteadt D, Walenga J M, Fareed J 1990 Comparative antithrombotic and hemorrhagic effects of dermatan sulfate, heparan sulfate and heparin. Thromb Res 60: 191–200

Hung D T, Vu T-K, Wheaton V I et al 1992 Cloned platelet thrombin receptor is necessary for thrombin-induced platelet activation. J Clin Invest 89: 1350–1353

Jorgensen L N, Wille-Jorgensen P, Hauch O 1993 Prophylaxis of postoperative thromboembolism with low molecular weight heparins. Br J Surg 80: 689–704

Krupski W C, Bass A, Cadroy Y et al 1992 Antihemostatic and antithrombotic effects of monoclonal antibodies against vWF in nonhuman primates. Surgery 112: 433–439

Leizorovicz A, Haugh M C, Chapuis F-R et al 1992 Low molecular weight heparin in prevention of perioperative thrombosis. Br Med J 305: 913–920

Leizorovicz A, Simonneau G, Decousus H, Boissel J P 1994 Comparison of efficacy and safety of low molecular weight heparins and unfractionated heparin in initial treatment of deep vein thrombosis: a meta-analysis. Br Med J 309: 299–304

Levi M, ten Cate H, Bauer K A et al 1994 Inhibition of endotoxin-induced activation of coagulation and fibrinolysis by pentoxifylline or by a monoclonal anti-tissue factor antibody in chimpanzees. J Clin Invest 93: 114–120

Lidon R-M, Theroux P, Lesperance J et al 1994 A pilot, early angiographic patency study using a direct thrombin inhibitor as adjunctive therapy to streptokinase in acute myocardial infarction. Circulation 89: 1567–1572

Maffrand J P, Bernat A, Delebassee D et al 1988 ADP plays a key role in thrombogenesis in rats. Thromb Haemost 59: 225–230

Magnani H N 1993 Heparin-induced thrombocytopenia (HIT): an overview of 230 patients treated with Orgaran (Org 10172). Thromb Haemost 70: 554–561

Maraganore J M, Bourdon P, Jablonski J et al 1990 Design and characterization of hirulogs: a novel class of bivalent peptide inhibitors of thrombin. Biochemistry 29: 7095–7101

Marbet G A, Verstraete M, Kienast J et al 1993 Clinical pharmacology of intravenously administered recombinant desulfatohirudin (CGP 39393) in healthy volunteers. J Cardiovasc Pharmacol 22: 364–372

Markwardt F 1994 The development of hirudin as an antithrombotic drug. Thromb Res 74: 1–23

Meyer B L, Fernandez-Ortiz A, Mailhac A et al 1994 Local delivery of r-hirudin by a double balloon perfusion catheter prevents mural thrombosis and minimizes platelet deposition after angioplasty. Circulation 90: 2474–2480

Miller J L, Thiam-Cisse M, Drouet L O 1991 Reduction in thrombus formation by PG-1 F(ab')2, an anti-guinea pig platelet glycoprotein Ib monoclonal antibody. Arterioscler Thromb 11: 1231–1236

Morio H, Hirai A, Terano T et al 1993 Effect of the infusion of OKY-046, a thromboxane A2 synthase inhibitor, on urinary metabolites of prostacyclin and thromboxane A2 in healthy human subjects. Thromb Haemost 69: 276–281

Neuhaus K L, von Essen R, Tebbe U et al 1994 Safety observations from the pilot phase of the randomized r-hirudin for improvement of thrombolysis (HIT-III) study. Circulation 90: 1638–1642

Nicholson N S, Panzer-Knodle S G, Salyers A K et al 1995 SC-54684A: an orally active inhibitor of platelet aggregation. Circulation 91: 403–410

Nicolini F A, Lee P, Rios G et al 1994 Combination of platelet fibrinogen receptor antagonist and direct thrombin inhibitor at low doses markedly improves thrombolysis. Circulation 89: 1802–1809

Nurmohamed M T, ten Cate J, Stevens P et al 1991 Long-term efficacy and safety of a low molecular weight heparin in chronic hemodialysis patients. A comparison with standard heparin. ASAIO Trans 37: M459–461

Nurmohamed M T, Roosendaal F R, Buller H R et al 1992 Low-molecular weight heparin in general and orthopedic surgery: a meta analysis. Lancet 340: 152–156

Olson S T, Bjork I, Sheffer R et al 1992 Role of the antithrombin-binding pentasaccharide in heparin acceleration of antithrombin-proteinase reactions. J Biol Chem 267: 12528–12538

Parent F, Bridey F, Dreyfus M et al 1993 Treatment of severe venous thrombo-embolism with intravenous hirudin (HBW 023): an open pilot study. Thromb Haemost 70: 386–388

Prandoni P, Meduri F, Cuppini S et al 1992 Dermatan sulfate: a safe approach to prevention of postoperative deep vein thrombosis. Br J Surg 79: 505–509

Reilly I A G, FitzGerald G A 1987 Inhibition of thromboxane formation in vivo and ex vivo: implications for therapy with platelet inhibitory drugs. Blood 69: 180–186

Roth G J, Calverley D C 1994 Aspirin, platelets, and thrombosis: theory and practice. Blood 83: 885–898

Rothrock J F, Hart R G 1994 Ticlopedine hydrochloride use and threatened stroke. West J Med 160: 43–47

Savi P, Bernat A, Dumas A et al 1994 Effect of aspirin and clopidogrel on platelet-dependent tissue factor expression in endothelial cells. Thromb Res 73: 117–124

Schiele F, Vuillemenot A, Kramarz Ph et al 1994 A pilot study of subcutaneous recombinant hirudin (HBW 023) in the treatment of deep vein thrombosis. Thromb Haemost 71: 558–562

Schumacher W A, Heran C L, Steinbacher T E et al 1993 Superior activity of a thromboxane receptor antagonist as compared with aspirin in rat models of arterial and venous thrombosis. J Cardiovasc Pharmacol 22: 526–533

Simoons M L, de Boer J M, Brand M et al 1994 Randomized trial of a GpIIb/IIIa platelet receptor blocker in refractory unstable angina. Circulation 89: 596–603

Szczeklik A, Gryglewski R J, Nizankowski R et al 1978 Circulatory and antiplatelet effects of intravenous protacyclin in healthy men. Pharmacol Res Commun 10: 545–556

Taylor F B Jr 1993 Role of tissue factor in the coagulant and inflammatory response to LD100 E. coli sepsis and in the early diagnosis of DIC in the baboon. In: Berghaus G M, Madlener K, Blomback M, ten Cate J W (eds) DIC. Pathogenesis, diagnosis and therapy of disseminated intravascular fibrin formation. Excerpta Medica, Amsterdam, pp 19–31

Tcheng J E, Ellis S G, Kleiman N S et al 1993 Outcome of patients treated with the GPIIb/IIIa inhibitor integrelin during coronary angioplasty: results of the IMPACT study. Circulation 88 (suppl II): I-595

ten Cate H, Henny C P, ten Cate J W et al 1987 Randomized double-blind, placebo controlled safety study of a low molecular weight heparinoid in patients undergoing transurethral resection of the prostate. Thromb Haemost 57: 92–96

ten Cate H, Henny C P, ten Cate J W, Buller H R 1988 Clinical studies with low-molecular-weight heparin(oid)s: an interim analysis. Am J Hematol 27: 146–153

The EPIC Investigators 1994 Use of a monoclonal antibody directed against the platelet glycoprotein IIb/IIIa receptor in high-risk coronary angioplasty. N Engl J Med 330: 956–961

The GUSTO IIa Investigators 1994 Randomized trial of intravenous heparin versus recombinant hirudin for acute coronary syndromes. Circulation 90: 1631–1637

The RAPT Investigators 1993 Randomized trial of Ridogrel, a combined thromboxane A2 synthase inhibitor and thromboxane A2/prostaglandin endoperoxide receptor antagonist, versus aspirin as adjunct to thrombolysis in patients with acute myocardial infarction. Circulation 89: 588–595

Theroux P, White H, David D et al 1994 A heparin-controlled study of MK-383 in unstable angina. Circulation 90: 1242 (abstract)

Topol E J 1995 Novel antithrombotic approaches to coronary artery disease. Am J Cardiol 75: 27B–33B

Topol E, Califf R M, Weisman H F et al 1994a Randomised trial of coronary intervention with antibody against platelet IIb/IIIa integrin for reduction of clinical restenosis: results at six months. Lancet 343: 881–886

Topol E J, Fuster V, Harrington R A et al 1994b Recombinant hirudin for unstable angina pectoris. Circulation 89: 1557–1566

Van den Bos A A, Deckers J W, Heyndrickx G R et al 1993 Safety and efficacy of recombinant hirudin (CGP 39393) versus heparin in patients with stable angina undergoing coronary angioplasty. Circulation 88: 2058–2066

Vogel G M T, van Amsterdam R G M, Kop W J, Meuleman D G 1993 Pentasaccharide and Orgaran arrest, whereas heparin delays thrombus formation in a rat arteriovenous shunt. Thromb Haemost 69: 29–34

Walenga J M, Petitou M, Lormeau J C et al 1987 Antithrombotic activity of a synthetic heparin pentasaccharide in a rabbit stasis thrombosis model using different thrombogenic challenges. Thromb Res 46: 187–198

Wilson H C, Coffman W, Killam A L, Cohen M L 1991 L Y 53587, a 5-HT2 receptor antagonist, delays occlusion and inhibits platelet aggregation in a rabbit model of carotid artery occlusion. Thromb Haemost 66: 355–360

Wun T-C 1992 Lipoprotein-associated coagulation inhibitor (LACI) is a cofactor for heparin: synergistic anticoagulant action between LACI and sulfated polysaccharides. Blood 79: 430–438

12. von Willebrand disease and its diagnosis

D. J. Bowen   K. K. Hampton

The German professor Erik von Willebrand first described a dominantly inherited bleeding diathesis distinct from the haemophilias in several members of a family from the Foglo island of the Åland archipelago in the Gulf of Bosnia (von Willebrand 1926). Since then, the disorder, eponymously named von Willebrand disease (vWD), has been extensively studied physiologically, biochemically and genetically. The implicated protein, von Willebrand factor (vWF), has been characterized and its interactions with other components of the haemostatic system have been defined. The gene encoding vWF has been cloned, the mRNA has been sequenced and expressed in vitro and, in recent years, mutations underlying vWD have been revealed. While our understanding of the molecular pathophysiology of the less common types of vWD has increased impressively and the list of mutations causing disease is expanding rapidly, there is decreasing certainty regarding the diagnosis, inheritance and molecular genetics of the commoner forms of vWD.

This chapter overviews the biology, diagnosis, classification and investigation of vWD and highlights some of the issues yet to be resolved in the study of this disorder. More detailed reviews include those of Coller (1987), Ruggeri & Ware (1992) and Tuddenham & Cooper (1994).

VON WILLEBRAND FACTOR

Protein biochemistry

vWF is a large, polymeric (multimeric) glycoprotein synthesized in endothelial cells (Jaffe et al 1974) and megakaryocytes (Nachman et al 1977), but also found in plasma, platelets and the subendothelial matrix. The primary translation product is 2813 amino acids and comprises a signal peptide (prepeptide) of 22 residues, a propolypeptide of 741 residues and a mature subunit of 2050 residues (Fig. 12.1A) (Verweij et al 1986, Bonthron et al 1986a). Pre-pro-vWF contains four types of internal homology: three copies of an A domain, three copies of a B domain, two copies of a C domain, and four copies plus one partial copy of a D domain (Fig. 12.1A)

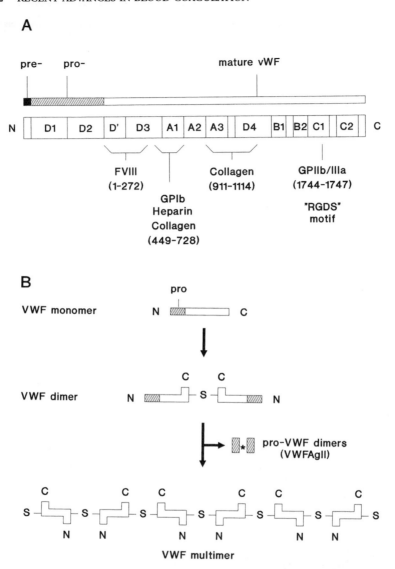

Fig. 12.1 von Willebrand factor. **A** Structural and binding domains. Structural domains are represented by A1 to D4 within the protein bar, binding domains are indicated below it. Bracketed numbers beneath the binding domains indicate the amino acid residues of mature vWF which contain the domains. 'RGDS' signifies arginine-glycine-aspartate-serine, the peptide motif common to platelet GPIIb/IIIa ligands. Pre-, pro- and mature vWF (■, ▨ and □ respectively) are delineated above the protein bar. **B** Schematic outline of vWF multimerization. vWF monomers form dimers covalently joined at their C-termini by disulphide bonds. Dimers polymerize via their N-termini and pro-vWF is proteolytically removed as dimeric units (vWF:AgII) leaving the mature vWF multimer.

(Shelton-Inloes et al 1987a). After cleavage of the signal peptide, pro-vWF undergoes dimerization through specific C-terminal cysteine residues, and the dimers then undergo polymerization (multimerization) through specific disulphide linkages at their N-termini (Fig. 12.1B) (Wagner & Marder 1984). Following multimerization, the propolypeptide is excised, becoming vWF antigen II (vWFAgII). The multimers, which contain upwards of 20 dimeric units, are constitutively secreted by endothelial cells into the subendothelium and plasma or are packaged into Weibel–Palade bodies, a storage organelle from which vWF can be released by physiological stress or desmopressin. In megakaryocytes, vWF is directed into the alpha-granules of forming platelets. The post-translational processing and multimerization of vWF have been reviewed in Wagner (1989) and Verweij (1988).

Biological activity

In primary haemostasis, vWF supports platelet interaction with exposed subendothelial matrices at sites of vascular damage by specific, high-affinity binding to both components. In addition, vWF acts as a carrier molecule for coagulation factor VIII, protecting it from premature proteolytic degradation and delivering it directly to the site of need. The half-life of factor VIII in the circulation is increased 4-fold by its non-covalent association with vWF (Tuddenham et al 1982).

vWF has four physiologically important binding activities which underlie the above functions: it binds subendothelial matrix (collagen) (Pareti et al 1987), platelet glycoprotein Ib (GPIb) (Martin et al 1980), platelet glycoprotein IIb/IIIa (GPIIb/IIIa) (Girma et al 1986) and factor VIII (Foster et al 1987). In addition, heparin-binding sites have been identified (Fujimura et al 1987) but their physiological importance is unclear. The binding sites have been localized within the mature subunit (Fig. 12.1A).

The order of molecular events during primary haemostasis is uncertain; however, the initial step is probably attachment of vWF to collagen (and possibly other matrix components). This induces a change in the GPIb-binding domain of vWF which permits its interaction with platelet GPIb. This interaction does not occur spontaneously in plasma, but can be induced by the obsolete antibiotic ristocetin (Howard & Firkin 1971) and the snake venom botrocetin (Read et al 1989), which are used diagnostically to test vWF-mediated platelet agglutination in vitro.

Binding of vWF to the second platelet receptor, GPIIb/IIIa, appears to be a subsequent event, occuring after the platelet is stimulated. The RGDS motif (see Fig. 12.1A, legend) via which vWF binds to GPIIb/IIIa is also found on fibrinogen, which is a second ligand for the platelet receptor. Although fibrinogen is present in far greater concentrations than vWF in plasma, it appears that vWF is important in GPIIb/IIIa binding at high shear-stress (Weiss et al 1978).

It has been suggested that the highest molecular weight multimers of vWF represent the most biologically active forms because (1) they represent the highest density of biological activities, (2) underpolymerized vWF is ineffective in platelet agglutination in vitro, and (3) some factor VIII concentrates contain predominantly lower molecular weight multimers and do not correct the bleeding time in vWD (Weinstein & Deykin 1979). However, data obtained using an ex vivo model system suggest that multimers of different size are equally capable of supporting the adhesion of platelets to the subendothelium (Sixma et al 1984).

The vWF GENE (*VWF*)

VWF is located distally on the short arm of chromosome 12 at 12p12–12pter (Verweij et al 1985). The gene is approximately 178 kb (kilobase) in length and contains 52 exons ranging in size from 40 bp (base pairs) to 1379 bp (Mancuso et al 1989). The 51 introns vary from 97 bp to 19.9 kb in length. A portion of the gene, spanning exons 23–34, is duplicated on chromosome 22 at 22q11.22–q11.23 (Shelton-Inloes et al 1987b). The duplicated region shares 97% nucleotide homology with *VWF* but contains splice site, frameshift and nonsense mutations, which prevent its expression and indicate that it represents an incomplete, unprocessed vWF pseudogene (Mancuso et al 1991). *VWF* is rich in polymorphisms; more than 20 have been reported, the majority being nucleotide dimorphisms giving rise to restriction fragment length polymorphisms (compiled in Sadler and Ginsburg 1993). These are scattered throughout the gene. Additionally, there are highly polymorphic variable number tandem repeat (VNTR) sequences: in the 5' promoter region a (GT)n VNTR (Zhang et al 1992) and in intron 40 an extensive (ATCT)n VNTR (Standen et al 1990, Ploos van Amstel & Reitsma 1990, Mercier et al 1991). This plethora of well-distributed polymorphic loci provide a highly informative foundation for linkage analyses in families affected with vWD.

Transcription of *VWF* takes place in endothelial cells and megakaryocytes – the sites of vWF synthesis. The mature transcript is 8825 nucleotides long and comprises an open reading frame of 8439 nucleotides (encoding the 2813 amino acids of pre-pro-vWF) flanked by a 5' untranslated region of 250 nucleotides and a 3' untranslated region of 136 nucleotides (Sadler et al 1985, Bonthron et al 1986b). vWF mRNA is also found in platelets, and provides a readily available source of message for molecular studies following reverse transcription to cDNA (Nichols et al 1991). This circumvents the problems of manipulating at the level of genomic DNA such a large gene with multiple exons and introns.

VON WILLEBRAND DISEASE

vWD results from a deficiency or dysfunction (or both) of vWF and is primarily an inherited disorder, although rare cases of acquired disease (acquired von Willebrand syndrome) have been reported. Inherited vWD is subdivided into three categories which reflect pathophysiology: type 1 vWD refers to partial quantitative deficiency of vWF; type 2 vWD refers to qualitative deficiency of vWF (with possible associated quantitative deficiency); type 3 vWD refers to virtually complete deficiency of vWF. Type 1 vWD is the most prevalent form, accounting for approximately 75% or so of patients. Types 2 and 3 vWD are much less common, respectively occurring in approximately 20% and 5% of patients (Colvin et al 1986).

Nomenclature

Until recently, the nomenclature used in the classification of vWD employed the Roman numerals I, II and III to denote the primary vWD types (Ruggeri & Zimmerman 1987a,b) and a combination of Arabic letters, numbers or toponyms to indicate a particular subtype. This nomenclature had certain strengths, for example the primary categories of type I, II and III bore a clear relationship to pathophysiology, vWF biochemistry, type of genetic lesion and clinical behaviour. Similarly, certain subcategories (e.g. IIA and IIB) were easily recognized and were clinically useful. However, the nomenclature did have a number of evolving problems. For example, the ever-increasing list of vWD variants had become a confusion of names with inconsistent derivations which often gave no insight into the pathophysiology. Additionally, the nomenclature did not accommodate compound heterozygosity nor did it have provision for the rapidly expanding molecular diagnosis of vWD.

A revised classification of vWD has recently been introduced (Sadler 1994) which addresses the problems of the previous system. The new classification defines vWD as a bleeding disorder caused by mutations at the vWF locus. The Arabic numerals 1, 2 and 3 respectively define the primary categories of partial quantitative, qualitative and virtually complete deficiency of vWF. Type 2 is subdivided into four categories: 2A refers to qualitative variants with decreased platelet-dependent function that is associated with the absence of high molecular weight vWF multimers; 2B refers to all qualitative variants with increased affinity for GPIb; 2M refers to qualitative variants with decreased platelet-dependent function that is not caused by the absence of high molecular weight vWF multimers; 2N refers to all qualitative variants with markedly decreased affinity for factor VIII. Toponyms may be added to identify individual families (e.g. vWD type 2A Miami). Compound heterozygosity is indicated by a double classification separated by a slash (e.g. 1/2N).

Molecular defects are specified by amino acid position, numbered 1–2813 from the initiator methionine of pre-pro-vWF to its carboxy-terminus, or by nucleotide number in the cDNA, assigning +1 to the major transcription cap site 250 nucleotides before the A of the initiator methionine

ATG. Genomic DNA numbering is not yet defined since this is expected to change with the prevailing state of knowledge. The representation of mutations essentially follows the standard nomenclature laid down for factor VIII and factor IX (Peake & Tuddenham 1994); for example, substitution of arginine 91 for glutamine is R91Q (single-letter amino acid code) or the substitution of thymine 4935 for cytosine is T4935C. Where known, the molecular defect can be appended to the phenotypic classification to give a full descriptor (e.g. vWD type 2M Vicenza R1308C; Randi et al 1993).

Related disorders, such as platelet-type vWD (Miller & Castella 1982) or pseudo-vWD (Weiss et al 1982), which are not due to a defect in the vWF gene are designated 'pseudo-vWD'. This can be prefixed by a qualifier if appropriate (e.g. platelet-type pseudo-vWD). Acquired, non-inherited disorders that mimic vWD are referred to as 'acquired von Willebrand syndrome'.

The new nomenclature greatly facilitates vWD classification and eliminates the confusion which was evolving with the previous system which had been introduced at a time when the need to standardize the naming of vWF variants did not exist.

Clinical diagnosis

vWD is classically characterized by the triad of a clinical history of mucocutaneous bleeding, a pattern of autosomal dominant inheritance and positive confirmatory laboratory tests. There are, however, significant problems apparent in each of these areas. The incidence of vWD is uncertain. Older studies only included patients with severe disease and so underestimated the incidence at 0.3–0.4 per thousand. Population screening studies have suggested an incidence of up to 1% (Rodeghiero et al 1987), although the incidence of symptomatic disease has been estimated at approximately one-eighth of this (Sadler & Gralnick 1994). The incidence of the severe autosomally recessive inherited type 3 disease is quoted at 0.5–5.3 per million (Mannucci et al 1984), suggesting that the heterozygous form of this condition will be present in approximately 1–5 per 1000 people. Whilst the diagnosis of vWD is relatively straightforward in the more severe forms (and especially in the less common type 2 and type 3 disease), there remains a very real problem of correct diagnosis in the commonest type 1 disease. It is obviously important not to diagnose incorrectly normal individuals who do not have a bleeding condition, but conversely it is important to diagnose and classify correctly those who do have a bleeding condition so they can be treated appropriately with desmopressin or concentrate if necessary.

In all forms of vWD, bleeding is lifelong and is usually first apparent during childhood, but in milder forms the disease may only become manifest at times of severe challenge to the haemostatic system. Bleeding tends to be primarily mucocutaneous, with epistaxis, gingival bleeding, easy bruising, menorrhagia and bleeding after dental extraction being common, while spontaneous bleeding into muscles or joints, as seen in severe haemophilia, is unusual except in the most severe, type 3, disease. However, clinical history alone has relatively poor sensitivity (65%) and specificity (75%) for the diagnosis of vWD, which is illustrated by the observation that a positive bleeding history has been found in 23% of unaffected persons (Miller et al 1979a).

As discussed later, inheritance in type 1, 2A and 2B disease is usually autosomal dominant, and autosomal recessive in type 2N and type 3. This does not take into account compound heterozygosity which may be far more common than previously supposed (Eikenboom et al 1993), and in studies in patients with type 1 disease it would appear that penetrance is variable since individuals with no bleeding history and normal laboratory tests exist who have both an affected parent and affected children (Miller et al 1979a).

Type 2N vWD mimics mild haemophilia. Factor VIII levels are low; however, bleeding time and phenotypic vWF parameters are all normal (see section on Phenotypic diagnosis). Indeed, this autosomal, recessively inherited condition is far removed from the classical phenotype of vWD (Mazurier 1992).

Differential diagnosis should include quantitative and qualitative platelet disorders together with deficiencies of most of the proteins of the coagulation cascade. The finding of vWD in the absence of a previous bleeding history and with negative family studies should raise the possibility of acquired von Willebrand syndrome and initiate a search for an associated underlying vascular disorder or lymphoproliferative condition.

Phenotypic diagnosis

Laboratory-based diagnosis of vWD comprises screening tests and specific investigations to confirm the diagnosis and allow correct classification. Screening tests are notoriously lacking in sensitivity and specificity, particularly in milder type 1 disease (Miller et al 1979b). In the presence of a positive bleeding history or family history the finding of normal screening tests, such as the bleeding time and KCCT (kaolin cephalin clotting time), does not exclude the diagnosis of vWD, and specific tests should be performed. Except in type 2B disease and platelet-type pseudo-vWD, platelet count and morphology should be normal. It must be remembered that both vWF and factor VIII are acute phase proteins and levels can be transiently elevated into the normal range by stress, exercise and also pregnancy and oestrogen-containing oral contraceptives. Consequently, repeated testing may be necessary before a diagnosis can be established. There does appear to be significant intrapatient variability in tests over time (Abildgaard et al 1980).

The following phenotypic tests are particularly informative in the diagnosis of vWD and in refining the vWD subtype: bleeding time, vWF anti-gen (vWF:Ag), ristocetin cofactor activity (RiCoF), multimeric profile of plasma and platelet vWF, factor VIII activity (VIII:C), factor VIII antigen (VIII:Ag), factor VIII binding capacity and ristocetin sensitivity (RIPA). It should be remembered that, with the exception of the bleeding time, the other phenotypic tests are static in vitro assays which do not reproduce the dynamic, high shear environment of the microcirculation in which vWF functions in vivo. The information provided by many of these tests is im-mediately apparent, however, RiCoF, RIPA, multimer profile and factor VIII binding activity are worthy of additional comment.

RiCoF.   vWF agglutinates platelets in the presence of ristocetin (Howard & Firkin 1971). The RiCoF assay measures the ability of a test plasma to induce agglutination of a standardized platelet suspension in a fixed con-centration of ristocetin which is in excess of the threshold required for agglutination. It is actually the rate of agglutination which is measured and this is expressed as the percentage dilution required of a standardized con-trol plasma to obtain the same rate. RiCoF is absent in type 3 vWD, de-creased in type 1, decreased in type 2A and variable in type 2B, 2M and 2N.

RIPA.   The RIPA assay (ristocetin-induced platelet agglutination) meas-ures the ability of a test plasma to induce platelet agglutination in decreas-ing concentrations of ristocetin. RIPA is altered in type 2B vWD due to the increased affinity of 2B vWF for GPIb; platelet agglutination is induced at a much lower concentration of ristocetin than is normally required (Ruggeri et al 1980). In other types of vWD, RIPA is generally not altered. The absence of vWF antigen in type 2 vWD makes RIPA a redundant assay for this vWD subtype.

Multimer profile.   The plasma vWF multimer profile is one of the major diagnostic criteria of vWD (Sadler 1994). In type 1 vWD the multimer profile is qualitatively normal but quantitatively decreased, each multimer band having reduced levels of antigen (Fig. 12.2). In type 2A vWD, me-dium to high molecular weight multimers are missing and there may be anomalies in the triplet structure – for example, a quantitative increase in the fastest migrating band of each triplet (Fig. 12.2). In type 2B vWD the high molecular weight multimers are absent and there may be a quantita-tive change in any of the three bands of each triplet (Fig. 12.2). In type 2M vWD all multimer size ranges are represented, but there is a qualitative change in the triplet pattern – for example, the satellite bands may be missing or a doublet and not a triplet may be observed. In type 2N vWD the multimer profile is normal. Type 3 vWD plasma gives no detectable vWF multimers.

Platelet vWF multimer profiles are not commonly requested for diagno-sis. Type 1 vWD can be either platelet-normal (plasma vWF:Ag low but platelet vWF:Ag and RiCoF normal), or platelet-low (plasma vWF:Ag low, platelet vWF:Ag and RiCoF low), or platelet-discordant (plasma vWF:Ag low, platelet vWF:Ag normal but platelet RiCoF decreased) (Mannucci

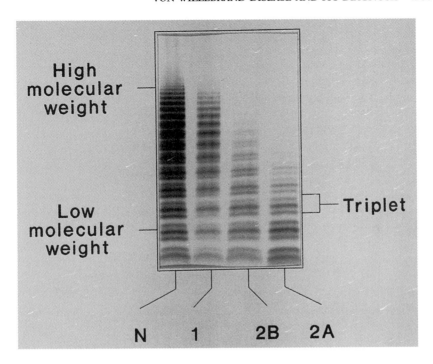

Fig. 12.2 Multimeric profiles of plasma vWF. N, normal plasma; 1, type 1 vWD plasma; 2B, type 2B vWD plasma; 2A, type 2A vWD plasma. Multimers were visualized by immunostaining with alkaline phosphatase conjugated antibody (Goodwin et al 1992).

et al 1985). The platelet multimer profile in type 2A vWD is similar to that observed in 2A plasma, with an absence of medium and high molecular weight forms (Ruggeri & Zimmerman 1980). In contrast, in 2B vWD the platelet multimer profile is normal and shows the high molecular weight forms which are missing in 2B plasma (Ruggeri & Zimmerman 1980). Platelet vWF antigen is not detected in type 3 vWD.

Factor VIII binding activity. The ability of vWF to bind factor VIII is mostly relevant in type 2N vWD. This subcategory was first recognized in a patient who possessed normal vWF parameters but decreased levels of circulating factor VIII (Nishino et al 1989). This was found to be due to a mutation in the factor VIII binding site of vWF and the mutant vWF was given the toponym 'Normandy variant' to reflect the geographic origin of the patient. Under the new nomenclature, the Normandy has been abbreviated to 'N'. The factor VIII binding assay measures the affinity of vWF for factor VIII and is illustrated in Figure 12.3. Anti-vWF antibody is coated on the wells of a microtitre plate and test plasma is added to the well. The factor VIII–vWF complex from the plasma is bound by the antibody following which factor VIII is removed from the complex by a high ionic

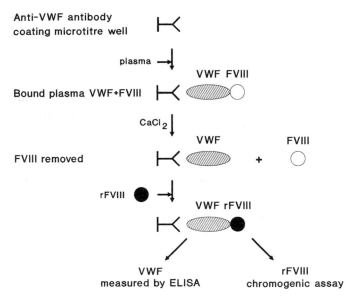

Fig. 12.3   Schematic representation of the factor VIII–vWF binding assay. Plasma factor VIII–vWF is immobilized in the well of a microtitre plate by anti-vWF antibody. Factor VIII is removed using a high ionic strength buffer and replaced by recombinant factor VIII (rVIII). vWF and bound rVIII are then respectively measured using ELISA and a chromogenic assay.

strength buffer. Excess recombinant factor VIII (rVIII) is then added and, after removal of unbound rVIII, the vWF and its bound rVIII are assayed. An ELISA (enzyme-linked immunosorbent assay) is used to measure vWF:Ag and a chromogenic assay is used to determine VIII:C. The ratio of VIII:C to vWF:Ag is decreased in type 2N vWD due to a decrease in the amount of factor VIII bound by vWF.

The factor VIII binding assay can permit type 2N vWD to be distinguished from mild to moderate haemophilia A. In the latter, the factor VIII binding capacity of vWF should be intact and a normal ratio of VIII:C to vWF:Ag should be obtained in the assay. There is a small but finite possibility of mild/moderate haemophilia A occurring in conjunction with type 2N vWD. Measurement of VIII:Ag in the patient's plasma may help resolve this since, in mild/moderate haemophilia A, VIII:Ag and VIII:C are usually not decreased in parallel.

In the phenotypic assessment of vWD, determination of bleeding time, vWF:Ag and RiCoF alone may yield a diagnosis; however, the inclusion of additional parameters where possible should provide a more precise picture of the patient's disorder. Accurate diagnosis is particularly relevant in type 2 disease since the four subcategories 2A, 2B, 2M and 2N have distinctive clinical implications which may influence treatment.

A further factor which is important in the assessment of the diagnosis of vWD is blood group. A number of studies have shown that plasma vWF:Ag levels differ significantly between blood groups, in the rank order O < A < B < AB (Gill et al 1987, Rodeghiero et al 1987). The significance of this is that the molecular basis for apparent type 1 vWD in symptomatic individuals of blood group O may not lie within the vWF gene and may actually not be due to a gene defect per se. This has implications for inheritance and for classification but should not influence the approach to treatment. It is noteworthy that, in one large study, the proportions of blood groups O (77%), A (18%), B (4%), and AB (0%) were significantly different among type 1 patients compared with those observed in the normal population (45%, 45%, 7% and 3% respectively) (Gill et al 1987).

Genetics

Inheritance

It is generally stated that type 1 and type 2 vWD show autosomal dominant inheritance, whilst type 3 vWD is recessive. It is becoming increasingly apparent that this represents an oversimplification of a more complicated reality. The inheritance patterns observed for vWD (especially type 1) can be confused by undetected compound heterozygosity, variable penetrance, and the effect of blood group on phenotypic expression.

Classical type 1 vWD shows autosomal dominant inheritance and significantly decreased vWF levels (Miller et al 1979a). However, the molecular defect(s) responsible for this form of disease remain undiscovered. Silent alleles, premature stop codons and partial/whole gene deletions have been forwarded as type 1 defects (Eikenboom et al 1993, compiled in Ginsburg & Sadler 1993); however, these probably represent type 3 defects which, in combination with a normal allele, may give rise to borderline or reduced vWF levels, and account for recessively inherited type 1 disease. Paradoxically, both dominant and recessive inheritance have been observed within single families with type 1 disease and this may be due to unrecognized compound heterozygosity. It still remains to be established that type 1 vWD is invariably a consequence of a defect of the vWF gene.

Type 2 vWD may be dominant or recessive. Type 2A and 2B are primarily dominant (Ginsburg 1991) and 2N is recessive, only being symptomatic in homozygous or compound heterozygous form (Mazurier 1992).

Type 3 vWD consistently shows recessive inheritance (Ginsburg 1991) and can result from homozygous or compound heterozygous gene defects which negate expression of a gene product (compiled in Ginsburg & Sadler 1993). As discussed above, carriers of type 3 defects may have borderline/decreased vWF levels, but usually they are asymptomatic with vWF levels within the normal range.

Gene defects

A heterogeneous mixture of mutations has been characterized in type 2 and type 3 vWD (compiled in Ginsburg & Sadler 1993). In type 2 vWD the majority of defects are missense point mutations. Those causing type 2A vWD are clustered in exon 28 and bring about amino acid substitutions in the A2 homologous domain of vWF. These amino acid substitutions may cause defective intracellular transport of vWF, resulting in a quantitative decrease in vWF secretion and selective loss of the larger multimers (group 1) (Dent et al 1990), or they may increase the sensitivity of vWF to proteolysis, also resulting in loss of larger multimers (group 2) (Lyons et al 1992). Type 2B mutations are also clustered within exon 28 and these bring about amino acid substitutions in the GPIb binding domain of the A1 homologous repeat of vWF. Surprisingly, 2B mutations do not result in loss of function but cause the mutant vWF to bind spontaneously to GPIb, with the consequential loss of high molecular weight multimers from the plasma. This explains the characteristic multimer profile in type 2B vWD (Fig. 12.2) and the tendency for thrombocytopenia, which is exacerbated by desmopressin.

Mutations underlying type 2N vWD are clustered within the factor VIII binding site of vWF (compiled in Ginsburg & Sadler 1993). They comprise missense point mutations whose resultant amino acid substitutions interfere with factor VIII–vWF interactions. A variety of mechanisms may explain this; for example, perturbation of protein structure, loss of binding interactions between vWF and factor VIII, or simple steric hindrance. Whatever the mechanism, type 2N vWF has decreased affinity for factor VIII and this results in decreased levels of circulating factor VIII.

Various mutations have been reported in type 3 vWD, including whole and partial gene deletions and nonsense point mutations (compiled in Ginsburg & Sadler 1993). These defects have in common lack of expression of a gene product. When inherited alongside a normal vWF allele, a normal or mild type 1 phenotype may result. However, when inherited in homozygous or compound heterozygous form with a second type 3 defect, type 3 disease results. Type 3 vWD appears to be consistent in showing recessive inheritance. The development of alloantibody inhibitors to vWF occurs, but not invariably, in patients with deletion mutations (Shelton-Inloes et al 1987b).

In type 1 vWD, heterozygosity for a type 3 gene defect and a normal vWF allele has been demonstrated in a small number of cases (Eikenboom et al 1993). However, the molecular basis for type 1 vWD in the majority of patients does not appear to be of the 'type 3 carrier' kind and remains to be revealed.

The accumulating list of mutations characterized in vWD is compiled and updated in a database which also contains information on polymorphisms of the vWF gene. The database is coordinated by Dr David Ginsburg of the University of Michigan Medical School and can be accessed on the World Wide Web (Internet WEB page: http://mmg2.im.med.umich.edu/vWF) or by E-Mail (address: vwfdb@umich.edu or vwfdb-help@umich.edu).

Genetic diagnosis

There are two main approaches to the genetic diagnosis of vWD: direct mutation detection (DMD) and linkage analysis. Neither represents a first-line investigation for diagnosis, but both can support a clinical and phenotypic diagnosis with considerable precision.

Direct mutation detection

DMD is most applicable in type 2A, type 2B and type 2N vWD, in each of which mutations cluster within a limited region of the vWF coding sequence: type 2A and 2B mutations cluster within exon 28, and type 2N mutations cluster within the first 272 codons of mature vWF. The latter are encoded across several exons spanning several kilobases of genomic DNA, but are contained within 816 nucleotides of the mRNA, which therefore represents an easier target for mutation screening following conversion to cDNA by reverse transcription.

A standard approach to DMD is to amplify the relevant target regions of genomic DNA (or cDNA) using the polymerase chain reaction (PCR) and then to screen the PCR products for the presence of a mutation using any of a number of techniques such as chemical mismatch cleavage. Once a mutation is located, the relevant stretch of DNA can be sequenced to determine the genetic change involved. This approach has the advantage of thoroughly screening for the presence of a mutation, but has the disadvantage that the work involved is considerable and far removed from a routine diagnostic test.

A second approach is the use of universal heteroduplex generator (UHG) technology, which has been applied successfully in type 2B vWD (Wood et al 1995) and which is being developed for type 2A vWD (Standen 1995). The principle of the approach is outlined in Figure 12.4. A synthetic strand of DNA corresponding to the target region of the gene acts as a UHG. This has built-in sequence changes which yield heteroduplexes of different mobilities when hybridized to a normal target sequence and a mutant target sequence. The target sequences are generated from the genomic DNA using the PCR.

UHG screening is extremely useful when a small number of mutations in a confined region of the gene account for the majority of patients. Such is the case in type 2A, 2B and 2N vWD: the 1993 edition of the vWF database (Ginsburg & Sadler 1993) lists 14 missense point mutations in type 2A vWD, of which four (Gly742Glu, Ser743Leu, Arg834Trp and Arg834Gln) account for 58% of patients characterized so far; in type 2B

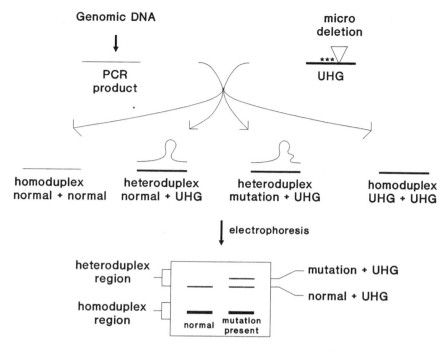

Fig. 12.4   The principle of direct mutation detection using universal heteroduplex genera-tors (UHG). A synthetic polynucleotide (UHG) corresponding to the target region of genomic DNA to be screened is synthesized containing specific sequence alterations (e.g. a microdeletion) vicinal to the mutation cluster site (***). The UHG is hybridized with PCR product amplified from the target region of a patient's genomic DNA. The heteroduplexes formed differ according to the presence or absence of a mutation and according to the location and nature of a mutation. These differences are reflected in the electrophoretic mobilities of the heteroduplexes in suitable gel systems. The sequence alterations introduced into the UHG magnify the change in electrophoretic mobility of a heteroduplex containing a mutation. The results obtained for autosomal genes, such as the vWF gene, usually reflect the presence of one normal and one mutant allele.

vWD, ten missense point mutations are compiled, of which four (Arg543Trp, Arg545Cys, Val553Met and Arg578Gln) are present in 75% of patients; and in type 2N vWD, five missense point mutations are listed, of which two are present in 75% of patients.

UHG screening does have a number of weaknesses:

- The target region screened is limited in size and is highly localized; there-fore mutations lying outside this region will be missed.

- A mutation may be detected within the target region, but a second mu-tation outside this region (which may attenuate or exacerbate the effect of the first) will be missed.

- Novel mutations, which the UHG is not designed to detect, may go undetected.

Linkage analysis

In the absence of a characterized mutation within a family, linkage analysis permits a defective vWF gene to be tracked, thereby corroborating phenotypic diagnosis. The most highly informative intragenic markers – the 5' (GT)nVNTR (Zhang et al 1992) and the intron 40 (ATCT)nVNTRs (Standen et al 1990, Ploos van Amstel & Reitsma 1990, Mercier et al 1991) – can be analysed using the PCR, as can many of the remaining RFLP loci; therefore linkage analysis in vWD can be achieved rapidly and efficiently from small quantities of DNA. Appropriate care should be taken in the interpretation of genetic data obtained from the portion of the vWF gene which is duplicated in the pseudogene. Genetic diagnosis of vWD using linkage is only possible in the context of a family study and could be used for prenatal diagnosis, although this is rarely requested.

CONCLUDING REMARKS

vWD has presented a great challenge to clinicians and scientists alike since its initial description by von Willebrand in 1926. The complexities of this disorder have really only just begun to be unravelled and we are still far from a comprehensive understanding of its molecular pathophysiology. Indeed, many basic questions remain unanswered. For example:

- Is the vWF in the subendothelium protected from collagen or bound by collagen and primed for interaction with GPIb?

- Whether bound or unbound to collagen, what is the turnover rate of vWF in the subendothelium and how is turnover achieved?

- Why do plasma vWF multimers apparently circulate in a range of sizes?

- How is the factor VIII load on vWF regulated? Type 1 vWD often shows normal VIII:C levels despite decreased vWF:Ag, suggesting an increased loading of factor VIII.

- What is the molecular basis for type 1 vWD in patients who do not appear to carry a type 3 defect?

- How does blood group affect vWF levels and could the answer to this question underlie classic type 1 vWD?

These apparently simple questions remind us that there are fundamental aspects of vWD which are yet to be understood. However, considerable progress has been made in many areas, especially in the molecular genetics of vWD. Both vWD and vWF promise many further insights to reward their continued investigation and they offer plenty of scope for quality research. The results should not only be clinically and scientifically relevant but should also greatly enhance our understanding of the haemostatic arena.

KEY POINTS FOR CLINICAL PRACTICE

- Diagnosis of vWD depends upon a history of mucocutaneous bleeding along with a family history consistent with dominant inheritance and characteristic laboratory investigations.

- The classification of vWD has recently been revised into types 1, 2 and 3 depending upon the results of investigative tests.

- Accurate identification of the type of vWD is important because treatment depends on the diagnosis, e.g. DDAVP may be useful for type 1, but not type 2A patients; it is contraindicated for those with type 2B.

- For diagnosis measurement of bleeding time, vWF antigen, ristocetin co-factor activity and FVIII are essential in all patients. The multimer profile of plasma vWF, ristocetin induced platelet agglutination, the binding of factor VIII to vWF and platelet vWF assessments may aid accurate diagnosis.

- A detailed pedigree may aid diagnosis as types 1 and 2 are usually dominantly inherited. Type 1 may, however, be due to compound heterozygosity and have variable penetrance. Type 2A and 2B are usually dominantly inherited whereas 2N is recessive. Type 3 may be homozygous or compound heterozygous.

- A large variety of different genetic mutations cause vWD. Those with type 2A and 2B are usually due to point mutations in exon 28; while 2N is due to a mis-sense mutation in the factor VIII binding site. Type 3 is characterised by whole, or partial, gene deletion and non-sense point mutations.

- Direct mutation detection and linkage analysis within a family can be used to support and clarify a clinical and phenotypic diagnosis.

REFERENCES

Abildgaard C F, Suzuki Z, Harrison J et al 1980 Serial studies in von Willebrand's disease: variability versus 'variants'. Blood 56: 712–716
Bonthron D T, Handin R I, Kaufman R J et al 1986a Structure of pre-pro-von Willebrand factor and its expression in heterologous cells. Nature 324: 270–273
Bonthron D, Orr E C, Mitsock L M et al 1986b Nucleotide sequence of pre-pro-vWF cDNA. Nucleic Acids Res 14: 7125–7127
Coller B S 1987 von Willebrand disease. In: Colman R W, Hirsh J, Marder V J, Salzman E W (eds) Haemostasis and thrombosis. Lippincott, Philadelphia, pp 60–96
Colvin B T, O'Callaghan U, Thomas U et al 1986 A survey of von Willebrand's disease in North London. Ric Clini Lab 16: 236 (abstract)
Dent J A, Berkowtiz S D, Ware J et al 1990 Identification of a cleavage site directing the immunochemical detection of molecular abnormalities in type IIA von Willebrand factor. Proc Natl Acad Sci USA 87: 6306–6310
Eikenboom J C J, Reitsma P H, Peerlink K M J, Briet E 1993 Recessive inheritance of von Willebrand's disease type I. Lancet 341: 982–986
Foster P A, Fulcher C A, Marti T et al 1987 A major factor VIII binding domain resides

within the amino-terminal 272 amino acid residues of von Willebrand factor. J Biol Chem 262: 8443–8446

Fujimura Y, Titani K, Holland L Z et al 1987 A heparin-binding domain of human von Willebrand factor. Characterisation and localisation of a tryptic fragment extending from amino acid residue VAL-449 to LYS-728. J Biol Chem 262: 1734–1739

Gill J C, Endres-Brooks J, Bauer P J et al 1987 The effect of ABO blood group on the diagnosis of von Willebrand disease. Blood 69: 1691–1695

Ginsburg D 1991 The von Willebrand factor gene and genetics of von Willebrand's disease. Mayo Clin Proc 66: 506–515

Ginsburg D, Sadler J E 1993 von Willebrand disease: a database of point mutations, insertions and deletions. Thromb Haemost 69: 177–184

Girma J P, Kalafatis M, Pietu G et al 1986 Mapping of distinct von Willebrand factor domains interacting with platelet GPIb and GPIIb/IIIa and with collagen using monoclonal antibodies. Blood 67: 1356–1366

Goodwin S G, Bowen D J, Webb C E, Bloom A L 1992 A facile method for analysis of von Willebrand factor multimer patterns. Abstracts of the International Society of Haematology, p 189 (abstract)

Howard M A, Firkin B G 1971 Ristocetin – a new tool in the investigation of platelet aggregation. Thromb Diath Haemorrh 26: 362–369

Jaffe E A, Hoyer L W, Nachman R L 1974 Synthesis of von Willebrand factor by cultured human endothelial cells. Proc Natl Acad Sci USA 71: 1906–1909

Lyons S E, Bruck M E, Bowie E J W, Ginsburg D 1992 Impaired intracellular transport produced by a subset of type IIA von Willebrand disease mutations. J Biol Chem 267: 4424–4430

Mancuso D J, Tuley E A, Westfield L A et al 1989 Structure of the gene for human von Willebrand factor. J Biol Chem 264: 19514–19527

Mancuso D J, Tuley E A, Westfield L A et al 1991 Human von Willebrand factor gene and pseudogene structural analysis and differentiation by polymerase chain reaction. Biochemistry 30: 253–269

Mannucci P M, Bloom A L, Larrieu M J et al 1984 Atherosclerosis and von Willebrand factor. I. Prevalence of severe von Willebrand's disease in Western Europe and Israel. Br J Haematol 57: 163–169

Mannucci P M, Lombardi R, Bader R et al 1985 Heterogeneity of type I von Willebrand disease: evidence for a subgroup with an abnormal von Willebrand factor. Blood 66: 796–802

Martin S E, Marder V J, Francis C W et al 1980 Enzymatic degradation of the factor VIII – von Willebrand protein: a unique tryptic fragment with ristocetin cofactor activity. Blood 55: 848–858

Mazurier C 1992 von Willebrand disease masquerading as haemophilia A. Thromb Haemost 67: 391–396

Mercier B, Gaucher C, Mazurier C 1991 Characterisation of 98 alleles in 105 unrelated individuals in the F8vWF gene. Nucleic Acids Res 19: 4800

Miller J L, Castella A 1982 Platelet-type von Willebrand's disease: characterisation of a new bleeding disorder. Blood 60: 790–794

Miller C H, Graham J B, Goldin L R, Elston R C 1979a Genetics of classic von Willebrand's disease. I. Phenotypic variation within families. Blood 54: 117–136

Miller C H, Graham J B, Goldin L R, Elston R C 1979b Genetics of classic von Willebrand's disease. II. Optimal assignment of the heterozygous genotype (diagnosis) by discriminant analysis. Blood 54: 137–145

Nachman R, Levin R, Jaffe E A 1977 Synthesis of FVIII antigen by cultured guinea-pig megakaryocytes. J Clin Invest 60: 914–921

Nichols W C, Lyons S E, Harrison J S et al 1991 Severe von Willebrand disease due to a defect at the level of von Willebrand factor mRNA expression: detection by exonic PCR-restriction fragment length polymorphism analysis. Proc Natl Acad Sci USA 88: 3857–3861

Nishino M, Girma J P, Rothschild C et al 1989 New variant of von Willebrand disease with defective binding to factor VIII. Blood 74: 1591–1599

Pareti F I, Niiya K, McPherson J M, Ruggeri Z M 1987 Isolation and characterisation of two domains of human von Willebrand factor that interact with fibrillar collagen types I and III. J Biol Chem 262: 13835–13841

Peake I, Tuddenham E 1994 A standard nomenclature for factor VIII and factor IX gene mutations and associated amino acid alterations. Thromb Haemost 72: 475–476

Ploos van Amstel H K, Reitsma P H 1990 Tetranucleotide repeat polymorphism in the vWF gene. Nucleic Acids Res 18: 4957

Randi A M, Sacchi E, Castaman G C et al 1993 The genetic defect of type I von Willebrand disease 'Vicenza' is linked to the von Willebrand factor gene. Thromb Haemost 69: 173–176

Read M S, Smith S V, Lamb M A, Brinkhous K M 1989 Role of botrocetin in platelet agglutination: formation of an activated complex of botrocetin and von Willebrand factor. Blood 74: 1031–1035

Rodeghiero F, Castaman G, Enrico D 1987 Epidemiological investigation of the prevalence of von Willebrand's disease. Blood 69: 454–459

Ruggeri Z M, Ware J 1992 The structure and function of von Willebrand factor. Thromb Haemost 67: 594–599

Ruggeri Z M, Zimmerman T S 1980 Variant von Willebrand's disease: characterisation of two subtypes by analysis of multimeric composition of factor VIII/von Willebrand factor in plasma and platelets. J Clin Invest 65: 1318–1325

Ruggeri Z M, Zimmerman T S 1987a von Willebrand factor and von Willebrand disease. Blood 70: 895–904

Ruggeri Z M, Zimmerman T S 1987b Classification of von Willebrand disease. J Clin Lab Anal 1: 353–362

Ruggeri Z M, Pareti F I, Mannucci P M et al 1980 Heightened interaction between platelets and factor VIII/von Willebrand factor in a new subtype of von Willebrand's disease. N Engl J Med 302: 1047–1051

Sadler J E 1994 A revised classification of von Willebrand disease. Thromb Haemost 71: 520–525

Sadler J E, Ginsburg D 1993 A database of polymorphisms in the von Willebrand factor gene and pseudogene. Thromb Haemost 69: 185–191

Sadler J E, Gralnick H R 1994 A new classification of von Willebrand disease. Blood 84: 676–679

Sadler J E, Shelton-Inloes B B, Sorace J M et al 1985 Cloning and characterisation of two cDNAs coding for human von Willebrand factor. Proc Natl Acad Sci USA 82: 6394–6398

Shelton-Inloes B B, Broze G J, Miletich J P, Sadler J E 1987a Evolution of human von Willebrand factor: cDNA sequence polymorphisms, repeated domains and relationship to von Willebrand antigen II. Biophys Biochem Res Commun 144: 657–665

Shelton-Inloes B B, Chehab F F, Mannucci P M et al 1987b Gene deletions correlate with the development of alloantibodies in von Willebrand disease. J Clin Invest 79: 1459–1465

Sixma J J, Sakariassen K J, Beeser-Visser N H et al 1984 Adhesion of platelet to human artery subendothelium: effect of factor VIII von Willebrand factor of various multimeric composition. Blood 63: 128–139

Standen G R 1995 Personal communication

Standen G R, Bignell P, Bowen D J et al 1990 Family studies in von Willebrand's disease by analysis of restriction fragment length polymorphisms and an intragenic variable number tandem repeat (VNTR) sequence. Br J Haematol 76: 242–249

Tuddenham E G D, Cooper D N 1994 The von Willebrand factor and von Willebrand disease. In: Motulsky A G, Bobrow M, Harper P S, Scriver C (eds) The molecular genetics of haemostasis and its inherited disorders. Oxford monographs on medical genetics 25. Oxford University Press, Oxford, ch 30: 374–401

Tuddenham E G D, Lane R S, Rotblat F et al 1982 Response to infusions of polyelectrolyte fractionated human factor VIII in human haemophilia A and von Willebrand's disease. Br J Haematol 52: 259–267

Verweij C L 1988 Biosynthesis of human von Willebrand factor. Haemostasis 18: 224–245

Verweij C L, de Vries C J M, Distel B et al 1985 Construction of cDNA coding for human von Willebrand factor using antibody probes for colony screening and mapping of the chromosomal gene. Nucleic Acids Res 13: 4699–4717

Verweij C L, Diergaarde P, Hart M, Pannekoek H 1986 Full length von Willebrand factor (VWF) cDNA encodes a highly repetitive protein, considerably larger than the mature VWF subunit. Eur Mol Biol Org J 5: 1839–1847

von Willebrand E A 1926 Hereditar Pseudohemifil. Fin Laekaresaallsk Handl 67: 87–112

Wagner D D 1989 Storage and secretion of von Willebrand factor. In: Zimmerman T S, Ruggeri Z M (eds) Coagulation and bleeding disorders. Marcel Dekker, New York, ch 8

Wagner D D, Marder V J 1984 Biosynthesis of von Willebrand protein by human endothelial cells: processing steps and their intracellular localisation. J Cell Biol 99: 2123–2130

Weinstein M, Deykin D 1979 Composition of factor VIII related von Willebrand factor proteins prepared from human cryoprecipitate and FVIII concentrate. Blood 53: 1095–1105

Weiss H J, Turitto V T, Baumgartner H R 1978 Effect of shear rate on platelet interaction with subendothelium in citrated and native blood. Shear rate dependent decrease in adhesion in von Willebrand's disease and the Bernard–Soulier syndrome. J Lab Clin Med 92: 750–764

Weiss H J, Meyer D, Rabinowitz R et al 1982 Pseudo-von Willebrand's disease: an intrinsic platelet defect with aggregation by unmodified human factor VIII/von Willebrand factor and enhanced adsorption of its high molecular weight multimers. N Engl J Med 306: 326–333

Wood N, Standen G R, Murray E W et al 1995 Rapid genotype analysis in type 2B von Willebrand's disease using a universal heteroduplex generator. Br J Haematol 89: 152–156

Zhang Z P, Deng L P, Blomback M, Anvret M 1992 Dinucleotide repeat polymorphism in the promoter region of the human von Willebrand factor gene (VWF gene). Hum Mol Genet 1: 780

13. Treatment of von Willebrand disease

P. M. Mannucci   A. B. Federici

Von Willebrand disease (vWD) is a bleeding disorder mainly characterized by mucocutaneous hemorrhages (e.g. epistaxis, gastrointestinal bleeding, menorrhagia; see Ch. 12). vWD is named after Erich von Willebrand, who first described this abnormality in a family from the Åland Islands (von Willebrand 1926). vWD is caused by quantitative or qualitative defects of von Willebrand factor (vWF), a high molecular weight glycoprotein that plays a key role in primary hemostasis by promoting platelet adhesion to the subendothelium and platelet aggregation under high shear-stress conditions (Ruggeri et al 1993). In most cases, vWD is inherited in an autosomal dominant fashion, although an autosomal recessive pattern of inheritance has been described in a few cases.

vWD is the most frequent of inherited bleeding disorders. In Sweden, a frequency of approximately 125 cases per million persons – twice that of hemophilia – has been reported (Holmberg & Nilsson 1985). In Italy, during a large epidemiological study, a frequency of 0.82% was found in the general population (Rodeghiero et al 1987). Studies in other countries also showed high frequencies (1–2%) (Werner et al 1991).

Patients with vWD are characterized by a mild or moderately severe bleeding tendency since early childhood. Usually one of the two parents is clinically affected (Cooney et al 1993); however, there are patients with no family history who have the hemostatic defects typical of vWD. This pattern may occur concomitantly with other acquired clinical conditions and is therefore called acquired von Willebrand syndrome (vWS).

DIAGNOSIS AND CLASSIFICATION OF vWD

vWD is diagnosed in three steps:

1. Identification of patients at risk for vWD, based on data from the clinical history and the results of hemostatic screening tests.
2. Diagnosis and definition of vWD type.
3. Characterization of the vWD subtype.

The clinical and laboratory parameters used in this three-step diagnostic work-up are summarized in Table 13.1.

Although vWD is an extremely heterogeneous disease, different forms can be differentiated by different patterns of genetic transmission and abnormalities of vWF in plasma and platelets. Since genetic mutations responsible for vWD have been identified in only a relatively limited number of cases (Ginsburg & Bowie 1992), phenotypic classification is still used. Recently, the Scientific and Standardization Committee of the International Society of Thrombosis and Hemostasis formulated a new classification (Sadler 1994), which is a modification of the previous classification

Table 13.1   Clinical and laboratory parameters used for diagnosis of vWD

A. Patients at risk for vWD
   1. Clinical history: lifelong mucocutaneous bleeding; symptoms are often present in other family members
   2. Screening tests: usually prolonged bleeding time with normal platelet count and prolonged APTT

B. Diagnosis of vWD type
   1. vWF antigen (vWF:Ag)
   2. Ristocetin cofactor (vWF:RiCoF)
   3. Factor VIII coagulant activity (factor VIII:C)
   4. Multimeric structure of plasma vWF

C. Diagnosis of vWD subtype
   1. Ristocetin-induced platelet agglutination
   2. Platelet vWF levels (vWF:Ag, vWF:RiCoF)
   3. Test of infusion with desmopressin

APTT, activated partial thromboplastin time.

Table 13.2   Laboratory classification of vWD patients

Laboratory parameters	Type 1	Type 2				Type 3
		2A	2B	2M	2N	
Bleeding time	More or less prolonged	├──── More or less prolonged ────┤				Very prolonged
Plasma levels						
vWF:Ag	Low/normal	Low/normal	Low/normal	Low/normal	Low/normal	Unmeasurable
vWF:RiCoF	Low	Low	Low/normal	Low	Low/normal	Unmeasurable
Factor VIII	Low/normal or normal	Low/normal	Low/normal	Low/normal	Low	Unmeasurable
vWF–platelet GPIb binding (i.e. RIPA)	Normal or low	Low	Higher	Low	Normal	Unmeasurable
Plasma HMW multimers	Present	Absent	Absent	Present	Present	Absent
Platelet HMW multimers	Present	Group 1: Absent Group 2: Present	Present	Present	Present	Absent

GP, glycoprotein; HMW, high molecular weight; RIPA, ristocetin-induced platelet agglutination.

proposed by Ruggeri & Zimmerman (1987). There are three main phenotypes of vWD: types 1, 2 and 3. Type 2 patients are further classified into four different subtypes (A, B, M, N). This classification system and the corresponding phenotypic patterns are summarized in Table 13.2.

Type 1 is the most frequent form of vWD (70–80%) and is usually inherited as an autosomal dominant trait. Patients with type 1 vWD are characterized by mild bleeding symptoms, which usually only occur after trauma or surgery. Laboratory testing shows normal or prolonged bleeding time (BT) and low levels (10–40 IU/dl) of factor VIII–vWF activities in plasma, with normal multimeric structure. Patients with type 1 vWD are heterogeneous, with a high degree of variability among affected members of the same family (Miller et al 1979, Abildgaard et al 1980). More recently, three subgroups have been differentiated based on a comparison between plasma and platelet vWF content and function (Weiss et al 1983, Mannucci et al 1985): in one group there is normal platelet vWF (type 1, platelet-normal), in another group low platelet vWF (type 1, platelet-low), and in a third group dysfunctional vWF in platelets (type 1, platelet-discordant).

Type 2 vWD is caused by qualitative abnormalities of vWF and is characterized by moderate bleeding diathesis and by lower values for vWF: RiCoF (ristocetin cofactor) than for vWF:Ag. High molecular weight multimers are lacking to various degrees in most cases. The prevalence of type 2 vWD is 15–20% of all vWD cases. Subtypes are indicated by capital letters and can be divided into two major (2A and 2B) and two minor (2M and 2N) groups.

Type 2A is the most frequent subtype of type 2 vWD (Ruggeri & Zimmerman 1980). It is inherited mainly as an autosomal dominant, but recessive inheritance has also been described (Asakura et al 1987). Patients with type 2A vWD have low to normal levels of vWF:Ag, contrasting with low vWF:RiCoF, and an abnormal multimeric pattern consisting of a severe deficiency of larger multimers. All the other vWD subtypes previously described as type II (C–I) should now be included in this subgroup of type 2A because they are deficient in larger multimers (Sadler 1994).

Type 2B is a peculiar variant with increased affinity of an abnormal vWF for platelets, in which there is enhanced ristocetin-induced platelet agglutination (RIPA) and a deficiency of large multimers in the plasma. The inheritance is mainly autosomal dominant, but cases with apparently recessive patterns have also been described (Federici et al 1986). The most typical features of type 2B vWD are mild thrombocytopenia with increased mean platelet volume, prolonged BT, low to normal factor VIII, low to normal vWF:Ag, low to normal vWF:RiCoF and enhanced RIPA. Type 2M vWD are qualitative variants with a low platelet-dependent function not caused by a deficiency of larger multimers. This category includes the previously described vWD type B, type I Vicenza, type IC and type ID (Cooney et al 1993).

Type 2N vWD are all qualitative variants with markedly low affinity for factor VIII. 'N' stands for Normandy because this particular variant was identified in 1989 in a patient from that region (Nishino et al 1989, Mazurier et al 1990). Type 2N vWD is characterized by normal levels of vWF:Ag and vWF:RiCoF, normal multimeric patterns in plasma and platelets, but slightly low factor VIII levels. The clinical features are similar to those observed in mild or moderate hemophilia A, but the inheritance pattern is autosomal dominant, not X-linked (Mazurier 1992).

Type 3 (severe) vWD is caused by severe impairment of the biosynthesis of vWF and there are unmeasurable levels of vWF in plasma and platelets. Since vWF is also the carrier of factor VIII, plasma levels of factor VIII are very low (1–5%). Patients with type 3 vWD have a severe bleeding tendency: they have not only mucocutaneous hemorrhages but also hemarthroses and hematomas, as in severe hemophilia. The inheritance of type 3 vWD is autosomal recessive and its prevalence is 1–5 per million population. Some cases of type 3 vWD are associated with gene deletions that predispose to the formation of alloantibodies against vWF in patients treated with blood products (Shelton-Inloes et al 1987). The prevalence of alloantibodies to vWF in this type is estimated to be approximately 7–8% (Mannucci & Federici 1995). Patients with type 3 vWD and antibodies can be identified by poor clinical responses to replacement therapy, as detected by low recovery of vWF in plasma, lack of correction of the prolonged BT and absence of a delayed rise in factor VIII. In some patients, replacement therapy is not only ineffective, it may also trigger life-threatening anaphylactic reactions (Mannucci et al 1987).

GENERAL PRINCIPLES OF THERAPY

The aim of therapy is to correct the dual defects of vWD, i.e. the prolonged BT due to the defective platelet adhesion and the abnormal blood coagulation due to low factor VIII levels. In general, superficial bleeding can be controlled with topical hemostatic agents, by application of pressure dressings and proper use of sutures. Antiplatelet drugs, especially aspirin, should be avoided. When an anti-inflammatory agent is required, a drug that does not affect platelet function (such as paracetamol) is preferable; if anti-inflammatory medication is required for an extended period, concurrent medication to protect the upper gastrointestinal tract is indicated.

There are two main options available for management of vWD: demopressin or transfusion therapy with blood products (Table 13.3). Since all currently available forms of transfusion therapy carry some risk of viral transmission, the initial approach to treatment should be to use the non-transfusion option (i.e. desmopressin) whenever possible.

DESMOPRESSIN

Desmopressin (1-deamino-8-D-arginine vasopressin) is a synthetic analog

Table 13.3   Management of different types and subtypes of vWD

vWD diagnosis	Minor bleeding	Major bleeding	Alternative and adjunctive therapies
Type 1	Desmopressin	Desmopressin or factor VIII–vWF concentrate	Antifibrinolytics Estrogens
Type 2A	Desmopressin (in some) Factor VIII–vWF concentrate	Factor VIII–vWF concentrate	
Type 2B	Factor VIII–vWF concentrate	Factor VIII–vWF concentrate	
Type 2M	Desmopressin	Factor VIII–vWF concentrate	
Type 2N	Desmopressin	Factor VIII–vWF concentrate	
Type 3	Factor VIII–vWF concentrate	Factor VIII–vWF concentrate	Desmopressin Platelet concentrate
Type 3 and alloantibodies	r VIII		
Acquired vWS	Desmopressin (in some) Factor VIII–vWF concentrate	Intravenous immunoglobulin	

r VIII, recombinant factor VIII.

of vasopressin that was originally produced to treat diabetes insipidus. Desmopressin increases plasma factor VIII and vWF concentrations without significant side-effects in healthy volunteers or patients with mild hemophilia and vWD (Cash et al 1974). It has little or no effect on smooth muscle V_1-vasopressin receptors, but it has a strong antidiuretic activity which is related to its stimulatory effect on V_2-receptors. The mode of action of desmopressin is not very well understood. Its addition to cultured endothelial cells has no effect on vWF synthesis or secretion and the agent is presumed to act through a second messenger (probably platelet-activating factor) derived from monocytes (Hashemi et al 1993). The first successful clinical trial of desmopressin was performed in 1977 with the aim of avoiding use of blood products in mild hemophiliacs and vWD patients who needed dental extractions and other surgical procedures (Mannucci et al 1977). Since then, desmopressin has become widely used to treat both vWD and mild hemophilia A (Rodeghiero et al 1991).

The obvious advantages of desmopressin are that it is inexpensive and carries no risk of transmitting blood-borne viruses. It is usually administered intravenously over 15–30 min at a dose of 0.3 µg/kg diluted in 50 ml of saline. This treatment can increase plasma factor VIII and vWF to 3–5 times above their basal levels within 30 min. In general, high factor VIII–vWF concentrations may last for 4–6 h, but there is a large between-patient variability. Since the responses in a given patient are consistent on different occasions, a test dose of desmopressin should be administered at the time of diagnosis to establish the response patterns. Infusions can be repeated every 8–12 h, depending on the type and severity of the bleeding episode. However, most patients treated repeatedly with desmopressin tend to become progressively less responsive to therapy (tachyphylaxis) (Mannucci et al 1992). The drug is also available in concentrated forms for subcutaneous and intranasal administration (Rodeghiero et al 1993), which can be convenient for home treatment.

Side-effects of desmopressin, which are usually limited to mild tachycardia, headache and flushing, are due to the vasomotor effects of the drug and can often be attenuated by slowing the rate of infusion. Hyponatremia and volume overload due to the antidiuretic effects of the drug are relatively rare. Some cases have been described in young children who were given closely repeated infusions (Smith et al 1989). Even though no thrombotic episodes have been reported in patients with vWD treated with desmopressin, the drug should be used cautiously for elderly patients with significant atherosclerotic disease because a few cases of myocardial infarction and stroke have occurred in hemophiliacs and uremic patients given the drug (Bond & Nevan 1988, Byrnes et al 1988).

Desmopressin is most effective in type 1 vWD patients, especially those who have normal vWF in storage sites (type 1, platelet-normal). In these patients factor VIII, vWF:Ag and vWF:RiCoF levels and the BT are usually corrected within 30 min and remain normal for 2–4 h. In the other vWD subtypes, responsiveness to desmopressin varies. A poor and short-lasting response is observed in type 1 platelet-low vWD (Mannucci et al 1985). In type 2A, factor VIII levels are usually increased by desmopressin, but the BT is shortened in only a minority of cases. It has been postulated that there is a correlation between the type of 2A molecular abnormality and positive effects of desmopressin on the BT (Gralnick et al 1986). Desmopressin is considered to be contraindicated in type 2B vWD because of the appearance of transient thrombocytopenia (Holmberg et al 1983). However, there have been sporadic reports of clinical usefulness of desmopressin in some type 2B cases (Fowler et al 1989, Casonato et al 1990). In type 2N vWD, high levels of factor VIII are observed following desmopressin (Mazurier et al 1994). Patients with type 3 vWD are usually unresponsive to desmopressin. However, there is a recently identified subgroup of type 3 patients in whom factor VIII levels became normal after desmopressin, even though the BT remained markedly prolonged (Castaman et al 1995).

OTHER NON-TRANSFUSION THERAPIES FOR vWD

Two other types of non-transfusion therapies are commonly used for management of vWD: antifibrinolytic agents and estrogens. Antifibrinolytic agents interfere with the lysis of newly formed clots by saturating the binding sites on plasminogen, preventing its attachment to forming fibrin and making plasminogen unavailable within the forming clot. Aminocaproic acid (50 mg/kg four times a day) and tranexamic acid (25 mg/kg three times a day) are the most widely used antifibrinolytic agents. Both medications can be administered orally, intravenously or topically and may be useful alone or as adjuncts in the management of oral cavity bleeding, epistaxis, gastrointestinal bleeding and menorrhagia. These drugs that inhibit the fibrinolytic system carry a potential risk for thrombosis in patients with underlying prethrombotic states. They are also contraindicated in the management of genitourinary bleeding. Estrogens increase plasma vWF but the response is variable and unpredictable. This effect is apparently due to direct stimulation of endothelial cells (Harrison & McKee 1984). Some reports have described the successful use of preoperative estrogen therapy in patients with type 1 vWD (Alperin 1982). It is common clinical experience that the continued use of oral contraceptives is very useful in reducing the severity of menorrhagia in women with vWD, even in those with type 3 in whom this treatment does not affect factor VIII–vWF levels.

TRANSFUSION THERAPY

Transfusion therapy with blood products containing factor VIII–vWF is the treatment of choice in all vWD patients who are unresponsive to desmopressin. Factor VIII–vWF may be infused with fresh frozen plasma, but the large volumes required to achieve hemostasis limit its use. Cryoprecipitate contains 5–10 times more vWF than fresh frozen plasma (each bag contains approximately 80–100 IU of factor VIII in 10 ml). An early study indicated that a dose of 15–20 IU/kg (1 bag per 5 kg body weight) administered every 12–24 h normalized plasma factor VIII levels, shortened the BT and stopped or prevented clinical bleeding in vWD patients (Perkins 1967). Based on these observations, cryoprecipitate has been the mainstay of vWD therapy for many years. However, a recent analysis of previously published reports revealed that the BT is not always corrected by cryoprecipitate (Rodeghiero et al 1992). In addition, virucidal methods cannot be applied to cryoprecipitate and thus this product carries a small but definite risk of transmitting blood-borne infections. Therefore, virus-inactivated concentrates, originally developed for therapy of hemophilia A, now play an important role in the management of vWD patients who are unresponsive to desmopressin. These concentrates can be classified according to their specific factor VIII activity into intermediate-purity concentrates (factor VIII 1–5 IU/mg) and high-purity concentrates (factor VIII 50–250 IU/mg). Very-high-purity concentrates, obtained by immunoaffinity chromatography (factor VIII > 2000 IU/mg), contain only small amounts of vWF and are therefore not suitable for vWD management. Recently, a solvent/detergent chromatographically purified concentrate particularly rich in vWF and with a low content of factor VIII has been produced and named very-high-purity vWF concentrate (Burnouf-Radosevich & Burnouf 1992).

This concentrate was effective when tested in a small cohort of type 3 vWD cases (Meriane et al 1993), and its efficacy and safety are now being evaluated in a large number of patients.

Since the intermediate- and high-purity factor VIII–vWF concentrates available commercially contain large amounts of both factor VIII and vWF, high postinfusion levels of these moieties are consistently obtained. In addition, unlike in hemophilia A, there is a sustained rise in factor VIII – higher than predicted from the doses infused – for 12–24 h. This pattern, already observed with cryoprecipitate, is due to the stabilizing effect of the exogenous vWF on endogenous factor VIII, which is synthesized at a normal rate in these patients (Cornu et al 1963). Therefore, all these products are able to correct factor VIII deficiency, but they are not always effective in correcting the BT (Rodeghiero et al 1992). There are probably several reasons for these inconsistent effects on the BT. So far, no concentrate has contained a completely functional vWF, as shown by an intact multimeric

Table 13.4 Doses of factor VIII–vWF concentrates in vWD unresponsive to desmopressin

Type of bleeding	Dose (IU/kg)	Number of infusions	Objective
Major surgery	50–100	Once a day or every other day	Maintain factor VIII >50 IU/dl for 10 days
Minor surgery	30–80	Once a day or every other day	factor VIII >50 IU/dl for 5 days
Dental extraction	30–80	Single	factor VIII >50 IU/dl for 6 h
Spontaneous or post-traumatic bleeding	20–40	Single	

Table 13.5 Clinical conditions more frequently associated with acquired vWS

- Malignant neoplasms
  - Adenocarcinoma
  - Squamous cell carcinoma
  - Hepatocellular carcinoma
  - Wilm's tumor
- Lymphoproliferative disorders
  - B-cell lymphomas
  - Chronic lymphocytic leukemia
  - Waldenstrom macroglobulinemia
  - Myeloma
  - Monoclonal gammopathies of uncertain significance
- Myeloproliferative disorders:
  - Chronic myelogenous leukemia
  - Thrombocythemia
- Systemic lupus erythematosus
- Hypothyroidism
- Congenital cardiac defects
- Angiodysplasia

pattern in vitro and by several functional assays, because vWF is proteolysed during purification by platelet proteases contaminating the fractionated plasma (Mannucci et al 1994). In addition, the action of platelet vWF is essential for a normal primary hemostasis in vWD (see below). Despite their limited and inconsistent effects on the BT, factor VIII–vWF concentrates are being successfully used to treat vWD patients unresponsive to desmopressin, especially for soft-tissue and postoperative bleeding (Rodeghiero et al 1992). Timing and dosage of concentrates in desmopressin-unresponsive patients are summarized in Table 12.4 according to the severity of surgery and bleeding episodes. When the BT remains prolonged and mucosal bleeding persists despite replacement therapy, other therapeutic options are available. Desmopressin given after cryoprecipitate, shortened or normalized the BT in type 3 vWD patients in whom cryoprecipitate failed to correct the BT (Cattaneo et al 1989). Platelet concentrates (given at doses usually used for patients with leukemia and thrombocytopenia) produced similar effects in patients unresponsive to cryoprecipitate, in terms of both BT correction and mucosal bleeding control (Castillo et al 1991). These data emphasize once more the important role of platelet vWF in establishing and maintaining primary hemostasis (Mannucci 1995).

TREATMENT AND vWD DURING PREGNANCY AND DELIVERY

During pregnancy, vWF:Ag and factor VIII levels tend to rise in type 1 and type 2 vWD but this rise does not occur until the 11th week of gestation. No significant changes occur in patients with type 3 vWD. Since the improvements of vWF:Ag and in factor VIII levels during pregnancy are variable, patients should be monitored during pregnancy and for several weeks after delivery when levels fall rapidly and late hemorrhages may ensue (Conti et al 1986). In type 1 vWD the factor VIII levels appear to be the best predictor of the risk of bleeding at delivery. The risk of bleeding is minimal when factor VIII is >50 IU/dl, but can be significant when it is <30 IU/dl. Careful surgical hemostasis along with effective uterine contraction will compensate for a prolonged BT. In type 2 and type 3 vWD, characterized by prolonged BT and low factor VIII levels, replacement therapy with concentrates is necessary. Patients with type 2B vWD have been reported to develop or aggravate thrombocytopenia during pregnancy (Rick et al 1987, Pareti et al 1990), but it is not clear whether thrombocytopenia exacerbates clinical bleeding.

TREATMENT OF PATIENTS WITH ALLO- AND AUTOANTIBODIES TO vWF

For patients with type 3 vWD complicated by alloantibodies, infusion of vWF concentrates is not only ineffective but may also cause postinfusion anaphylaxis due to formation of immune complexes (Mannucci et al 1981). These reactions may be life-threatening (Mannucci et al 1987). To avoid the development of such reactions, one of these patients undergoing emergency abdominal surgery was treated with recombinant factor VIII (rVIII), which will not cause an anaphylactic response as it does not contain vWF. Because of the very short half-life of factor VIII without its vWF carrier, rVIII had to be administered by continuous intravenous infusion at very large doses sufficient to maintain factor VIII levels above 50 IU/dl for 10 days after surgery (Bergamaschini et al 1995).

Since acquired vWS occurs concomitantly with several clinical disorders (Table 13.5), treatment of the underlying disorder may improve the bleeding diathesis and sometimes result in a cure. Desmopressin and vWF concentrates are sometimes useful but are not always as effective as in congenital vWD, because the half-lives of both endogenous and exogenous vWF are shorter (Mannucci et al 1984, 1987). Treatment with high-dose intravenous immunoglobulin (1 g/kg/day for 2 consecutive days) may temporarily control bleeding (Macik et al 1988). In refractory cases, plasma exchange can also be considered (Silberstein et al 1987).

KEY POINTS FOR CLINICAL PRACTICE

- Make sure to use appropriate tests to characterise every new patient with vWD by differentiating between type 1, 2 and 3 and their specific subtypes. Exclude a diagnosis of acquired von Willebrand syndrome.

- Give a test infusion of DDAVP to all newly diagnosed types 1 and 2 vWD. Measure bleeding time, platelet count and FVIII and vWF before and 30 min, 1, 2 and 4 h following DDAVP.

- Idenfity vWD patients who are responsive or unresponsive to DDAVP. DDAVP-responsive patients are characterised by normalisation of FVIII and vWF:RiCo and correction or significant shortening of the prolonged bleeding time within 2 h.

- In responsive patients, DDAVP is useful against post-traumatic bleeding and before dental extractions and other minor surgery. Antifibrinolytic agents should also be given.

- Major surgery can be carried out in DDAVP-responsive patients with close monitoring of FVIII. When DDAVP is not able to maintain FVIII levels higher than 50 U/dl and post-surgical bleeding occurs, FVIII–vWF concentrates should be given.

- Use intermediate or high purity FVIII–vWF concentrates for all DDAVP-unresponsive patients. Give single infusions (20–50 U/kg) for spontaneous or post-traumatic bleeding and before dental extractions.

- Consider larger doses (50–100 U/kg) and repeated infusions of FVIII–vWF concentrate for cases of major bleeding and surgery. Adjust the dosage to keep FVIII levels above 50 U/dl for 3 days (minor surgery) or for 7–10 days (major surgery).

- For type 3 with alloantibodies, consider continuous infusion of recombinant FVIII. For acquired vWS, administer i.v. immunoglobulin (1 g/kg/day for 2 days) or consider DDAVP and FVIII–vWF concentrates after immunoabsorption techniques.

- Recommend oral contraceptives for all women with menorrhagia. Monitor FVIII-vWF levels during pregnancy, use DDAVP or FVIII–vWF concentrates during delivery and *post partum.*

REFERENCES

Abildgaard C F, Suzuki Z, Harrison J et al 1980 Serial studies in von Willebrand disease: variability versus variants. Blood 56: 712–716

Alperin J B 1982 Estrogen and surgery in women with von Willebrand disease. Am J Med 73: 367–371

Asakura A, Harrison J, Gompertz E, Abildgaard C 1987 Type IIA vWD with apparent recessive inheritance. Blood 69: 1419–1420

Bergamaschini L, Mannucci P M, Federici A B et al 1995 Postransfusion anaphylactic reaction in a patient with severe von Willebrand disease: role of complement and alloantibodies to von Willebrand factor. J Lab Clin Med 125: 348–355

Bond L, Bevan D 1988 Myocardial infarction in a patient with hemophilia A treated with DDAVP. N Engl J Med 318: 121

Burnouf-Radosevich M, Burnouf T 1992 Chromatographic preparation of a therapeutic highly purified von Willebrand factor concentrate from human cryoprecipitate. Vox Sang 62: 1–11

Byrnes J J, Larcada A, Moake J L 1988 Thrombosis following desmopressin for uremic bleeding. Am J Hematol 28: 63–65

Cash J D, Garder A M A, Da Costa J 1974 The release of plasminogen activator and factor VIII by LVP, AVP, DDAVP, ATIII and OT in man. Br J Haematol 27: 363–364

Casonato A, Fabris F, Girolami A 1990 Platelet aggregation and pseudothrombocytopenia induced by 1-desamino-8-D-arginine vasopressin (DDAVP) in type IIB von Willebrand disease. Eur J Haematol 45: 36

Castaman G, Lattuada A, Mannucci P M, Rodeghiero F 1995 Factor VIII:C increases after desmopressin with autosomal recessive severe von Willebrand disease. Br J Haematol 89: 849–854

Castillo R, Monteagudo J, Escolar G et al 1991 Hemostatic effect of normal platelet transfusion in severe von Willebrand disease. Blood 77: 1901–1905

Cattaneo M, Moia M, Della Valle P et al 1989 DDAVP shortens the prolonged bleeding time of patients with severe von Willebrand disease treated with cryoprecipitate. Evidence for a mechanism of action independent of released von Willebrand factor. Blood 74: 1972–1975

Conti M, Mari D, Conti E et al 1986 Pregnancy in women with different types of von Willebrand disease. Obstet Gynecol 68: 282–285

Cooney K A, Ginsburg D, Ruggeri Z M 1993 von Willebrand disease. In: Loscalzo J, Schafer A I (eds) Thrombosis and hemorrhage. Blackwell Scientific, Oxford, pp 657–682

Cornu P, Larrieu M J, Caen J, Bernard J 1963 Transfusion studies in von Willebrand disease: effect on bleeding time and factor VIII. Br J Haematol 9: 189–202

Federici A B, Mannucci P M, Bader R et al 1986 Heterogeneity in type IIB vWD: two unrelated cases with no family history and mild abnormalities of ristocetin-induced interactions between vWF and platelets. Am J Hematol 23: 381–390

Fowler W E, Berkowitz L R, Roberts H R 1989 DDAVP for type IIB von Willebrand disease. Blood 74: 1859–1860

Ginsburg D, Bowie E J W 1992 Molecular genetics of von Willebrand disease. Blood 79: 2507–2519

Gralnick H R, Williams S B, McKeown L P et al 1986 DDAVP in type IIA von Willebrand disease. Blood 66: 796–802

Harrison R L, McKee P A 1984 Estrogen stimulates von Willebrand factor production by cultured endothelial cells. Blood 63: 657–665

Hashemi S, Palmer D S, Aye M T, Ganz P R 1993 Platelet-activating factor secreted by DDAVP-treated monocytes mediates von Willebrand factor release from endothelial cells. J Cell Physiol 154: 496–505

Holmberg L, Nilsson I M 1985 Von Willebrand's disease. Clin Hematol 14: 461–488

Holmberg L, Nilsson I M, Borge L et al 1983 Platelet aggregation induced by 1-desamino-8-D-arginine vasopressin (DDAVP) in type IIB von Willebrand disease. N Engl J Med 309: 816–821

Macik B G, Gabriel D A, White G C et al 1988 The use of high-dose intravenous gammaglobulin in acquired von Willebrand disease. Arch Pathol Lab Med 112: 143–146

Mannucci P M 1995 Platelet von Willebrand factor in inherited and acquired bleeding disorder. Proc Natl Acad Sci USA 92: 2428–2432

Mannucci P M, Federici A B 1995 Antibodies to von Willebrand factor in von Willebrand disease. In: Inhibitors to coagulation factors. Pergamon Press, Oxford (in press)

Mannucci P M, Ruggeri Z M, Pareti F I, Capitanio A 1977 A new pharmacological approach to the management of hemophilia and von Willebrand disease. Lancet i: 869–872

Mannucci P M, Ruggeri Z M, Ciavarella N et al 1981 Precipitating antibodies to FVIII/von Willebrand factor in von Willebrand disease: effects on replacement therapy. Blood 57: 25–31

Mannucci P M, Lombardi R, Bader R et al 1984 Studies of the pathophysiology of acquired von Willebrand disease in seven patients with lymphoproliferative disorders or benign monoclonal gammopathies. Blood 64: 614–621

Mannucci P M, Lombardi R, Bader R et al 1985 Heterogeneity of type I von Willebrand disease: evidence for a subgroup with an abnormal von Willebrand factor. Blood 66: 796–802

Mannucci P M, Tamaro G, Narchi G et al 1987 Life-threatening reaction to FVIII concentrate in a patient with severe vWD and alloantibodies to vWF. Eur J Haematol 39: 467–470

Mannucci P M, Bettega D, Cattaneo M 1992 Consistency of responses to repeated DDAVP infusions in patients with von Willebrand disease and haemophilia A. Br J Haematol 82: 87–93

Mannucci P M, Lattuada A, Ruggeri Z M 1994 Proteolysis of von Willebrand factor in therapeutic plasma concentrates. Blood 83: 3018–3027

Mazurier C 1992 von Willebrand disease masquerading as hemophilia A. Thromb Haemost 67: 391–396

Mazurier C, Dieval J, Jorieux S et al 1990 A new von Willebrand factor (vWF) defect in a patient with factor VIII (FVIII) deficiency but with normal level and multimeric patterns of both plasma and platelet vWF. Characterization of abnormal vWF/FVIII interaction. Blood 75: 20–26

Mazurier C, Gaucher C, Jorieux S, Goudemand M and the Collaborative Group 1994 Biological effect of desmopressin in eight patients with type 2N ('Normandy') von Willebrand disease. Br J Haematol 88: 849–854

Meriane F, Zerhouni L, Djeha N et al 1993 Biological effects of a S/D-treated, very high purity, von Willebrand factor concentrate in five patients with severe von Willebrand disease. Blood Coagulat Fibrinol 4: 1023–1029

Miller C H, Graham J B, Goldin L R, Elston R C 1979 Genetics of classic von Willebrand's disease. I. Phenotypic variations within families. Blood 54: 117–145

Nishino M, Girma J P, Rothschild C et al 1989 New varient of von Willebrand disease with defective binding to FVIII. Blood 74: 1591–1599

Pareti F I, Federici A B, Cattaneo M, Mannucci P M 1990 Spontaneous platelet aggregation during pregnancy in a patient with vWD type IIB can be blocked by monoclonal antibodies to both platelet glycoproteins Ib and IIb/IIIa. Br J Haematol 75: 86

Perkins H A 1967 Correction of the hemostatic defects in von Willebrand disease. Blood 30: 375–380

Rick M E, Williams S B, Sacher R A, McKeown L P 1987 Thrombocytopenia associated with pregnancy in a patient with type IIB vWD. Blood 69: 786–789

Rodeghiero F, Castaman G, Dini E 1987 Epidemiological investigation of the prevalence of von Willebrand's disease. Blood 69: 454–459

Rodeghiero F, Castaman G, Mannucci P M 1991 Clinical indications for desmopressin (DDAVP) in congenital and acquired von Willebrand disease. Blood Rev 5: 155–161

Rodeghiero F, Castaman G, Meyer D, Mannucci P M 1992 Replacement therapy with virus-inactivated plasma concentrates in von Willebrand disease. Vox Sang 62: 193–199

Rodeghiero F, Castaman G, Giustolisi R, Mariani G 1993 Multicenter evaluation of a new concentrated desmopressin preparation (Emosint) administered intravenously or subcutaneously: analysis of biological responses and side-effects in 49 patients with hemophilia A and von Willebrand's disease. In: Mariani G, Mannucci P M, Cattaneo M (eds) Desmopressin in bleeding disorders (NATO ASI Series A, vol 242). Plenum Press, New York, pp 261–266

Ruggeri Z M, Zimmerman T S 1980 Variant von Willebrand's disease. Characterization of two subtypes by analysis of multimeric composition of FVIII/vWF in plasma and platelets. J Clin Invest 65: 1318

Ruggeri Z M, Zimmerman T S 1987 von Willebrand factor and von Willebrand disease. Blood 71: 895–904

Ruggeri Z M, Ware J L, Ginsburg D 1993 von Willebrand factor. In: Loscalzo J, Schafer A I (eds) Thrombosis and hemorrhage Blackwell Scientific, Oxford, pp 305–329

Sadler J E 1994 A revised classification of von Willebrand disease. Thromb Haemost 71: 520–525

Shelton-Inloes B B, Chehab F F, Mannucci P M et al 1987 Gene deletions correlate with the development of antibodies in von Willebrand disease. J Clin Invest 79: 1459–1465

Silberstein L E, Abraham J, Shattil S J 1987 The efficacy of intensive plasma exchange in acquired von Willebrand disease. Transfusion 27: 234–237

Smith T J, Gill J C, Ambroso D R, Hathaway W E 1989 Hyponatremia and seizures in young children given DDAVP. Am J Hematol 31: 199–202

von Willebrand E A 1926 Hereditary pseudohemofilii. Fin Laekaresaellsk Handl 67: 7–112

Weiss H J, Pietu G, Rabinowitz R et al 1983 Heterogeneous abnormalities in the multimeric structure, antigenic properties, and plasma-platelet content of factor VIII/von Willebrand factor in subtypes of classic (type I) and variant (IIA) von Willebrand's disease. J Lab Clin Med 101: 411–425

Werner E J, Broxson E H, Tucker E L et al 1991 Prevalence of von Willebrand disease in children: a multiethnic study. Blood 78: 68a

14. Treatment of haemophilia

C. A. Ludlam

Haemophilia treatment over the past 40 years has been revolutionized by the availability of clinically effective coagulation factor concentrates, but this new era has been punctuated by the disastrous effects of virus transmission by blood products. The prospects for the future are now much brighter as plasma-derived concentrates have a higher degree of viral safety, because recombinant coagulation factor concentrates are becoming available and because progress is being made with gene therapy. This chapter will describe recent developments in the production of coagulation factor concentrates, including those manufactured by recombinant technology, as well as review novel approaches to improve the efficacy of therapy. New ways of managing patients with anti-factor VIII antibodies are described. Strategies for preventing virus transmission are reviewed. The consequences of hepatitis C virus (HCV) and human immunodeficiency virus (HIV) that are more specifically related to haemophilia are considered. There have been several recent good general reviews on haemophilia therapy (Mannucci 1993, Furie et al 1994, Hoyer 1994, Lusher 1995).

THERAPEUTIC PRODUCTS FOR TREATMENT OF HAEMOPHILIA A

In the past few years the use of more highly purified concentrates has become widespread. The initial impetus for this was the view that intermediate-purity products may modulate the immune system (Ludlam et al 1983) more than those of higher purity and that the latter were therefore more suitable for HIV positive patients (see below). Evidence has now accumulated that in HIV negative haemophiliacs concentrate may affect immune function (Goudemand et al 1993, Smid et al 1993) but that the immune abnormalities may be secondary to chronic liver disease (Makris & Preston 1993).

High-purity concentrates are usually manufactured by one of three technologies. Plasma-derived (pd) factor concentrates can be prepared by use of anti-factor VIII or anti-vWF (von Willebrand factor) monoclonal columns (Hemofil M and Monoclate P, respectively) or by ion-exchange chromatography. Although during the preparation of monoclonally prepared concentrates factor VIII reaches a specific activity of 2–3000 IU/mg, it is diluted in albumin solution to give a final purity of approximately 10–30 IU/mg. The ion-exchange concentrates, however, have a much higher final purity of approximately 50–150 IU/mg protein in the final vial. There has been considerable controversy as to how concentrates of differing purity should be described. Those with a specific activity of less than about 5 IU of factor VIII per mg of protein are usually considered to be of intermediate purity and in these only 0.1–1% is factor VIII, the remainder being fibrinogen, immunoglobulins and other plasma proteins. The problem of terminology arises when considering ion-exchange and monoclonally prepared concentrates, particularly as to whether vWF is seen as a contaminant, or impurity, in those prepared by ion-exchange and whether albumin is seen as an inert non-contaminant component. It should be noted that the albumin is derived from plasma, and the concentration of non-factor VIII non-albumin protein may in fact be greater in the monoclonally derived concentrates than in the ion-exchange concentrates (Schoppmann et al 1994). Rather than use terms such as high-purity, or ultra-high-purity, it is more informative to describe the mode of preparation of the concentrate and details of any additive (e.g. albumin).

These high-purity factor VIII concentrates are not suitable for treating von Willebrand's disease because they contain relatively low concentrations of vWF. They are preferred to intermediate-purity concentrates by patients (and staff) because they are easier and quicker to reconstitute, and because they have a higher potency (IU of factor VIII per ml) smaller infusion volumes are needed. They are thus more suitable for continuous infusion therapy than intermediate concentrates.

Recombinant factor VIII (rVIII) has been licensed in many countries after careful and thorough clinical trials. These have demonstrated that Kogenate (Cutter) and Recombinate (Baxter) are effective clinically, probably do not result in more anti-factor VIII inhibitors than pdVIII and have not transmitted viruses (Schwartz et al 1990, Lusher et al 1993, Bray et al 1994). The initial two rVIIIs are of the complete factor VIII molecule and are apparently very similar to pdVIII except that Kogenate has reduced glycosylation. A further rVIII has been produced which lacks the B domain; following synthesis the polypeptide spontaneously hydrolyses to give a light and a heavy chain which then associate to produce an active molecule. Clinical studies, which are well advanced, demonstrate that it is efficacious and that it probably does not contain neoantigens as none of the previously heavily treated severe haemophiliacs who have received it has developed an inhibitor. One intriguing difference from pdVIII that has emerged is that its coagulant activity in a one-stage factor VIII assay is almost half that when measured by a chromogenic method; the reason for this remains obscure (Oswaldsson et al 1994).

Initially clinicians were a little hesitant to use rVIII concentrates because of the possibility that they might lead to a higher incidence of anti-factor

VIII inhibition. Despite some reservations, because comparable data are not available for plasma-derived concentrates, many believe that existing licensed rVIIIs are probably not associated with a greater risk of inhibitor formation (see below). The widespread use of recombinant concentrates is partly checked, however, by the relatively high price. As availability is restricted it could be argued that initially they should be used in new patients with severe haemophilia and in others with mild haemophilia who only require infusions infrequently (e.g. to cover surgery) if desmopressin is not considered suitable.

For a review of progress in gene therapy for haemophilia A and B see Chapter 15.

Concentrates for the treatment of patients with anti-factor VIII inhibitors

Although human factor VIII can be used to treat individuals with low-level inhibitors, it is unsuitable alone for treating patients in whom the inhibitor titre is greater than 5 Bethesda units/ml. For treatment of patients with moderate- and high-titre anti-factor VIII inhibitors (>10 Bethesda units/ml), the main products used are prothrombin complex concentrates, activated prothrombin complex concentrate (FEIBA), porcine factor VIII and recombinant factor VIIa (rVIIa).

FEIBA, now virally attenuated by pressurized steam, has been in clinical use for treatment of inhibitor patients for many years and is moderately effective in promoting haemostasis. Its principal drawback is that it has occasionally been associated with arterial and venous thromboembolism and haemorrhagic myocardial infarcts (Thompson 1993). It should therefore be used with caution in patients with known vascular disease.

Polyelectrolyte-fractionated porcine factor VIII (Hyate C) is a high-purity concentrate which contains, in addition to factor VIII, some porcine vWF. This latter protein may cause acute transient thrombocytopenia although this is rarely clinically significant (Hay et al 1994). The frequency of this complication is now much less than with the previous lower-purity porcine concentrate which contained relatively large amounts of vWF. Occasionally, some patients experience a reaction to an infusion of porcine factor VIII; such reactions do not usually recur with subsequent infusions and they are not a contraindication to its continued use.

After initial studies (Hedner et al 1989) demonstrated that pdVIIa could promote haemostasis in severe haemophilia in the presence of an anti-factor VIII inhibitor, an VIIa was developed by Novo-Nordisk. The mechanism by which rVIIa stops bleeding remains uncertain, although it may act in combination with tissue factor and phospholipids at the site of injury to activate factor X and hence promote haemostasis. Its localization in this way would explain why it only rarely causes disseminated intravascular coagulation. rVIIa has a median half-life of 3.0 h in non-bleeding patients, and 2.3 h in those with active haemorrhage, suggesting that it is consumed in the haemostatic process (Lindley et al 1994). Using therapeutic doses of 70–90 µg/kg results in plasma factor VII:C levels that are 10–20 times normal; because of the short half-life, repeat infusions need to be given every 2–3 h. The resultant very high factor VII:C level leads to a 1–2-s shortening of the prothrombin time; it is possible, if monitoring is eventually considered necessary, that this might be a simple way in which it could be accomplished. Currently therapy with rVIIa is not routinely monitored by coagulation tests. Clinical studies are at an advanced stage and demonstrate that rVIIa can be safely used for the treatment of inhibitor patients (Schulman et al 1994a).

Fibrin sealant

Preparations of human fibrinogen and thrombin are available which, when applied together on bleeding surfaces, stop haemorrhage. This fibrin glue has found many potential applications, particularly when bleeding cannot be controlled by other means. For example, it is currently in trial in patients undergoing second, or subsequent, coronary artery bypass graft operations, when bleeding from previous scar tissue can be troublesome. In the management of haemophilia it may be of particular value in securing haemostasis following dental extraction by its application to the tooth socket (Martinowitz & Schulman 1995).

THERAPEUTIC PRODUCTS FOR TREATMENT OF HAEMOPHILIA B

Soon after the introduction of prothrombin complex concentrates, occasional cases of both arterial and venous thromboembolism began to be reported (Aronson 1979, Chistolini et al 1990, Conlan & Hoots 1990, Lusher 1991). It became clear that venous thromboembolism was particularly likely to occur in those individuals given large doses, especially in the postoperative setting; a number of patients are known to have died directly from pulmonary embolism. These concentrates are likely to precipitate thromboembolism in those predisposed either through severe atherosclerosis, or because of impaired hepatic function leading to poor clearance of activated clotting factor from the circulation, or in individuals with sepsis or crush injuries.

The mechanism by which these prothrombin complex concentrates cause thromboembolism is unclear. As they contain appreciable amounts of factors II and X, in addition to IX, it is possible that the high plasma concentration of these former proteins in the recipient's plasma after infusion may induce a hypercoagulable state. Alternatively, and perhaps more likely, the concentrates are thrombogenic because they contain significant amounts of activated procoagulant proteins (e.g. factor Xa). The results of a recent study indicate that factor IXa is the component which promotes activation in the recipient (Limentani et al 1995, Gray et al 1995, Philippou et al 1995). Another possible explanation is that it is the procoagulant phospholipids in these concentrates which promote intravascular thrombosis (Giles et al 1982, Kemball-Cook et al 1988).

With the development of reliable techniques for demonstrating activation of the haemostatic mechanism in vivo, it has been possible to assess this potential of prothrombin complex concentrates in both animals and humans. Fibrinopeptide A, prothrombin fragment 1.2 and thrombin–antithrombin III complexes have been measured following infusion of both prothrombin complex concentrates and high-purity factor IX concentrates. In dogs a marked elevation of fibrinopeptide A has been observed following infusion of prothrombin complex, with the peak level occurring at about 6 h (MacGregor et al 1991). Studies in individuals with haemophilia B have demonstrated that many have raised levels of fibrinopeptide A, prothrombin 1.2 and thrombin–antithrombin III complexes for many hours after infusion of prothrombin complex concentrates (Mannucci et al 1990, 1991a, Kim et al 1991). Although the concentrates themselves may contain significant amounts of activation markers (e.g. prothrombin 1.2), the magnitude and duration of their elevation is much greater than can be explained purely in terms of passive infusion.

High-purity factor IX concentrate

The preparation of high-purity single factor IX concentrates has been made possible through chromatography on monoclonal antibodies, ion-exchange resins, heparin, dextran sulphate, or metal chelate gels (Philippou et al 1995, Burnouf et al 1989, Hrinda et al 1991, Kasper et al 1991, Thomas et al 1995). Such processes allow the purification of factor IX to greater than 100 IU/mg of protein.

When compared to prothrombin complex concentrates, the single factor IX products have very similar in vivo recovery and half-life, the former being 30–60% and the latter 17–27 h. The results, however, depend upon the frequency and duration of sampling as well as the factor IX assay technique (Zauber & Levin 1977, Kohler et al 1988, Thomas et al 1994). When compared by the model independent techniques, similar factor IX kinetic parameters are observed for both types of concentrates. There is thus no evidence that the factor IX molecule is adversely modified during the manufacture of the highly purified concentrates.

There is now a substantial accumulation of evidence to demonstrate that high-purity factor IX concentrates do not cause significant activation of the haemostatic system and they are therefore less likely to induce clinical thromboembolism (Mannucci et al 1990, 1991b, Kim et al 1991, Thomas et al 1994).

High-purity factor IX concentrates are as clinically efficacious as prothrombin complex concentrates for promoting haemostasis in individuals with haemophilia B (Bardin & Sultan 1990, Goldsmith et al 1992, Thomas et al 1995). Furthermore, there are enough reports of their use in surgery to demonstrate that they probably have a much lower propensity to cause thromboembolism. Kasper (1992) has reported that only 4% of her patients have postoperatively developed a clinical thromboembolic episode with high-purity factor IX concentrate compared with 28% who received prothrombin complex. Furthermore, the high-purity concentrate IXMC (Bioproducts Laboratory), available in the UK, has been used successfully to cover surgery in 13 patients, four of whom had previously had clinical episodes of thromboembolism following surgery. When treated with IXMC none had a clinical thromboembolic episode despite very high doses being given to some patients who had previously had such a complication.

It is now generally agreed that all individuals with haemophilia B requiring surgery, or large doses of factor IX to cover major bleeds or injuries, should be treated with high-purity factor IX concentrate. As thromboembolism has been associated with prothrombin complex concentrate use in apparent non-high-risk situations, it seems prudent also to have a policy of moving towards treating all bleeds in haemophilia B with high-purity concentrate.

PROPHYLACTIC THERAPY

The pioneering studies to introduce prophylactic therapy for haemophilia A and B were undertaken in Malmö and these have demonstrated that if this form of treatment is started in very small children there is maintenance of good joint function to adult life (Nilsson 1993). That such an approach is justified is supported by the Orthopaedic Outcome Study which followed the radiological status of joints over a 6-year period. This study revealed that joint damage could not be prevented by on-demand therapy but was when prophylactic treatment was used for more than 40 weeks per year (Aledort et al 1994).

The aim of prophylactic treatment is to reduce bleeding frequency substantially in severe haemophilia by regular transfusions of factor VIII or IX such that the plasma level does not fall below 1 IU/dl. This can be achieved by infusions of 25–40 IU of factor VIII per kg three times weekly, or 25–40 IU of factor IX per kg twice weekly; it is good practice to measure the trough level from time to time to ensure that it is just above 1 IU/dl.

Although there are clear benefits of prophylactic schedules, such therapy is not without difficulty. Regular infusions twice weekly starting in babies at 1–2 years of age pose the difficulty of venous access. Almost invariably an indwelling central venous catheter is needed. Hickman and Broviac lines have been used but are associated with more infections than with indwelling Port-A-Caths. With one of these in situ, treatment can be given at home three times weekly by parents. The success of such systems depends upon their careful maintenance and scrupulous attention to aseptic technique

(Girvan et al 1994). Infected catheters – which occur more frequently in patients with inhibitors – should be removed, but they can be replaced by one on the contralateral side.

The other drawback of prophylactic therapy is that factor VIII consumption is greater than with on-demand treatment. Using thrice weekly injections of factor VIII for prophylaxis the annual use is in the region of 5000 IU/kg, compared perhaps to 2000 IU/kg with on-demand therapy. Swedish studies have demonstrated that the amount of factor VIII/IX required can be reduced if careful pharmacokinetic studies are undertaken in each patient (Carlsson et al 1993, Bjorkman et al 1994). Consumption can also be radically reduced if daily injections are given because it is not necessary to achieve such high peak levels. When implantable, or other, devices become available to give a continuous infusion, the factor VIII requirements will enable prophylaxis to be given with very modest factor VIII use, i.e. less than is currently used with on-demand regimens.

The overall benefits of prophylactic therapy have been objectively assessed and it was found that children spent more time at school, or adults at work, and that they were hospitalized less often (Bohn et al 1993). There is, therefore, now a consensus that prophylactic therapy with factor VIII/IX is the treatment of choice for children with severe haemophilia. For those with haemophilia B this should be with high-purity factor IX; for those with haemophilia A a high-purity product is preferable (Roberts 1994).

Continuous infusion

Traditionally replacement therapy for those undergoing surgery, or with severe bleeds, has been by repeated bolus infusions of concentrate. Recent studies have demonstrated that some reconstituted preparations of factor VIII concentrate are stable at room temperature for up to 15 days (Schulman et al 1994b). Treatment is started with an initial bolus to raise the level of factor VIII to 80–100 IU/dl and the infusion is commenced at 2 IU/kg/h (Martinowitz et al 1992, Schulman et al 1994b, Doughty et al 1995). Children require higher infusion doses because factor VIII has a shorter half-life compared to adults. After a few days of continuous infusion the clearance of factor VIII diminishes and the rate of infusion can often be reduced. When used in this way the amount of factor VIII required to cover surgery is reduced to a half or two-thirds that needed by bolus injection because it is not necessary to have high peak levels to ensure that there is an appropriate trough concentration. Porcine factor VIII is reported to be stable in an infusion system after reconstitution and it has been given by this means for the treatment of bleeding, and to cover surgery, in inhibitor patients (McKernan et al 1995). Although there has been some anxiety about giving factor IX by continuous infusion in case it becomes activated while in the infusion pump, a recent report indicates that this reservation may be unfounded (Schulman et al 1995).

ANTI-FACTOR VIII ANTIBODIES

There has always been intense interest in anti-factor VIII antibodies because their clinical consequences are so detrimental (Hoyer & Scandella 1994, Hay 1995). Anti-factor VIII antibodies have also been reported in 17% of normal blood donors at low titre and in these individuals the factor VIII:C levels are no different from those in whom antibodies cannot be detected (Algiman et al 1992). In addition to antibodies that neutralize the factor VIII activity, it is now clear that there are also anti-factor VIII antibodies which bind but do not reduce its coagulant function (Gilles et al 1993). Anti-idiotypic antibodies have been reported to be present in some individuals, and these may be responsible for keeping the production of anti-factor VIII antibodies suppressed. It is possible that acquired haemophilia results from an imbalance in anti-factor VIII and its anti-idiotypic antibody (Tiarks et al 1989). Interest in this field has intensified recently because of the possibility that use of rVIII may be more antigenic than those derived from plasma. There may also be a genetic predisposition to antibody formation (Aly et al 1990). Interferon use may predispose to the development of antibodies (Castenskiold et al 1994). Inhibitors are also of topical interest because there are new therapeutic strategies to promote their suppression.

There is still controversy as to whether high-purity or recombinant concentrates are associated with a higher incidence of neutralizing antibodies than with cryoprecipitate or intermediate-purity concentrates. Whilst it can be readily understood that there may be differences between studies in incidence of low-level and transient inhibitors (because they may not be diagnosed), it is harder to find rational explanations for the very large difference in incidence rate for high-titre inhibitors as it is unlikely that these would be overlooked either clinically or on laboratory testing. For high-titre inhibitors (>10 Bethesda units/ml), the cumulative incidence ranges from 2% to 46% in severe haemophiliacs treated with cryoprecipitate or intermediate-purity concentrate. The mean cumulative incidence was 20% at 18 years but there was a very wide confidence level on this estimate. There are well-designed prospective studies assessing inhibitor incidence in previously untransfused patients receiving recombinant products and smaller numbers in receipt of plasma-derived monoclonal products. If there is a true difference in incidence of inhibitor development between cryoprecipitate, intermediate-purity, ion-exchange and monoclonally prepared concentrate and those manufactured by recombinant technology, it is likely to be relatively small and will only be demonstrable by very large prospective studies. The subject has been well reviewed and critically analysed (Briet & Rosendaal 1994, Briet et al 1994).

One clear example of a factor VIII concentrate being particularly immunogenic has been reported, and demonstrates that quite subtle changes in the fractionation process may lead to neoantigen formation. A recent outbreak of inhibitors was reported in Belgium and The Netherlands in which previously extensively treated adult patients were found to have developed neutralizing antibodies (Peerlinck et al 1993, Rosendaal et al 1993). This was observed after patients were converted from a dry-heated intermediate-purity concentrate to one of similar purity that had been pasteurized. The antibodies had different characteristics from classical inhibitors, being relatively slow-acting when tested in vitro and with activity against the factor VIII light chain. Unlike the usual haemophilic inhibitors they disappeared when the patients were treated with a different brand of factor VIII concentrate.

Whilst it is well established that anti-factor VIII antibodies develop predominantly in severe haemophiliacs, they do occasionally appear in those with mild disease. Whereas previously it was considered that many of these were low-level and often transient, there is now evidence that they can be of high titre, persistent and lead to uncontrollable haemorrhage. Many arise following large doses of concentrate to cover surgery even though the patient may have been transfused on numerous previous occasions for haemorrhagic episodes (Hay & Ludlam 1996).

MANAGEMENT OF PATIENTS WITH INHIBITORS

Treatment of bleeding episodes in inhibitor patients depends upon the severity of the bleed and the level of the inhibitor against both human and porcine factor VIII. It is generally agreed that better clinical results are obtained if a measurable increase in factor VIII is obtained after infusion of concentrate. With an anti-human factor VIII level of up to 5 Bethesda units/ml, it is often possible, using large doses of human factor VIII concentrate, to obtain measurable post infusion levels, particularly after the second or third infusion. Those with an anti-porcine level up to 15 Bethesda units/ml may respond to porcine factor VIII concentrate at 100 IU/kg. Above these inhibitor levels it is necessary to use either prothrombin complex, activated prothrombin complex (FEIBA) or factor VIIa. Much interest is accruing in rVIIa as clinical studies demonstrate its efficacy and safety, including to cover surgery (Schulman et al 1994a). Contrary to prior preconceptions this product has proved to be remarkably safe, particularly from inducing intravascular coagulation.

An important aspect of the management of patients with inhibitors is to consider whether it might be possible to suppress anti-factor VIII synthesis. The infusion of large daily doses of factor VIII concentrate over a period of many months often leads to the inhibitor concentration falling to levels at which it cannot be detected in vitro and does not shorten the survival time of infused factor VIII. It is becoming clear that the success of tolerization regimens is highest if regular factor VIII infusions are started early after the appearance of an inhibitor. Success is also greater for those with a low, compared to a high, level of antibodies. Although daily infusions of less than 100 IU of factor VIII per kg will suppress the inhibitor in 70% of those with <10 Bethesda units/ml, doses over 100 IU/kg will give success in 95% of patients. For those with high initial levels of inhibitor (i.e. > 50 Bethesda units/ml), it is necessary to give 100–200 IU of factor VIII per kg daily, and this will be successful in about 90% of patients (Mariani et al 1994, Kreuz et al 1995). Tolerization has also been reported using porcine factor VIII (Hay et al 1990).

Tolerization should be continued until the inhibitor is no longer detectable and the half-life of infused concentrate has normalized. It is important that tolerizing treatment should not be interrupted as this reduces its efficacy. If the inhibitor is still detectable at 18 months there is little to be gained by further therapy. Once patients are tolerized, inhibitors usually do not reappear, thus allowing the patient to revert to on-demand or prophylactic factor VIII therapy.

Some tolerizing regimens have included other blood products and immunosuppressives. That of Brackman included daily high-dose FEIBA therapy in addition to factor VIII; the value of this activated prothrombin complex remains unproven (Brackmann 1992). The Malmö regimen has additional components (extracorporeal antibody adsorption on protein A, intravenous IgG and cyclophosphamide), each of which individually has a rationale for use, but whether the success of the overall regimen is dependent on anything other than factor VIII remains uncertain (Nilsson et al 1988). Data from the International Registry, and other studies, indicate that a low starting inhibitor level aids success; in the Malmö protocol this is achieved by immunoadsorption using an extracorporeal protein A column to reduce the anti-factor VIII antibody. The 5-day course of intravenous IgG not only replaces antibodies removed by adsorption but its anti-idiotypic antibodies may contribute to the overall success of the therapy (Dietrich et al 1992). A similar protocol has been used successfully to treat anti-factor IX inhibitors in haemophilia B (Nilsson et al 1995). Further studies to demonstrate the value of immunosuppressive chemotherapy with cyclophosphamide in reducing the level of remaining alloantibodies are needed to prove the efficiency of this therapy.

The mechanism by which these tolerizing regimens suppress the inhibitor level remains obscure. Possible mechanisms include a change in antibody specificity such that it becomes non-inhibitory and may be present as an immune complex with factor VIII (Nilsson et al 1990). It is possible that there may be an increased production of anti-idiotypic antibodies. These may be stimulated by immunizing patients with immune complexes, and preliminary results demonstrate suppression of anti-factor VIII titres by such means (Gilles et al 1994).

VIRAL SAFETY OF FACTOR VIII AND IX CONCENTRATE

The overall safety of all blood products depends not only upon careful donor selection and the screening of donations for infectious viruses, but also on the efficacy of specific antiviral steps in the manufacturing process (Mannucci 1993).

The viruses transmissible by coagulation factor concentrates derived from plasma are listed in Table 14.1. The recently described hepatitis G virus may also be transmissible by blood products (Simons et al 1995, Zuckerman 1995). Intracellular pathogenic viruses (e.g. Epstein–Barr virus (EBV), cytome-galovirus, human T-cell lymphoma virus 1), although potentially transmissible by fresh cellular blood components, are not transmitted by cell-free products.

The techniques currently employed for viral inactivation of factor VIII/ IX concentrates are listed in Table 14.2. Of the viruses tested in Table 14.1, those that are lipid-coated are sensitive to solvent/detergent, and several are also heat-sensitive. Although some concentrates have undergone systematic assessment for viral safety using guidelines of the Scientific and Standardization Committee (SSC) of the International Society of Thrombosis and Hemostasis (Mannucci & Colombo 1989), many products have not (Laurian et al 1994) and are presumed to present a low risk of virus transmission on the basis of experience with the virucidal process used for other concentrates and anecdotes rather than properly conducted studies.

Hepatitis A virus (HAV) has only recently been found to be transmitted by factor VIII concentrates. The initial four outbreaks in Italy, Germany, Belgium and Ireland were all linked to a single manufacturing technique (Mariani et al 1991, Gerritzen et al 1992a, Mannucci 1992, Temperley et al 1992, Peerlinck & Vermylen 1993, Mannucci et al 1994). The concentrate was a high-purity ion-exchange product treated by solvent/detergent. Although HAV infection in non-haemophiliacs is often asymptomatic, many

Table 14.1 Viruses potentially transmissible by coagulation factor concentrates

	Lipid coat	Solvent/detergent-sensitive	Heat-sensitive
Hepatitis A (HAV)	No	No	Yes
Hepatitis B (HBV)	Yes	Yes	Yes
Hepatitis C (HCV)	Yes	Yes	Yes
Hepatitis D (HDV)	No	Yes	Yes
Human immuno-deficiency virus (HIV)	Yes	Yes	Yes
Parvovirus	No	No	No

Table 14.2 Current single viral inactivation methods

• Dry heat	80°C for 72 h
• Pasteurization	60°C for 10 h
• Steam heat	60°C for 10 h + 80°C/1h
• Solvent/detergent	TNBP + Tween 80 or Triton X-100

TNBP, tri(n-butyl) phosphate

haemophiliacs infected in these outbreaks became clinically unwell and jaundiced, presumably because of pre-existing liver disease due to hepatitis C virus (HCV). HAV infection may therefore be of serious consequence, unlike in the majority of non-haemophiliacs. A further outbreak in South Africa has recently been reported in association with the use of an intermediate-purity, solvent/detergent concentrate (Cohn et al 1994). Why after many years when factor VIII has not transmitted hepatitis A should it suddenly do so now? One explanation is that there has been a change in the epidemiology of hepatitis A in the community. Previously many individuals became infected as children and thereafter became immune. Now acute infection in Western countries tends to occur in young adults; thus blood donors are likely to have a higher incidence of viraemia and fever will have specific humoral immunity which will contribute neutralizing antibodies to the plasma pools. In an attempt to prevent HAV infection of haemophiliacs in the UK, hepatitis A vaccination has been recommended.

Hepatitis B virus (HBV) was transmitted by some batches of factor VIII/ IX concentrate prior to the mid 1980s, despite screening of individual donations for HBsAg (Stirling et al 1983). Since then, transmission has been rare, partly because all potential recipients are vaccinated against hepatitis B and also because of viral inactivation steps in the manufacturing process. As HBV has a lipid coat it is susceptible to the solvent/detergent virucidal process. As a result of vaccinating recipients it is now very difficult to assess the safety of current concentrates for HBV, but the virus may withstand pasteurization at 60°C for 10 h (Brackmann & Egli 1988). An outbreak has recently been reported in which HBV has been transmitted by a prothrombin complex concentrate pasteurized at 60°C for 10 h (Arzneimittelkommission 1994).

Hepatitis C virus (HCV) was probably transmitted by all batches of factor VIII/IX concentrates prior to the introduction of virucidal procedures (Fletcher et al 1983, Kernoff et al 1985). Furthermore, HCV RNA could be detected in the early concentrates, particularly those from commercial sources (Simmonds et al 1990, Makris et al 1993, Guo & Yu 1995). As it is a lipid-coated, relatively heat-labile virus, it is susceptible to solvent/ detergent (Horowitz et al 1994). Although HCV is heat-sensitive, at least three cases of HCV transmission have been reported as being from pasteurized concentrates (Gerritzen et al 1992b, Schulman et al 1992, Koehler-Vajta et al 1993). Heat treatment at 80°C for 72 h is particularly effective at reducing infectivity (Rizza et al 1993).

Hepatitis D virus (HDV) is an incomplete virus, being a passenger within HBV; individuals only become infected, therefore, by HDV if they are not immune to HBV. This occurs if a non-HBV-immune patient is exposed to the HBV with HDV, or if an individual is HBsAg positive (and therefore not immune) and becomes superinfected by HBV possessing HDV. In some series, up to 65% of HBsAg positive haemophiliacs may be anti-HDV positive (Wagner et al 1992).

Human immunodeficiency virus (HIV) is a lipid-coated, heat-sensitive virus and is therefore also susceptible to heat and solvent/detergent treatment. The currently used virucidal techniques appear to be extremely effective in ensuring that concentrates have an exceedingly low HIV infectivity, although the early heat treatment processes were relatively ineffective (Van den Berg et al 1986, White et al 1986, Mariani et al 1987, Weisser 1988, Dietrich et al 1990, Remis et al 1990, Williams et al 1990b). Following an outbreak of HIV in ten haemophiliacs reported in 1990, the β-propiolactone and ultraviolet (UV) light virucidal process used for factor IX concentrates (Kleim et al 1990, Karcher 1991) was withdrawn. Further investigation revealed that the safety margin for this technique was small (Norley et al 1993).

Parvovirus is a small single-stranded DNA virus lacking a lipid envelope (Young 1995), the genome can be detected in factor VIII concentrates (Kerr et al 1995). Its heat resistance is demonstrated by transmission by pasteurized concentrates and following dry heat treatment at 80°C for 72 h as well as at 100°C for 30 min (Lyon et al 1989, Williams et al 1990a, Azzi et al 1992, Santagostino et al 1994). There is therefore a high seroprevalence for parvovirus in young children with haemophilia (Mortimer et al 1983, Kluiber & Wolff 1994). As it lacks a lipid envelope, solvent/detergent is ineffective in preventing infection (Lefrere et al 1994, Santagostino et al 1994). In children, parvovirus causes a self-limiting acute erythematous illness, but in some adults it may cause serious sequelae (e.g. chronic arthropathy or severe systemic illness) and may result in persistent viraemia (Kerr et al 1995, Musiani et al 1995). Infection is pregnancy may cause hydrops fetalis. Because of its ability to infect erythroblasts it can caused red cell aplasia, particularly in those individuals who already have a haemolytic state or who are actively bleeding. HIV-infected individuals may fail to clear the virus following infection and become chronically viraemic, which may result in persistent anaemia. There is no plasma-derived coagulation factor concentrate with a proven safety record for parvovirus.

The sporadic instances of viral infection, as described above, are often difficult to investigate because they are rare, discovered retrospectively, usually only involve a single batch of concentrate and may be difficult to distinguish from an outbreak of the same virus in the community (e.g. hepatitis A). Why are some viruses still being transmitted by blood products? Failure of good manufacturing practice could lead to virus transmission, as may a virucidal process with a low safety margin (e.g. HIV transmission by β-propiolactone and UV light-treated concentrate). Changes in the seroprevalence of viruses in the donor community may potentially result in an increased likelihood of transmission (e.g. hepatitis A; see above). The level of viraemia in the plasma pools may vary markedly over time; the incidence of parvovirus is high in the Spring and Autumn with a result that 1:3300 donations may be infectious, whereas at other times of the year it may be as low as 1:20 000 (McOmish et al 1993).

As a result of the episodes of virus transmission by currently available concentrates there have been calls for all manufacturing processes to include two viral inactivation procedures. Such concentrates are available from several manufacturers (see Table 14.3). There have been no clinical studies, however, to demonstrate that these products have enhanced viral safety. A variety of other virucidal techniques are under evaluation (Table 14.4). Although it is tempting to include additional virucidal procedures in the manufacturing process, these may not be innocuous as demonstrated by the recent outbreak of anti-factor VIII antibodies developing in haemophiliacs treated with a recently introduced intermediate-purity pasteurized concentrate in The Netherlands and Belgium as described above (Peerlinck et al 1993, Rosendaal et al 1993).

How should the viral safety of coagulation factor VIII/IX concentrates be assessed? The use of model viruses in scaled-down bench-top fractionation models has provided a sound basis for the initial assessment of virucidal processes. Screening the final vial to detect viral RNA/DNA sequences by PCR (polymerase chain reaction) will not prove sufficiently sensitive to detect all infectious batches; products that are PCR negative may still transmit virus. Those that are PCR positive are likely to be infectious, although it should be remembered that this detection technique only identifies viral RNA/DNA sequences and not infectious virus. The SCC guidelines for monitoring the treatment of previously untransfused patients were a very valuable step forward in the systematic appraisal of viral safety (Mannucci et al 1989). The difficulty with the protocol is that fortnightly blood samples are required for 16 weeks and monthly ones until 26 weeks, and as most patients are newly diagnosed severe haemophiliacs this has put a major burden on these babies and their parents. A way forward may be a form of postmarketing surveillance or 'pharmacovigalence' in which large numbers of haemophiliacs are routinely screened for known transmissible viruses and the data systematically collected (Vermylen & Briet 1993).

Table 14.3 Double viral inactivation methods

• Sodium thiocyanate	plus	ultrafiltration
• Solvent/detergent	plus	dry heat at 80°C for 72 h
• Solvent/detergent	plus	dry heat at 100°C for 30 min

Table 14.4 Viral reduction processes under evaluation

- Nanofiltration
- Irradiation ± photosensitive chemicals
- Ozone treatment
- Chemical treatments
  - phenanthroline – Cu^{2+} complex
  - long-chain fatty acids

HEPATITIS C INFECTION

It is now generally agreed that many individuals with haemophilia who were treated with non-virally inactivated concentrates prior to the mid-1980s, have significant liver disease due to HCV (Watson et al 1992), and the genome can be detected in factor VIII/IX concentrates manufactured prior to 1985 (Simmonds et al 1990). Whereas formerly the persistent transmission of non-A and non-B hepatitis was considered by many as benign, there is now substantial evidence that those with hepatitis C infection have chronic progressive liver disease (Hay et al 1985). In the UK, deaths from liver disease are as frequent as those from intracranial haemorrhage and are now only surpassed in incidence by fatalities directly due to HIV. Although hepatitis C infection in haemophiliacs is similar to that in non-haemophiliacs, the former has a number of distinctive features. Most individuals with severe haemophilia will have been infected lifelong as all concentrates prior to the mid-1980s were infectious for HCV. Many haemophiliacs are also coinfected with HIV and there is evidence that in such circumstances the level of hepatitis C viraemia is higher and the progression to symptomatic liver disease quicker (Eyster et al 1994). Additionally, 8% of haemophiliacs have chronically replicating HBV which suppresses HCV replication (Hanley et al 1993). Haemophiliacs are likely to have been exposed to multiple genotypes of HCV and have become infected with more than one, unlike non-haemophiliacs who almost exclusively appear to be infected with a single genotype (Jarvis et al 1994). Longitudinal studies in haemophiliacs, however, reveal that one genotype is predominantly expressed, except in those who are HIV positive in whom there is a greater propensity for the principal genotype in the serum to change over a period of years. Transmission to household and sexual contacts, particularly if HIV negative, has been reported but is uncommon (Brackmann et al 1993).

HCV has been subdivided into six major genotypes and some of these have a marked geographical restriction (Dusheiko & Simmonds 1994). Genotypes 1, 2 and 3 are present in Western Europe, while type 4 is found almost exclusively in Egypt, type 5 in South Africa and type 6 in South-East Asia. Haemophiliacs treated with coagulation factor concentrates prepared from local blood donors have a spectrum of HCV genotypes which clearly mirror the distribution of genotypes in the donors. Thus haemophiliacs in Hungary have almost exclusively type 1 and in South Africa predominantly type 5, whereas in Scotland types 1, 2 and 3 are present in haemophiliacs in proportions almost identical to those in the local population (Jarvis et al 1996).

Systematic study of haemophiliacs has revealed that many have progressed to have significant liver pathology. In one recent study of 86 anti-HCV positive patients, 15% had oesophageal varices and 17% splenomegaly (Hanley et al 1996b). Laparoscopic inspection and/or biopsy revealed severe inflammatory change and fibrosis in 34%. The severity of liver disease in this study was not related to the circulating HCV genotype although in another report genotype 3 was associated with more advanced disease (Preston et al 1995b). Other studies suggest that genotype 1b may be associated with more severe disease in non-haemophiliacs (Nousbaum et al 1995).

A further complication of HCV-induced liver disease is hepatocellular carcinoma. The observed incidence in haemophiliacs is 20 times that expected. In a report of 13 cases, at least four arose in mild haemophiliacs and one individual only had a single infusion of concentrate (Colombo et al 1991, Preston et al 1995a). If hepatocellular carcinoma arises as a single lesion and is diagnosed early, treatment by injection of ethanol or liver transplantation can be lifesaving. For this reason it is now recommended policy in the UK that haemophiliacs over the age of 45 years should have liver ultrasound examinations every 4 months.

The only licensed treatment for HCV infection is interferon-α. Initial studies in haemophiliacs (Table 14.5) indicated that the response, as judged by normalization of alanine aminotransferase (AIT), was similar to other individuals and that this was not adversely affected by HIV infection (Makris et al 1991, Bresters et al 1992). More recent investigations of larger numbers has indicated that the response, as judged by normalization of the ALT, is observed in only about 25–45% (Peerlinck et al 1994, Telfer et al 1995, Hanley et al 1996a). If serum HCV RNA is quantitated it becomes undetectable in only 20–25% when assessed by a sensitive PCR assay which can detect 80 copies of HCV per ml. The response rate is closely related to genotype. Those of genotype 3 (and probably 2) have a better prognosis in that seven out of 11 individuals with genotypes 2 or 3 cleared HCV RNA compared to none out of 18 with genotype 1. After therapy was discontinued, five of seven patients relapsed rapidly, with HCV RNA becoming detectable again in the serum.

These results are similar to the findings of another recent study (Telfer et al 1995) and indicate that the chance of long-term cure with modest doses of interferon-α is small. There is some evidence in non-haemophiliacs that treatment with doses greater than 3 million units three times weekly or for periods of longer than 6 months may result in a modest enhancement in the response rate (Poynarad et al 1995).

Table 14.5 Interferon treatment for HCV in haemophilia

	n	Response (%)		Sustained response (%)
		ALT	HCV RNA	
Makris et al 1991	16	44	–	25
Bresters et al 1992	8	40	50	50
Peerlinck et al 1994	13	53	53	7
Telfer et al 1995	20	45	25	5
Hanley et al 1996a	32	35	25	6

ALT, alanine aminotransferase.

HIV IN HAEMOPHILIA

Between 1979 and 1985 HIV was transmitted by factor VIII and IX concentrates. The seroprevalence for HIV in recipients depends upon the frequency of transfusion and the source and type of blood products (Darby et al 1989). Treatment of patients with cryoprecipitate or concentrate prepared from local donors in whom there was a low prevalence of HIV resulted in few patients becoming infected, whereas treatment with plasma products from a donor population in which HIV was more common resulted in a high proportion of infected patients, even when cryoprecipitate was used. It is well established that the HIV prevalence is much higher in those who received frequent infusions (i.e. severe haemophiliacs), whereas those only occasionally transfused, especially if treated with cryoprecipitate, had a much lower incidence. The prognosis of HIV-infected haemophiliacs is age-dependent and is similar to that of other HIV positive risk groups (Darby et al 1990, Phillips et al 1994).

The manifestations, treatment and prognosis of HIV infection in haemophiliacs is similar to non-haemophiliacs with some important exceptions. Kaposi's sarcoma is rarely observed in haemophiliacs (or intravenous drug abusers) and the reason for this remains uncertain. It is possible that Kaposi's sarcoma is due to another virus cotransmitting with HIV, which can be passed on sexually but which cannot be transmitted by blood. The recent proposal that it may be due to a human herpes-like virus may offer an explanation in that such viruses are not transmitted by cell-free coagulation factor concentrates (Chang et al 1994).

Non-Hodgkin's lymphomas are a feature of AIDS infection and evidence is accumulating that their incidence may be higher in haemophiliacs than in others (Kaplan, 1990, Levin 1992, Ragni et al 1993). The risk of non-Hodgkin's lymphoma in HIV positive haemophiliacs is 30–100-fold greater than in those who are HIV negative. The risk increases with age and is probably not influenced by antiviral therapy. The lymphomas are characteristically aggressive, high-grade B-cell tumours often involving extranodal sites, especially in the gastrointestinal tract. About one-third are associated with EBV. An 11-fold increase in basal cell carcinoma in HIV positive haemophiliacs has also been reported.

There has been an extensive debate about whether the use of less pure coagulation factor concentrates may modulate the immune system of HIV infected haemophiliac recipients such that they develop manifestations of AIDS sooners. This was of major concern following the initial studies in the early 1980s which demonstrated that HIV negative haemophiliacs also had immune abnormalities, including reduced CD4 counts. These abnormalities were considered to be due either to non-A and non-B hepatitis or to non-factor VIII constituents in the relatively impure factor VIII concentrates in use at that time (Prowse 1992, Watson & Ludlam 1992). These have been shown to have a range of effects on lymphocytes, monocytes and natural killer cells when tested in vitro, but to what extent these are responsible for the immune modulation observed in patients is uncertain. There is now evidence that immune changes in HIV negative haemophiliacs may in part be due to HCV. More recent studies in patients treated exclusively with virally inactivated intermediate-purity concentrates, who are both HIV and HCV negative, reveal that the recipients have normal CD4 counts, supporting the concept that the previously reduced levels were secondary to chronic liver disease (Makris & Preston 1993).

As a result of the initial studies demonstrating immune abnormality, possibly resulting from the non-factor VIII components of the concentrates, concern has been expressed at to whether their use in HIV-infected individuals might hasten its progression (Berntorp 1994). That the prognosis is apparently the same for severe and mild haemophilia suggests that the large amounts of concentrate used by the former patients to treat frequent bleeds does not hasten HIV progression (Goedert et al 1989).

Several studies have compared serial CD4 cell counts in patients treated with high- and intermediate-purity concentrates. All studies suffer from the disadvantage of small numbers of patients and in some there was an appreciable loss of individuals during follow-up, making interpretation of the results problematic. An unusual feature of these reports is that CD4 counts remained stable in recipients of high-purity monoclonal concentrates compared to intermediate-purity concentrates, over a 2-year period; thus it appears that such concentrates are able to prevent the gradual decline in CD4 numbers which is characteristic of HIV infection (de Biasi et al 1991). A similar observation was made in another 3-year study (Seremetis et al 1993). A further study compared an intermediate-purity with a high-purity ion-exchange concentrate; the CD4 count declined gradually and equally in the recipients of both products, thus not demonstrating any benefit of the high-purity concentrate (Mannucci et al 1991b). A recent study comparing a high-purity ion-exchange concentrate with a monoclonal concentrate reported that the CD4 count declined more rapidly with the former (Varon et al 1994). This study suggested that it was not the purity that was important but that a constituent in the ion-exchange product is detrimental to those with HIV infection. Unfortunately in this study the two groups of patients were not comparable as the initial CD4 count in the recipients of ion-exchange concentrate was twice that of those who received the monoclonal product. It is reported that CD4 counts fall more rapidly early in HIV infection and hence the differences observed in this study may merely be due to the patients in the ion-exchange concentrate-treated group being at an earlier stage of their HIV infection. A further study to assess prospectively HIV progression in recipients of ion-exchange and monoclonal purified concentrates is under way in the UK.

The evidence is therefore inconclusive, but there is a consensus that high-purity products should be used for the treatment of HIV positive patients, but whether a monoclonal concentrate is better than an ion-exchange prepared concentrate remains uncertain. The studies reported above have emphasized the differences in CD4 cell count which has been used as a surrogate marker for HIV progression. None of the studies has demonstrated that use of high-purity concentrates delays progression to clinical AIDS.

KEY POINTS FOR CLINIC PRACTICE

- Recently new plasma derived coagulation factor concentrates have been developed, e.g. IX, which are of higher purity than formerly and their use is associated with fewer side effects, e.g. thromboembolism. Recombinant factor VIIa and VIII are available and other synthetic products are under development.

- Prophylactic therapy with factor VIII and IX, thrice and twice weekly respectively, in young children with severe haemophilia, prevents most bleeds and maintains normal joint structure and function to adulthood.

- Continuous infusions of factor VIII intravenously, to cover the postoperative period or treatment of a severe bleed results in effective haemostatic cover and saves considerable quantities of concentrate compared to the use of regular bolus injections.

- For patients developing anti-factor VIII antibodies tolerisation with 200 U/kg/day factor VIII often leads to eradication of the inhibitor, this is most likely to occur if tolerisation is started shortly after the antibody is first detected and if it is <10 BU/ml.

- Currently available concentrates derived from human plasma are all manufactured with a single, and in some cases a double, viral inactivation step. All have a high degree of demonstrable safety for HIV and HCV. Parvovirus is resistant to both heat and solvent/detergent and can result in serious symptomatic infection particularly in adults.

- Infection with persistent viruses, e.g. HIV and HCV, requires regular monitoring of patients for the development of clinical sequelae, use of anti-viral drugs and prophylaxis against opportunistic infections.

REFERENCES

Aledort L M, Haschmeyer R H, Pettersson H 1994 A longitudinal study of orthopaedic outcomes for severe factor-VIII-deficient haemophiliacs. Intern Med 236: 391–399
Algiman M, Dietrich G, Nydegger U E et al 1992 Natural antibodies to factor VIII (anti-hemophilic factor) in healthy individuals. Proc Natl Acad Sci USA 89: 3795–3799
Aly A M, Aledort L M, Lee T D, Hoyer L W 1990 Histocompatibility antigen patterns in haemophilic patients with factor VIII antibodies. Br J Haematol 76: 238–241
Aronson D L 1979 Factor IX complex. Semin Thromb Hemost 7: 28–43
Arzneimittelkommission 1994 Information. Beriplex HS250 and 500. Pharm Ztg 139: 2192–2193
Azzi A, Ciappi S, Zakvrzewska K et al 1992 Human parvovirus B19 infection in

hemophiliacs first infused with two high-purity, virally attenuated factor VIII concentrates. Am J Hematol 39: 228–230

Bardin J M, Sultan Y 1990 Factor IX concentrate versus prothrombin complex concentrate for the treatment of hemophilia B during surgery. Transfusion 30: 441–443

Berntorp E 1994 Impact of replacement therapy on the evolution of HIV infection in hemophiliacs. Thromb Haemost 71: 678–683

Bjorkman S, Carlsson M, Berntorp E 1994 Pharmacokinetics of factor IX in patients with haemophilia B. Methodological aspects and physiological interpretation. Eur J Clin Pharmacol 46: 325–332

Bohn R L, Avorn J, Aledort L M et al 1993 Cost-effectiveness – can it be measured? Semin Hematol 30: 20–25

Brackmann H H 1992 16 years experience with the immunotolerance induction in hemophilia patients at the Bonn Hemophilia Centre. XX International Congress of the World Federation of Hemophilia, Athens, Greece (abstract)

Brackmann H H, Egli H 1988 Acute hepatitis B infection after treatment with heat-inactivated factor VIII concentrate. Lancet ii: 967 (letter)

Brackmann S A, Gerritzen A, Oldenburg J et al 1993 Search for intrafamilial transmission of hepatitis C virus in hemophilia patients. Blood 81: 1077–1082

Bray G L, Gomperts E D, Courter S et al 1994 A multicenter study of recombinant factor VIII (recombinate): safety, efficacy, and inhibitor risk in previously untreated patients with hemophilia A. Blood 83: 2428–2435

Bresters D, Mauser Bunschoten E P, Cuypers H T et al 1992 Disappearance of hepatitis C virus RNA in plasma during interferon alpha-2B treatment in hemophilia patients. Scand J Gastroenterol 27: 166–168

Briet E, Rosendaal F R 1994 Inhibitors in hemophilia A: are some products safer? Semin Hemat 31: 11–15

Briet E, Rosendaal F R, Kreuz W et al 1994 High titer inhibitors in severe haemophilia A. A meta-analysis based on eight long-term follow-up studies concerning inhibitors associated with crude or intermediate purity factor VIII products (4). Thromb Haemost 72: 162–164

Burnouf T, Michalski C, Goudemand M, Huart J J 1989 Properties of a highly purified human plasma factor IX:C therapeutic concentrate prepared by conventional chromatography. Vox Sang 57: 225–232

Carlsson M, Berntorp E, Bjorkman S, Lindvall K 1993 Pharmacokinetic dosing in prophylactic treatment of hemophilia A. Eur J Haemat 51: 247–252

Castenskiold E C, Colvin B T, Kelsey S M 1994 Acquired factor VIII inhibitor associated with chronic interferon-alpha therapy in a patient with haemophilia A. Br J Haematol 87: 434–436

Chang Y, Cesamab E, Pessin M S 1994 Identification of herpesvirus-like DNA sequences in AIDS-associated Kaposi's sarcoma. Science 26: 1865–1869

Chistolini A, Mazzucconi M G, Tirindelli M C et al 1990 Disseminated intravascular coagulation and myocardial infarction in a haemophilia B patient during therapy with prothrombin complex concentrates. Acta Haematol (Basel) 83: 163–165

Cohn R J, Schwyzer R, Field S P et al 1994 Acute hepatitis A in haemophiliacs. Thromb Haemost 72: 785–786

Colombo M, Mannucci P M, Brettler D B et al 1991 Hepatocellular carcinoma in hemophilia. Am J Hematol 37: 243–246

Conlan M G, Hoots W K 1990 Disseminated intravascular coagulation and hemorrhage in hemophilia B following elective surgery. Am J Hematol 35: 203–207

Darby S C, Rizza C R, Doll R et al 1989 Incidence of AIDS and excess of mortality associated with HIV in haemophiliacs in the United Kingdom: report on behalf of the directors of haemophilia centres in the United Kingdom. BMJ 298: 1064–1068

Darby S C, Doll R, Thakrar B et al 1990 Time from infection with HIV to onset of AIDS in patients with haemophilia in the UK. Stat Med 9: 681–689

de Biasi R, Rocino A, Miraglia E et al 1991 The impact of a very high purity factor VIII concentrate on the immune system of human immunodeficiency virus-infected hemophiliacs: a randomized, prospective, two-year comparison with an intermediate purity concentrate. Blood 78: 1919–1922

Dietrich S L, Mosley J W, Lusher J M et al 1990 Transmission of human immunodeficiency virus type 1 by dry-heated clotting factor concentrates. Vox Sang 59:

129–135

Dietrich G, Algiman M, Sultan Y et al 1992 Origin of anti-idiotypic activity against anti-factor VIII autoantibodies in pools of normal human immunoglobulin G (IVIg). Blood 79: 2946–2951

Doughty H A, Coles J, Parmar K et al 1995 The successful removal of a bleeding intracranial tumour in a severe haemophiliac using an adjusted dose continuous infusion of monoclonal factor VIII. Blood Coagulat Fibrinol 6: 31–34

Dusheiko G, Simmonds P 1994 Sequence variability of hepatitis C virus and its clinical relevance. J Viral Hepatitis 1: 3–15

Eyster M E, Fried M W, Di B, Goedert J J 1994 Increasing hepatitis C virus RNA levels in hemophiliacs: relationship to human immunodeficiency virus infection and liver disease. Blood 84: 1020–1023

Fletcher M L, Trowell J M, Craske J et al 1983 Non-A non-B hepatitis after transfusion of factor VIII in infrequently treated patients. Br Med J 287: 1754–1757

Furie B, Limentani S A, Rosenfield C G 1994 A practical guide to the evaluation and treatment of hemophilia. Blood 84: 3–9

Gerritzen A, Schneweis K E, Brackmann H H et al 1992a Acute hepatitis A in haemophiliacs. Lancet 340: 1231–1232

Gerritzen A, Scholt B, Kaiser R et al 1992b Acute hepatitis C in haemophiliacs due to 'virus-inactivated' clotting factor concentrates. Thromb Haemost 68: 781

Giles A R, Nesheim M E, Hoogendoorn H et al 1982 Stroma free human platelet lysates potentiate the in vivo thrombogenicity of factor Xa by the provision of coagulant-active phospholipid. Br J Haematol 51: 457–468

Gilles J G G, Arnout J, Vermylen J, SaintRemy J M R 1993 Anti-factor VIII antibodies of hemophiliac patients are frequently directed towards nonfunctional determinants and do not exhibit isotypic restriction. Blood 82: 2452–2461

Gilles J G, Arnout J, Peerlinck K et al 1994 Antigen–antibody complexes made of FVIII and autologous specific antibodies down regulate the production of anti-factor VIII antibodies. World Federation of Haemophilia Proceedings, Mexico City, 1994, abstract no. 85

Girvan D P, DeVeber L L, Inwood M J, Clegg E A 1994 Subcutaneous infusion ports in the pediatric patient with hemophilia. J Pediatr Surg 29: 1220–1223

Goedert J J, Kessler C M, Aledort L M et al 1989 A prospective study of human immunodeficiency virus type 1 infection and the development of AIDS in subjects with hemophilia. N Engl J Med 321: 1141–1148

Goldsmith J C, Kasper C K, Blatt P M et al 1992 Coagulation factor IX: successful surgical experience with a purified factor IX concentrate. Am J Hematol 40: 210–215

Goudemand J, Parquet Gernez A, Goudemand M 1993 Purity of factor VIII concentrates. Blood Coagulat Fibrinol 4: 499–500

Gray E, Tubbs J, Thomas S et al 1995 Measurement of activated factor IX in factor IX concentrates: correlation with in vivo thrombogenicity. Thromb Haemost 73: 675–679

Guo Z P, Yu M W 1995 Hepatitis C virus RNA in factor VIII concentrates. Transfusion 35: 112–116

Hanley J P, Dolan G, Day S et al 1993 Interaction of hepatitis B and hepatitis C infection in haemophilia. Br J Haematol 85: 611–612

Hanley J P, Jarvis L M, Andrews J et al 1996a Interferon treatment for chronic hepatitis C infection in haemophiliacs – influence of virus load, genotype and liver pathology on response. Blood 87: 1704

Hanley J P, Jarvis L M, Andrews J et al 1996b Investigation of haemophiliacs with chronic hepatitis C infection – assessment of invasive and non-invasive methods. Br J Haematol (in press)

Hay C R M 1995 Factor VIII inhibitors. Haemophilia 1(suppl): 14–21

Hay C R M, Ludlam C A 1996 Antifactor VIII antibodies arising in mild haemophiliacs. (in preparation)

Hay C R, Preston F E, Triger D R, Underwood J C 1985 Progressive liver disease in haemophilia: an understated problem? Lancet i: 1495–1498

Hay C R, Laurian Y, Verroust F et al 1990 Induction of immune tolerance in patients with hemophilia A and inhibitors treated with porcine VIIIC by home therapy. Blood 76: 882–886

Hay C R M, Lozier J N, Lee C A et al 1994 Porcine factor VIII therapy in patients with congenital hemophilia and inhibitors: efficacy, patient selection, and side effects. Semin Hematol 31: 20–25

Hedner U, Bjoern S, Bernvil S S et al 1989 Clinical experience with human plasma-derived factor VIIa in patients with hemophilia A and high titer inhibitors. Haemostasis 19: 335–343

Horowitz B, Prince A M, Hamman J, Watklevicz C 1994 Viral safety of solvent/detergent-treated blood products. Blood Coagulat Fibrinol 5: S21–S28

Hoyer L W 1994 Hemophilia A. N Engl J Med 330: 38–47

Hoyer L W, Scandella D 1994 Factor VIII inhibitors: structure and function in autoantibody and hemophilia A patients. Semin Hematol 31: 1–5

Hrinda M E, Huang C, Tarr G C et al 1991 Preclinical studies of a monoclonal antibody-purified factor IX, Mononine. Semin Hematol 28: 6–14

Jarvis L M, Watson H G, McOmish F et al 1994 Frequent reinfection and reactivation of hepatitis C virus genotypes in multitransfused hemophiliacs. J Infect Dis 170: 1018–1022

Jarvis L M, Ludlam C A, Ellender J A et al 1996 Investigation of the relative infectivity and pathogenicity of different hepatitis C virus genotypes in haemophiliacs. Blood 87: 3007–3011

Kaplan L D 1990 AIDS-associated lymphoma. Baillières Clin Haematol 3: 139–151

Karcher H 1991 German haemophilic patients infected with HIV. BMJ 303: 1352–1353

Kasper C K 1992 Unpublished observation

Kasper C K, Abramson S B, Goldsmith J C, Herring S 1991 In vivo recovery, half-life and safety of affinity purified solvent-detergent coagulation factor IX. Blood 78: 58a (abstract)

Kemball-Cook G, Edwards S J, Sewerin K et al 1988 Factor VIII procoagulant protein interacts with phospholipids vesicles via its 80 kDa light chain. Thromb Haemost 60: 442–446

Kernoff P B, Lee C A, Karayiannis P, Thomas H C 1985 High risk of non-A non-B hepatitis after a first exposure to volunteer or commercial clotting factor concentrates: effects of prophylactic immune serum globulin. Br J Haematol 60: 469–479

Kerr J R, Curran M D, Moore J E et al 1995 Persistent parvovirus B19 infection. Lancet 345: 1118

Kim H C, Matts L, Eisele J et al 1991 Monoclonal antibody-purified factor IX – comparative thrombogenicity to prothrombin complex concentrate. Semin Hematol 28: 15–19

Kleim J P, Bailly E, Schneweis K E et al 1990 Acute HIV-1 infection in patients with hemophilia B treated with beta-propiolactone-UV-inactivated clotting factor. Thromb Haemost 64: 336–337

Kluiber R M, Wolff B G 1994 Evaluation of anemia caused by hemorrhoidal bleeding. Dis Colon Rectum 37: 1006–1007

Koehler-Vajta K, Guertier L, Schaetzl H 1993 Frequency of HCV-RNA in anti-HCV positive hemophilic children and young adults. Thromb Haemost 69: 853 (abstract 1115)

Kohler M, Seifried E, Hellstern P et al 1988 In vivo recovery and half-life time of a steam-treated factor IX concentrate in hemophilia B patients. The influence of reagents and standards. Blut 57: 341–345

Kreuz W, Ehrenforth S, Funk M et al 1995 Immune tolerance therapy in paediatric haemophiliacs with factor VIII inhibitors: 14 years follow up. Haemophilia 1: 24–32

Laurian Y, Lusher J M, Kessler C M 1994 Viral safety and clotting factor concentrates. Thromb Haemost 72: 649

Lefrere J J, Mariotti M, Thauvin M 1994 B19 parvovirus DNA in solvent/detergent-treated anti-haemophilia concentrates. Lancet 343: 211–212

Levin A M 1992 Acquired immunodeficiency syndrome-related lymphoma. Blood 80: 8–20

Limentani S A, Gowell K P, Deitcher S R 1995 In vitro characterization of high purity factor IX concentrate for the treatment of hemophilia B. Thromb Haemost 73: 584–591

Lindley C M, Sawyer W T, Macik B G et al 1994 Pharmacokinetics and pharmacodynamics of recombinant factor VIIa. Clin Pharmacol Ther 55: 638–648

Ludlam C A, Carr R, Veitch S E, Steel C M 1983 Disordered immune regulation in haemophiliacs not exposed to commercial factor VIII. Lancet i: 1226 (letter)

Lusher J M 1991 Thrombogenicity associated with factor IX complex concentrates. Semin Hematol 28: 3–5

Lusher J M 1995 Considerations for current and future management of haemophilia and its complications. Haemophilia 1: 2–10

Lusher J M, Arkin S, Abildgaard C F et al 1993 Recombinant factor VIII for the treatment of previously untreated patients with hemophilia A – safety, efficacy, and development of inhibitors. N Engl J Med 328: 453–459

Lyon D J, Chapman C S, Martin C et al 1989 Symptomatic parvovirus B19 infection and heat-treated factor IX concentrate. Lancet i: 1085 (letter)

MacGregor I R, Ferguson J M, McLaughlin L F et al 1991 Comparison of high purity factor IX concentrates and a prothrombin complex concentrate in a canine model of thrombogenicity. Thromb Haemost 66: 609–613

Makris M, Preston F E 1993 Chronic hepatitis in haemophilia. Blood Rev 7: 243–250

Makris M, Preston F E, Triger D R et al 1991 A randomized controlled trial of recombinant interferon-α in chronic hepatitis C in hemophiliacs. Blood 78: 1672–1677

Makris M, Garson J A, Ring C A et al 1993 Hepatitis C viral RNA in clotting factor concentrates and the development of hepatitis in recipients. Blood 81: 1898–1902

Mannucci P M 1992 Outbreak of hepatitis A among Italian patients with haemophilia. Lancet 339: 819

Mannucci P M 1993 Modern treatment of hemophilia: from the shadows towards the light. Thromb Haemost 70: 17–23

Mannucci P M, Colombo M 1989 Revision of the protocol recommended for studies of safety from hepatitis of clotting factor concentrates. International Society for Thrombosis and Hemostasis. Thromb Haemost 61: 532–534

Mannucci P M, Colombo M on behalf of the factor VIII and IX SubCommittee 1989 Revision of the protocol recommended for studies of safety from hepatitis of clotting factor concentrates. Thromb Haemost 61: 532–534

Mannucci P M, Bauer K A, Gringeri A et al 1990 Thrombin generation is not increased in the blood of hemophilia B patients after the infusion of a purified factor IX concentrate. Blood 76: 2540–2545

Mannucci P M, Bauer K A, Gringeri A et al 1991a No activation of the common pathway of the coagulation cascade after a highly purified factor IX concentrate. Br J Haematol 79: 606–611

Mannucci P M, Gringeri A, Debiasi R 1991b Immune status of HIV-positive haemophiliacs: a randomized prospective comparison of treatment with a high-purity or an intermediate-purity factor VIII concentrate. Thromb Haemost 65: 824

Mannucci P M, Gdovin S, Gringeri A et al 1994 Transmission of hepatitis A to patients with hemophilia by factor VIII concentrates treated with organic solvent and detergent to inactivate viruses. Ann Intern Med 120: 1–7

Mariani G, Ghirardini A, Mandelli F et al 1987 Heated clotting factors and seroconversion for human immunodeficiency virus in three hemophilic patients. Ann Intern Med 107: 113 (letter)

Mariani G, Di Paolantonio T, Baklaja R, Mannucci P M 1991 Prospective hepatitis C safety evaluation of a high purity solvent detergent treated FVIII concentrate. Blood 78 (suppl): 55a

Mariani G, Ghirardini A, Bellocco R 1994 Immune tolerance in hemophilia–principal results from the International Registry: Report of the Factor VIII and IX Subcommittee. Thromb Haemost 72: 155–158

Martinowitz U, Schulman S 1995 Fibrin sealant in surgery of patients with a haemorrhagic diathesis. Thromb Haemost 74: 486–492

Martinowitz U, Schulman S, Gitel S et al 1992 Adjusted dose continuous infusion of factor VIII in patients with haemophilia A. Br J Haematol 82: 729–734

McKernan A M, Hay C R M, Bolton-Maggs P B M et al 1995 Continuous infusion of porcine factor VIII in patients with severe haemophilia A and inhibitors. Thromb Haemost 73: 1025 (abstract)

McOmish F, Yap P L, Jordan A et al 1993 Detection of parvovirus B19 in donated blood: a model system for screening by polymerase chain reaction. J Clin Microbiol 31: 323–328

Mortimer P P, Luban N L, Kelleher J F, Cohen B J 1983 Transmission of serum parvovirus-like virus by clotting-factor concentrates. Lancet ii: 482–484

Musiani M, Zerbini M, Gentilomi G et al 1995 Persistent B19 parvovirus infections in haemophilic HIV-1 infected patients. J Med Virol 46: 103–108

Nilsson I M 1993 Experience with prophylaxis in Sweden. Semin Hematol 30: 16–19

Nilsson I M, Berntorp E, Zettervall O 1988 Induction of immune tolerance in patients with hemophilia and antibodies to factor VIII by combined treatment with intravenous IgG, cyclophosphamide, and factor VIII. N Engl J Med 318: 947–950

Nilsson I M, Berntorp E, Zettervall O, Dahlback B 1990 Noncoagulation inhibitory factor VIII antibodies after induction of tolerance to factor VIII in hemophilia A patients. Blood 75: 378–383

Nilsson I M, Berntorp E, Rickard K A 1995 Results in three Australian haemophilia B patients with high-responding inhibitors treated with the Malmö model. Haemophilia 1: 59–66

Norley S G, Lower J, Kurth R 1993 Insufficient inactivation of hiv-1 in human cryo poor plasma by beta-propiolactone: results from a highly accurate virus detection method. Biologicals 21: 251–258

Nousbaum J B, Pol S, Nalpas B et al and the Collaborative Study Group 1995 Hepatitis C virus type 1B(II) infection in France and Italy. Ann Intern Med 122: 161–168

Oswaldsson U, Mikaelsson M, Frank L 1994 Comparison of factor VIII:C methods and reagents in the assay of factor VIII concentrates and post-injection patient plasma samples. Proceedings of the International Congress of the World Federation of Haemophilia, Mexico City (abstract)

Peerlinck K, Vermylen J 1993 Acute hepatitis A in patients with haemophilia A (10). Lancet 341: 179

Peerlinck K, Arnout J, Gillies J G et al 1993 A higher than expected incidence of factor VIII inhibitors in multitransfused haemophilia A patients treated with an intermediate purity pasteurized factor VIII concentrate. Thromb Haemost 69: 115–118

Peerlinck K, Willems M, Sheng L et al 1994 Rapid clearance of hepatitis C virus RNA in peripheral blood mononuclear cells of patients with clotting disorders and chronic hepatitis C treated with alpha-2b interferon is not a predictor for sustained response to treatment. Br J Haematol 86: 816–819

Philippou H, Adami A, Lane D et al 1995 Pharmacokinetic evaluation of a high purity factor IX compared to a prothrombin complex concentrate: study of coagulation activation markers provides evidence for mechanism of thrombogenic potential of the latter. (in press)

Phillips A N, Sabin C A, Elford J et al 1994 Use of CD4 lymphocyte count to predict long term survival free of aids after HIV infection. Br Med J 309: 309–313

Poynarad T, Bedossa P, Chevallier M et al and the Multicentre Study Group 1995 A comparison of three interferon alfa-2b regimens for the long-term treatment of chronic non-A, non-B hepatitis, N Engl J Med 322: 1457–1462

Preston F E, Dusheiko G, Giangrande P L F et al on behalf of UK Haemophilia Centre Directors Organisation 1995a Hepatocellular carcinoma in UK haemophiliacs. Br J Haematol 89: 9 (abstract)

Preston F E, Jarvis L M, Makris M et al 1995b Heterogeneity of hepatitis C virus genotypes in hemophilia: relationship with chronic liver disease. Blood 85: 1259–1262

Prowse C 1992 The effects of type of factor VIII concentrate used in haemophilia on T-helper cell number and inhibitor incidence. Blood Coagul Fibriol 3: 597–604

Ragni M V, Belle S H, Jaffe R A et al 1993 Acquired immunodeficiency syndrome-associated non-Hodgkin's lymphomas and other malignancies in patients with hemophilia. Blood 81: 1889–1897

Remis R J, O'Shaughnessy M V, Tsoukas C et al 1990 HIV transmission to patients with hemophilia by heat-treated, donor-screened factor concentrate. Can Med Assoc J 142: 1247–1254

Rizza C R, Fletcher M L, Kernoff P B A 1993 Confirmation of viral safety of dry heated factor VIII concentrate (8Y) prepared by Bio Products Laboratory (BPL): a report on behalf of UK Haemophilia Centre Directors. Br J Haematol 84: 269–272

Roberts H R 1994 A comparison of the European accord and the recommendations of the American National Hemophilia Foundation. Blood Coagulat Fibrinol 5: S89–S90

Rosendaal F R, Nieuwenhuis H K, Van B et al 1993 A sudden increase in factor VIII inhibitor development in multitransfused hemophilia A patients in The Netherlands. Blood 81: 2180–2186

Santagostino E, Mannucci P M, Griggeri A et al 1994 Eliminating parvovirus B19 from blood products. Lancet 343: 798

Schoppmann A, Weber A, Hondl F, Linnau Y 1994 Factor VIII concentrate: what is 'high purty'? Thromb Haemost 72: 483–484

Schulman S, Lindgren A C, Petrini P, Allender T 1992 Transmission of hepatitis C with pasteurised factor VIII. Lancet 340: 305–306

Schulman S, Lindstedt M, Alberts K A, Agren P H 1994a Recombinant factor VIIa in multiple surgery. Thromb Haemost 71: 154–161

Schulman S, Varon D, Keller N et al 1994b Monoclonal purified f VIII for continuous infusion: stability, microbiological safety and clinical experience. Thromb Haemost 72: 403–407

Schulman S, Gitel S, Zivelin A et al 1995 The feasibility of using concentrates containing factor IX for continuous infusion. Haemophilia 1: 103–110

Schwartz R S, Abildgaard C F, Aledort L M et al 1990 Human recombinant DNA-derived antihemophilic factor (factor VIII) in the treatment of hemophilia A. Recombinant Factor VIII Study Group. N Engl J Med 323: 1800–1805

Seremetis S V, Aledort L M, Bergman G E et al 1993 Three-year randomised study of high-purity or intermediate-purity factor VIII concentrates in symptom-free HIV-seropositive haemophiliacs: effects on immune status. Lancet 342: 700–703

Simmonds P, Zhang L Q, Watson H G et al 1990 Hepatitis C quantification and sequencing in blood products, haemophiliacs and intravenous drug users. Lancet 336: 1469–1472

Simons J N, Leary T P, Dawson G J et al 1995 Isolation of novel virus-like sequences associated with human hepatitis. Nature Med 1: 564–569

Smid W M, Van M, Smit J W, Halie M R 1993 The course of preexistent immune abnormalities in HIV negative haemophiliacs treated for two years with a monoclonal purified factor VIII concentrate. Thromb Haemost 69: 306–310

Stirling M L, Murray J A, Mackay P et al 1983 Incidence of infection with hepatitis B virus in 56 patients with haemophilia A 1971–1979. J Clin Pathol 36: 577–580

Telfer P, Devereux H, Colvin B et al 1995 Alpha interferon for hepatitis C virus infection in haemophilic patients. Haemophilia 1: 54–58

Temperley I J, Cotter K P, Walsh T J et al 1992 Clotting factors and hepatitis A. Lancet 340: 1466

Thomas D P, Hampton K K, Dasani H et al 1994 A cross-over pharmacokinetic and thrombogenicity study of a prothrombin complex concentrate and a purified factor IX concentrate. Br J Haematol 87: 782–788

Thomas D P, Lee C A, Colvin B T et al 1995 Clinical experience with a highly purified factor IX concentrate in patients undergoing surgical operations. Haemophilia 1: 17–23

Thompson A R 1993 Factor IX concentrates for clinical use. Semin Thromb Hemost 19: 25–35

Tiarks C, Pechet L, Humphreys R E 1989 Development of anti-idiotypic antibodies in a patient with factor VIII autoantibody. Am J Hematol 32: 217–221

Van den Berg W, ten Cate J W, Breederveld C, Goudsmit J 1986 Seroconversion to HTLV-III haemophiliac given heat-treated factor VIII concentrate Lancet i: 803–804 (letter)

Varon D, Schulman S, Dardik R et al 1994 High versus ultra high purity factor VIII concentrate therapy: prospective evaluation of immunological and clinical parameters in HIV seronegative and seropositive hemophiliacs. Thromb Haemost 72: 359–362

Vermylen J, Briet E 1993 Factor VIII preparations: need for prospective pharmacovigilance. Lancet 342: 693–694

Wagner N, Rotthauwe H W, Becker M et al 1992 Correlation of hepatitis B virus, hepatitis D virus and human immunodeficiency virus type 1 infection markers in hepatitis B surface antigen positive haemophiliacs and patients without haemophilia with clinical and histopathological outcome of hepatitis. Eur J Pediatr 151: 90–94

Watson H G, Ludlam C A 1992 Immunological abnormalities in haemophiliacs. Blood Rev 6: 26–33

Watson H G, Ludlam C A, Rebus S et al 1992 Use of several second generation serological assays to determine the true prevalence of hepatitis C virus infection in haemophiliacs treated with non-virus inactivated factor VIII and IX concentrates. Br J Haematol 80: 514–518

Weisser J 1988 Probable transmission of human immunodeficiency virus (HIV) by dry heat-treated factor VIII coagulation substances? Ubertragung von Human-Immunodeficiency-Virus (HIV) durch trocken-hitzebehandelte Faktor-VIII-Gerinnungspraparate? Klin Padiatr 200: 375–378

White G C, Matthews T J, Weinhold K J et al 1986 HTLV-III seroconversion associated with heat-treated factor VIII concentrate. Lancet i: 611–612 (letter)

Williams M D, Cohen B J, Beddall A C et al 1990a Transmission of human parvovirus B19 by coagulation factor concentrates. Vox Sang 58: 177–181

Williams M D, Skidmore S J, Hill F G 1990b HIV seroconversion in haemophilic boys receiving heat-treated factor VIII concentrate. Vox Sang 58: 135–136

Young N S 1995 B/9 parvovirus. Baillières Clin Haematol 8: 25–56

Zauber N P, Levin J 1977 Factor IX levels in patients with hemophilia B (Christmas disease) following transfusion with concentrates of factor IX or fresh frozen plasma (FFP). Medicine (Baltimore) 56: 213–224

Zuckerman A J 1995 The new GB hepatitis virus. Lancet 345: 1453–1454

15. Gene therapy for haemophilia

N. Salooja   E. G. D. Tuddenham

Currently available replacement therapy for the haemophilias is unsatisfactory. It is costly, short-lived and inconvenient to administer. Furthermore, most factor concentrates currently available carry the risk of transmitting human viruses, and the practice of initiating treatment only when bleeding has started results in considerable long-term orthopaedic morbidity. Prophylactic treatment of severe haemophiliacs with recombinant products could reduce the morbidity from joint disease (Nilsson et al 1992) and viral transmission. However, a recombinant factor IX has only recently entered clinical trials and the high cost of recombinant factor VIII restricts its use, particularly in poorer countries. In theory, gene therapy could permanently cure a patient with haemophilia and even a low level of unregulated expression could transform a clinically severe phenotype into a mild one. Many different forms of gene therapy for factor VIII and factor IX DNA have been proposed and significant progress has been made. The clinical use of advances in gene therapy, however, for haemophilia are currently limited. In this chapter the major developments over the last few years will be reviewed.

OVERVIEW OF APPROACH TO GENE THERAPY

Haemophilia A and B arise because of mutations in the genes encoding factors VIII and IX respectively. The genetic defects responsible are varied and include deletions, point mutations, inversions and insertions (Tuddenham et al 1994). In theory the ideal form of gene therapy for haemophilia A or B would involve removing the mutant gene sequence and replacing it with its normal counterpart. In practice, however, attempts toward gene therapy for haemophilia have focused on inserting an additional copy or gene augmentation. This involves the addition of non-targeted but functional genetic information into non-specific sites of the genome. The physical length of the factor VIII and IX genes exceeds the capacity of most available gene delivery systems, but in the case of factor IX it seems that most non-coding regions of the gene are dispensable and the cDNA at 2.8 kb (kilobase) is used instead. At 8.8 kb factor VIII cDNA is overlarge for viral vectors and a B-domain deleted form can be used. This shortened form of factor VIII has similar activity and survival, and is more easily processed in vitro than the full-length protein (Burke et al 1986, Eaton et al 1986, Toole et al 1986, Pavirani et al 1987, Pittman & Kaufman 1989). There are two main ways in which genetic material can be introduced into somatic cells of a haemophiliac, namely in vivo or ex vivo. The former approach involves direct introduction of genetic material into the blood stream or host tissues and the genetic modification takes place in vivo. An ex vivo approach involves genetically manipulating cells in vitro and then implanting, injecting or infusing them back into the host. Factor VIII and factor IX synthesis occurs predominantly in the liver (Wion et al 1985) and this would therefore be the ideal target organ. Hepatocytes are not readily removed and retransplanted, however, and the majority are mitotically inactive. These factors impose limitations on the methods which can be used to transfer genetic material to the liver and research has inevitably explored the use of other tissues. Once the gene has been successfully transferred it is necessary to establish that the protein is expressed, secreted into the plasma at a clinically significant level and that it is functionally active. For therapy to be effective in the long term it is also necessary to show that the plasma levels are maintained, or, if they decline, that repeated administration of the genetic material results in restoration of an adequate plasma protein concentration.

GENE DELIVERY SYSTEMS

Addition of genetic information into a cell in vitro or in vivo requires a highly efficient system of gene delivery. The ideal vector should be non-toxic to the cell/host and lead to stable expression of introduced genetic material to a clinically relevant level. Furthermore, when considering in vivo gene delivery the vector should be easily targeted to the desired tissue and should not be susceptible to immune inactivation.

Several methods are applicable to human gene transfer (Table 15.1) but the ideal gene delivery system does not yet exist. The advantages of different systems have to be exploited depending on the gene and target tissue in question. For haemophilia A and B most published work has involved use of retroviral and adenoviral vectors and receptor-mediated endocytosis for gene delivery, so these techniques will be discussed in detail.

Retroviral vectors

These are the best characterized and to date most widely used vectors for

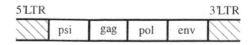

Fig. 15.1 Wild-type retrovirus genome.

Table 15.1   Gene delivery systems

Delivery system	Advantages	Disadvantages
Viral		
Retrovirus	Highly efficient transduction	Random insertion
	Permanent gene integration	Integration requires mitosis
	and long-term expression	
Adenovirus episomal	Transduces non-dividing cells	Only transient expression as
	High viral titre activity	Host immune response to viral antigens
		Toxic inflammatory reactions
Adeno associated virus	Inserts in chromosome 19	Second virus needed for replication
	Non-immunogenic	Size limit to exogenous DNA
	Tranduces non-dividing cells	
Non-viral		
CaPO$_4$ precipitation	Safety and possibility of transferring large amounts of DNA	Low efficiency of transfection
Direct injection of DNA	Safety and possibility of transferring large amounts of DNA	Low efficiency of transfection
Lipofection	Safety and possibility of transferring large amounts of DNA	Low efficiency of transfection
Ligand–DNA conjugates	Tissue specificity possible	Low efficiency of transfection

gene delivery. Their popularity is a result of their high (close to 100%) efficiency of transduction of dividing cells in culture. Furthermore, they infect many cell types without causing lysis and since the DNA integrates into the chromosomal DNA, transferred genetic information is not lost as the recipient cell divides. The vectors used for transferring factors VIII and IX have been derived from murine leukaemia viruses (MLV). A schematic representation of a typical wild-type retrovirus genome is shown in Figure 15.1.

The long terminal repeat (LTR) sequences are involved in transcription regulation. The 5′LTR contains promoter and enhancer elements which drive transcription and the 3′LTR contains signals required for RNA polyadenylation. *Gag* and *env* genes encode capsid proteins and *pol* encodes reverse transcriptase and integrase enzymes. A packaging signal, *psi*, is required to package viral genomic RNA into a mature virion. In order to serve as a vector the retrovirus needs to be modified to accommodate the therapeutic gene and to insert a suitable dominant selectable marker. In addition, regulatory elements from other genes may be inserted to drive transcription in preference to the viral LTR. Deleting *gag*, *env* and *pol* genes creates space for approximately 7 kb of exogenous material (Eglitis & Anderson 1988). Removing these genes serves the additional desirable effect of making the virus replication deficient, thus rendering it non-transmissible and therefore unable to transduce cells. Infectivity can be restored by transfecting the truncated virus into a packaging cell line (Miller

1990) containing helper virus sequences. These produce *gag*, *pol* and *env* proteins constitutively and so replication deficient but infective vector is shed from the packaging cell surface. Safety aspects remain one of the major concerns using retroviruses as vectors for gene transfer in humans. Retroviral genes are inherently unstable and can undergo recombination within their own genome, with helper virus sequences or the endogenous DNA of the host, and, as with any gene transfer technique resulting in random integration of new sequences, there remains the theoretical possibility of activating an oncogene. Donohue et al (1992) transfected bone marrow stem cells from rhesus monkeys with a retroviral vector contaminated with replication competent virus which had arisen through recombination. Three out of eight monkeys had a productive infection with the replication competent virus and subsequently went on to develop a rapidly progressive T-cell lymphoma. Second- and third-generation packaging lines include modifications to decrease the chance of generating a replication competent virus (Miller & Buttimore 1986, Danos & Mulligan 1988, Markowitz et al 1988, Muenchau et al 1990). Extensive in vivo testing, therefore, is required to establish safety.

A consequence of these modifications is that the number of infectious particles obtained is considerably lower than with wild-type retroviruses, and this limits the transfection efficiency that can be achieved. A further limitation of retroviral vectors are that they only infect dividing cells. Various techniques have been employed to facilitate transfection of mitotically inactive tissues. Hepatocytes can be stimulated to divide by surgically removing part of the liver, and muscle cells can be stimulated to divide by intramuscular injection of cardiotoxin (d'Albis et al 1989). Transduction efficiency can be improved in vitro by using cytokines and growth factors to facilitate cell division (Axelrod et al 1990).

Adenoviral vectors

Replication deficient vectors are derived from the wild-type adenovirus by deleting portions of the E1 and/or E3 regions of the genome. The E1 sequences are necessary to activate other adenoviral genes and in order to propagate the vector it is necessary to supplement E1 functions in trans. This is done by transfecting the vector into a cell line producing E1 proteins (Jones & Shenk 1979). Adenoviral vectors can infect a wide variety of cells and their safety for human use is implied by the lack of side-effects seen after vaccinating US military recruits with wild-type adenovirus. Furthermore, they have been used to transfer the transmembrane conductance regulator gene in patients with cystic fibrosis (Zabner et al 1993, Crystal et al 1994). The virus particle is relatively stable and amenable to purification and concentration and it can be prepared with higher high viral titre activity than retroviral vectors (up to 10^{11} compared to 10^6 infectious viral particles per millilitre). Another advantage of adenoviral vectors is that the latter can infect non-dividing or slowly dividing cells such as hepatocytes, muscle cells and respiratory endothelium. However, integration of DNA is not part of the adenoviral life cycle so gene expression is likely to be transient and persistent expression will require repeated administration. Since current adenoviral vectors carry many immunogenic sequences repeated therapy is likely to be ineffective (Smith et al 1993).

Other viral vectors

Other viral vector systems are less well developed for human gene transfer. Adeno-associated virus (AAV) has several potentially useful features: it is not immunogenic, it transduces non-dividing cells and the wild type integrates into human DNA in a site-specific manner on chromosome 19. However, vectors derived from AAV appear to integrate randomly (Kotin 1994), they accommodate less than 5 kb exogenous DNA and they require a second virus for replication.

Non-viral methods

Physical methods of gene delivery to cells are attractive because of their relative safety and their potential to transfer large amounts of DNA. As with adenoviral DNA transfer, the genetic material remains episomal and so expression is likely to be transient. However, repeated administration may be more feasible with these methods than with adenoviral delivery. The main limitations with all these methods are the low efficiency of transfection, cytotoxicity and lack of site-specific targeting. Various strategies have been developed in order to circumvent these problems: for example, the use of DNA ligand conjugates, which exploits physiological mechanisms to target and internalize exogenous DNA. Synthetic molecules are constructed which link a ligand binding moiety with a DNA binding domain. DNA to be transferred links electrostatically to the DNA binding domain and is internalized by cells bearing appropriate cell surface receptors for the attached ligand via receptor-mediated endocytosis. Asialoglycoprotein has been used as a ligand to target DNA specifically to the liver (Wu et al 1991) and transferrin has been used as a ligand to target DNA to haematopoietic cells (Zenke et al 1990). One of the problems with receptor-mediated endocytosis for DNA delivery has been the presumed lysosomal degradation of the endosome contents. Cytoplasmic delivery of DNA is enhanced if the endosome is disrupted by codelivery of adenovirus (Curiel et al 1991). Chemical conjugation of adenovirus to polylysine reduces the titre of adenovirus which has to be given for the desired endosomal lysis (Cristiano et al 1993).

A simpler strategy for directing DNA is to inject DNA directly into the desired site. Injection of plasmid DNA, adenoviral or retroviral vectors directly into muscles has resulted in expression of a number of recombinant genes (Thomason & Booth 1990, Wolff et al 1990, Stratford-Perricaudet et al 1992, Wells & Goldspink 1992, Davis et al 1993a,b).

TARGET TISSUES AND CHOICE OF TRANSFER STRATEGY

Provided the proteins are fully expressed, functionally active and have direct access to plasma, the site of production of factor VIII or factor IX is probably not critical, so several cells/tissues have been evaluated. A number of post-translational modifications need to be carried out for full functional activity and it is important that host cells can carry them out correctly and efficiently. In the case of factor VIII these consist of glycosylation and sulphation of tyrosine residues. Factor IX requires γ-carboxylation of 12 glutamic acid residues, β-hydroxylation of an aspartate residue (Fernlund & Stenflo 1983) and glycosylation of at least two asparagine residues. Cell types other than hepatocytes are capable of performing these modifications correctly albeit not as efficiently. γ-Carboxylase activity in skin, for example, is only one-fifth that of the liver. In fibroblast cell culture it has been demonstrated that the percentage of factor IX which is γ-carboxylated decreases as the amount of factor IX antigen increases (Palmer et al 1989). It remains to be seen whether non-hepatic cells can carry out adequate post-translational modifications when therapeutic levels of factor IX are produced. Glycosylation of recombinant factor IX has been shown to vary with its site of production (Yao et al 1994). Although factor IX activity would remain, antigenicity may be altered and this could affect survival of the protein in vivo.

Either an in vivo or an ex vivo approach could be considered for transfer of factor VIII or factor IX cDNA. An ex vivo approach allows transduction and expression to be assessed before implantation. The choice of target cell is governed by practical considerations such as accessibility, maintaining and manipulating cells in culture and their viability after a retransplant.

Table 15.2 Gene therapy for haemophilia A

Transduced cell	Species	Ex vivo transfer	Reference
Transformed fibroblasts	Mouse	–	Israel & Kaufman 1990
	Mouse	–	Hoeben et al 1990
	Mouse	+	Hoeben et al 1993
	Rat	+	Hoeben et al 1993
Primary fibroblasts	Mouse	–	Hoeben et al 1990
	Mouse	+	Zatloukal et al 1994
	Mouse	+	Dwarki et al 1995
	Human	–	Hoeben et al 1990
		–	Lynch et al 1990
		+	Hoeben et al 1993
Primary myoblasts	Mouse	+	Zatloukal et al 1994
Primary endothelial cells	Human	–	Lynch et al 1990
Haematopoietic tissue	Mouse	+	Hoeben et al 1992

Potential host cells which meet these criteria include haematopoietic cells, fibroblasts, keratinocytes, endothelial cells, lymphocytes and muscle cells. An in vivo system for gene transfer is theoretically more attractive than an ex vivo approach because it eliminates the cell culture, transduction and transplantation steps. However, such a system requires that the vector is not inactivated by antibodies and, to ensure that sufficient cells are transduced, targeting of genetic material to the relevant tissue is necessary. Animal models are of central importance in evaluating an in vivo strategy. Well-characterized canine models of haemophilia A and B are already in existence and a mouse model of haemophilia A has recently been reported (Bi et al 1995).

FACTOR VIII GENE TRANSFER

To date B-domainless factor VIII cDNA has been effectively transferred into a number of different cells in culture using retroviral vectors (Table 15.2).

The results of ex vivo transfer of factor VIII secreting cells have been disappointing. Hoeben and colleagues transplanted factor VIII secreting fibroblasts into immunodeficient mice but were unable to detect factor VIII in the recipient's plasma. The transduced cells were explanted and regrown in culture 4–8 weeks later and were found to still be capable of secreting active factor VIII (Hoeben et al 1993). Similarly when factor VIII transfected bone marrow was infused to lethally irradiated mice, no factor VIII was detected (Hoeben et al 1992). In the latter experiment the presence of vector proviral sequences in haematopoietic tissue was confirmed by Southern analysis but no RNA could be detected. Expression of active factor VIII has been observed in vitro but in comparison to other genes introduced into retroviruses the titres obtained have been low (Israel & Kaufman 1990, Lynch et al 1993). Lynch and colleagues found an approximately 100-fold reduction in vector titre when the vector carried factor VIII cDNA compared to other cDNAs. Deletion analysis enabled them to localize an inhibitory signal within the factor VIII coding region to a 1.2 kb stretch. However, there appeared to be other inhibitory signals over a wide distribution which could not be further localized. To avoid the problem of factor VIII sequences interfering with viral production, Zatloukal et al (1994) used receptor-mediated gene delivery to transfect mouse primary fibroblasts and myoblasts in vitro. When these cells were delivered to the spleens of syngeneic mice, therapeutic levels of factor VIII were transiently (<48 h) observed. No circulating factor VIII was detected when autologous myoblasts were transplanted into skeletal muscle. Very recently highly encouraging results have been reported using the MGF retroviral vector containing B-domain deleted factor VIII cDNA to transfect murine fibroblasts. When transplanted into the peritoneum, factor VIII could be found in the plasma of recipient mice at therapeutic levels for more than a week (Dwarki et al 1995).

FACTOR IX GENE TRANSFER

Progress involving factor IX has been more rapid than for factor VIII, but long-term clinically relevant levels of factor IX have not been achieved. The normal plasma factor IX level is 4 µg/ml but a level as low as 100–150 ng/ml may be of clinical benefit to severe haemophiliacs (Evans et al 1989). Prior to 1993 all studies involved ex vivo transfer of factor IX using retroviral vectors based on MoMLV (Moloney murine leukaemia virus) to transduce cells (Table 15.3). Several transformed cell lines have also been shown to synthesize functional factor IX after transduction by retroviral vectors, but they are unsuitable for gene therapy because their growth is uncontrollable and they often form tumours in their hosts. Primary fibroblasts, myoblasts, endothelial cells, hepatocytes and keratinocytes have all been transduced and shown to produce functionally active factor IX. in vitro. Following transfer to experimental animal in vivo, plasma levels observed have been low and usually transient. In some cell types at least the choice of promoter used to regulate transcription is relevant to the level and duration of factor IX expression (Palmer et al 1989, Dai et al 1992). In vivo work has focused on the liver as a target organ. Retroviral vectors and receptor-mediated endocytosis have been used to transfer factor IX (Table 15.4), but the most promising results by far have been achieved using adenoviral vectors.

Fibroblasts

Ex vivo transfer of factor IX secreting fibroblasts has led in each case to low, transient levels of factor IX in the plasma of recipient animals. Palmer et al (1989) transfected transformed fibroblast cell lines and primary fibroblasts from rat and human sources. The retroviral vectors used carried human factor IX, and one of three sets of regulatory elements: viral LTR, CMV (cytomegalovirus) immediate/early (IE) promoter/enhancer and SV40 early promoter. They found that the most effective regulatory region depended on the cell type being evaluated. For human diploid fibroblasts it was the CMV promoter. Ex vivo transfer of human diploid fibroblasts into nude mice resulted in peak factor IX levels of 190 ng/ml, but expression ceased within 1 week. Expression of longer duration (>40 days) was achieved using rat fibroblasts and a syngeneic host, but peak levels were lower at 23 ng/ml. Factor IX antibodies were detected in only one of six rats evaluated, and it was considered unlikely that an immune mechanism could explain the transient expression observed. The authors addressed the problem further by transplanting rat fibroblasts transduced with the adenosine deaminase (ADA) gene into syngeneic rats (Palmer et al 1991). Because ADA is intracellular it is unlikely to be immunogenic and its detection is not dependent on systemic distribution. Furthermore, sensitive assays are

Table 15.3   Ex vivo transfer of factor IX via primary cells

Transduced cell	Host	Reference
Fibroblasts		
Rat	Rat	Palmer et al 1989
Mouse	Nude mice	Scharfmann et al 1991
Human	Nude mice	Palmer et al 1989
Human	Human	Lu et al 1993
Myoblasts		
Mouse	Nude mice	Dai et al 1992
Mouse	Mice	Yao et al 1994
Keratinocytes		
Human	Nude mice	Gerard et al 1993

Table 15.4   In vivo transfer of factor IX

Gene delivery system	Recipient cell	Host	Reference
Adenovirus	Hepatocyte	Mouse	Smith et al 1993
Retrovirus	Hepatocyte	Dog	Kay et al 1993
Adenovirus	Hepatocyte	Dog	Kay et al 1994
Receptor-mediated endocytosis	Hepatocyte	Rat	Ferkol et al 1993
Receptor-mediated endocytosis	Hepatocyte	Rat	Perales et al 1994

available for its detection. Cells containing vector sequences persisted for at least 8 months, but in vivo expression decreased dramatically (>1500-fold) after 1 month. Expression was not restored after explanting cells and regrowing in culture. Because an immune response could not be detected, the authors hypothesized that the transferred gene was being inactivated in vivo. Sharfmann et al (1991) used different promoters to evaluate in vivo expressing using β-galactosidase activity as a marker. They found that they could achieve long-term expression (>3 months) with the promoter of a housekeeping gene, dihydrofolate reductase, but not with the CMV IE promoter (<10 days).

To date, there has been only one ex vivo study involving human subjects. Lu et al (1993) have transferred factor IX via skin fibroblasts to two mildly affected haemophilia B subjects. They used two retroviral vectors: one driven by viral LTR and the other by the CMV IE promoter. Transduced cells were selected for high expression of factor IX in vitro, embedded onto a collagen matrix and subcutaneously injected back into the patients. One patient achieved an increase in plasma factor IX from 71 ng/ml to 240 ng/ml, the clotting activity increased from 2.9% to 6.3% and a clinical improvement was noted. The other patient achieved an increase from 130 ng/ml to 280 ng/ml. Expression of recombinant factor IX was seen for 6 months and 5.5 months, respectively, at the time of the report.

Keratinocytes

Only low level transient expression has been observed after ex vivo transfer. Gerard et al (1993) transduced primary human keratinocytes with a retroviral vector carrying human factor IX using the viral 5'LTR promoter. When transduced cells were transplanted into nude mice, human factor IX was detected for only 7 days and peak levels of 3 ng/ml were achieved. The authors estimated that only 2.6% of the estimated factor IX secreted by the graft reached the circulation. Another problem was that γ-carboxylation was inefficient, contributing further to the low factor IX activity.

Myoblasts

Like fibroblasts and keratinocytes, myoblasts are easily accessible for biopsy and reimplantation and produce functionally active factor IX. Primary myoblasts injected into skeletal muscle can survive for more than 1 year while retaining myogenic capacity (Yao & Kurachi 1993). As with ex vivo transfer using fibroblasts, the choice of regulatory sequences in the vector appears to influence level and duration of expression of the transferred gene (Dai et al 1992, Yao et al 1994). Using a myoblast cell line and retroviral vectors driven by viral LTR, Yao & Kurachi (1992) transferred human factor IX into homologous cyclosporin-treated mice. Peak factor IX levels of 1 μg/ml were seen, but levels decreased over a 4-week period and this was accompanied by an increase in antibodies against human factor IX. Dai et al (1992) transferred canine factor IX cDNA into nude mice via primary myoblasts. Three different retroviral vectors were constructed using combinations of the CMV IE promoter, mouse muscle creatine kinase (MCK) enhancer and globin gene regulatory elements. In most cases plasma levels of canine factor IX peaked on day 2–4 but then returned to control levels. An exception was the CMV promoter, used in conjunction with the MCK enhancer, where a plateau level of 10 ng/ml was maintained for more than 180 days. Yao et al (1994) transfected primary mouse myoblasts with human factor IX using retroviral vectors with different promoters. Either the retroviral LTR or the MCK enhancer with the B-actin promoter was used to drive factor IX transcription. Transduced myoblasts were injected into skeletal muscles of SCID mice. By giving two successive injections of transduced fibroblasts at day 0 and day 95, they achieved plasma factor IX levels of 10–30 ng/ml for more than 5 months. In vivo factor IX production was actually higher with the viral LTR than with the CMV promoter. However, the viral LTR vector contained a selectable marker which ensured high transduction efficiency so the two vectors were not directly comparable. Even so, the results demonstrate that viral control elements were not inactivated in transplanted myoblasts. The study also demonstrated that significantly higher plasma factor IX levels could be achieved if transduced myoblasts were coinjected with basic fibroblast growth factor, though the average plasma concentration was still less than 20 ng/ml. Skeletal muscle is also amenable to an in vivo approach of gene transfer. Initial attempts at this approach for the factor IX gene have not demonstrated measurable factor IX, presumably because of low transfection efficiency (Yao & Kurachi 1992). The use of regenerating rather than mature muscle may help (Davis et al 1993b).

Hepatocytes

The liver represents the natural target for gene replacement therapy in haemophilia A and B because it is the major organ of factor IX synthesis. Hepatocytes transduced in vitro can be infused into the portal or intrasplenic vasculature and transfer of recombinant genes in this way has been achieved (Ferry et al 1991, Ponder et al 1991). Primary rabbit hepatocytes have been transduced in vitro with factor IX cDNA (Armentano et al 1990), but expression was lower by 6–10-fold than that reported for human and rat diploid fibroblasts (Palmer et al 1989). Hepatocytes undergo a limited number of cell divisions in culture and use of growth factors in the culture medium may increase transduction efficiency in the future. Successful ex vivo transfer of factor IX producing heptocytes has not yet been described.

In vivo transduction of the liver with factor IX cDNA has been reported using several methods. Retroviral vectors have been used to transfer canine factor IX into haemophiliac dogs (Kay et al 1993). Despite carrying out partial hepatectomy to stimulate cell division, transfection efficiency was low at 1% and 0.3% in two animals evaluated. Low plasma levels of factor IX were achieved (2–6 ng/ml) although in one animal expression was seen for over 5 months. Interestingly this low level of expression shortened the whole blood clotting time significantly. While this protocol for in vivo gene transfer may be useful for some disorders, it is clearly inapplicable to haemophilic patients. Adenoviral vectors and receptor-mediated endocytosis have been used with the surgically intact liver. Smith et al (1993) used an adenoviral vector carrying human factor IX under control of Rous sarcoma virus (RSV) to transduce the liver in vivo. The recombinant vector was injected into the tail veins of mice. They achieved factor IX levels greater than 250 ng/ml in all mice and factor IX remained at a therapeutic level for 4–5 weeks. Subsequently there was a decline in factor IX levels which was paralleled by loss of vector sequences from the liver as determined by Southern analysis. Antibodies to factor IX were detected after the first injection and levels rose 32-fold following a second injection. Kay et al (1994) infused a recombinant adenoviral vector carrying canine factor IX into the portal vasculature of haemophilic dogs. Transduction efficiency was 20–50%. Supranormal levels of factor IX were achieved in the first 4 days postinfusion. By 3 weeks levels were 1% of normal and by 2 months 0.1%. Transient expression was attributed to loss of DNA from transduced cells. It was not clear whether transduced cells were being slowly replaced or if the episomal DNA was being slowly degraded in hepatocytes. Ferkol et al (1993) constructed a plasmid vector using the PEPCK (phosphoenolpyruvate carboxykinase) promoter from rat which has a high level of expression in the liver and can be induced by glucocorticoids or a protein-rich diet. The plasmid was complexed to a neoglycoprotein carrier and infused into the heptic portal vein of adult rats. Human factor IX DNA was detected by PCR (polymerase chain reaction) for 30 days. Factor IX expression was inferred by measuring clotting times and lasted for 60 days. Perales et al (1994) condensed PEPCK with galactosylated polylysine and injected the complex into the caudal vena cava of adult rats. Episomal plasmid DNA was detected in the liver 32 days later. DNA, mRNA and protein were detected for the duration of the experiment (140 days).

FUTURE DIRECTIONS

Existing gene therapy protocols for haemophilia A and B all have limitations. Regulatory sequences affecting expression of both genes, but particularly factor VIII, need to be better defined. The use of cytokines to facilitate uptake of genetic material and immunoisolation devices (Carr-Brendel et al 1993, Liu et al 1993) to protect factor VIII or factor IX producing cells may increase the level and duration of response possible with existing methods. More sophisticated engineering of existing vectors may further increase gene transfer efficiency and stability of expression, but new methodology will probably be required to achieve clinically relevant levels of factor VIII and factor IX in vivo. A novel vector described recently (Forstova et al 1995) is a pseudocapsid derived from mouse polyoma virus. This offers the potential for efficient transfer of genetic material without cytotoxicity or transfer of viral genes. A mouse model for haemophilia A has recently been described (Bi et al 1995) which will facilitate evaluation of new gene transfer techniques. The ability to carry out cross-breeding experiments with well-characterized immunological mutant mice should allow the phenomenon of transient protein expression to be investigated further.

REFERENCES

Armentano D, Thompson A R, Darlington G, Woo S L 1990 Expression of human factor IX in rabbit hepatocytes by retrovirus mediated gene transfer: potential for gene therapy of haemophilia B. Proc Natl Acad Sci USA 87: 6141–6145

Axelrod J H, Read M S, Brinkhous K M, Verma I M 1990 Phenotypic correction of factor IX deficiency in skin fibroblasts of haemophiliac dogs. Proc Natl Acad Sci USA 87: 5173–5177

Bi L, Lawler A M, Antonarakis S E et al 1995 Targeted disruption of the mouse factor VIII gene produces a model of haemophilia A. Nature Genet 10: 119

Burke R L, Pachl C, Quiroga M et al 1986 The functional domains of coagulation factor VIII:C. J Biol Chem 261: 12574–12578

Carr-Brendel V, Lozier J N, Thomas T J et al 1993 An immunoisolation device for implantation of genetically engineered cells: long term expression of factor IX in rats. J Cell Biochem 17E: 224 (abstract)

Cristiano R J, Smith L C, Kay M A et al 1993 Hepatic gene therapy: efficient gene delivery and expression in primary hepatocytes utilizing a conjugated adenovirus–DNA complex. Proc Natl Acad Sci USA 90: 11548–11552

Crystal R G, McElvaney N G, Rosenfeld M A et al 1994 Administration of an adenovirus containing the human CFTR cDNA to the respiratory tract of individuals with cystic fibrosis. Nature Genet 8: 42–50

Curiel D T, Agarwal S, Wagner E et al 1991 Adenovirus enhancement of transferrin-polylysine-mediated gene delivery. Proc Natl Acad Sci USA 88: 8850–8854

Dai Y, Roman M, Naviaux R et al 1992 Gene therapy via primary myoblasts: long-term expression of factor IX protein following transplantation in vivo. Proc Natl Acad Sci USA 89: 10892–10895

d'Albis A, Couteaux R, Janmot C et al 1989 Myosin isoform transitions in regeneration of fast and slow muscles during postnatal development of the rat. Dev Biol 135: 320–325

Danos O, Mulligan R C 1988 Safe and efficient generation of recombinant retroviruses with amphotropic and ecotropic host ranges. Proc Natl Acad Sci USA 85: 6460–6464

Davis H L, Whalen R G, Demeneix B A 1993a Direct gene transfer into skeletal muscle in vivo: factors affecting efficiency of transfer and stability of expression. Human Gene Ther 4: 151–159

Davis H L, Demeneix B A, Quantin B et al 1993b Plasmid DNA is superior to viral vectors for direct gene transfer into adult mouse skeletal muscle. Human Gene Ther 4: 733–740

Donohue R E, Kessler S W, Bodine D et al 1992 Helper virus induced T-cell lymphoma in non human primates after retroviral mediated gene transfer. J Exp Med 176: 1125

Dwarki V J, Belloni P, Mijjar T et al 1995 Gene therapy for haemophilia A: production of therapeutic levels of human factor VIII in vivo in mice. Proc Natl Acad Sci USA 92: 1023–1027

Eaton D L, Wood W I, Eaton E et al 1986 Construction and characterization of an active factor VIII variant lacking the central one third of the molecule. Biochemistry 225: 8343–8347

Eglitis M A, Anderson W F 1988 Retroviral vectors for introduction of genes into mammalian cells. Biotechniques 6: 608–614

Evans J P, Watzke H H, Ware J L et al 1989 Molecular cloning of a cDNA encoding canine factor IX. Blood 74: 207–221

Ferkol L, Lindberg G L, Chen J et al 1993 Regulation of the phosphoenolpyruvate carboxykinase/human factor IX gene introduced into the livers of adult rats by receptor-mediated gene transfer. FASEB J 7: 1081–1091

Fernlund P, Stenflo J 1983 Beta-hydroxyaspartic acid in vitamin K-dependent proteins. J Biol Chem 258: 12509–12512

Ferry N, Duplessis O, Houssin D et al 1991 Retroviral-mediated gene transfer into hepatocytes in vivo. Proc Natl Acad Sci USA 88: 8377–8381

Forstova J, Kraizewicz N, Sandig V et al 1995 Polyoma virus pseudocapsids as efficient carriers of heterologous DNA into mammalian cells. Human Gene Ther 6: 297–306

Gerard A G, Hudson D L, Brownlee G G et al 1993 Towards gene therapy for haemophilia B using primary human keratinocytes. Nature Genet 3: 180–183

Hoeben R C, van der Jagt R C M, Schoute F et al 1990 Expression of functional factor VIII in primary skin fibroblasts after retrovirus-mediated gene transfer. J Biol Chem 265: 7318–7323

Hoeben R C, Einerhand M P W, Briet E et al 1992 Toward gene therapy in haemophilia A: retrovirus-mediated transfer of a factor VIII gene into murine haematopoietic progenitor cells. Thromb Haemost 67: 341–345

Hoeben R C, Fallaux F J, Tilburg N H V et al 1993 Toward gene therapy for haemophilia A: long term persistence of factor VIII secreting fibroblasts after transplantation into immunodeficient mice. Human Gene Ther 4: 179–186

Israel D I, Kaufman R J 1990 Retroviral-mediated transfer and amplification of a functional human factor VIII gene. Blood 75: 1074–1080

Jones N, Shenk T 1979 Isolation of adenovirus type S host range deletion mutants defective for transformation of rat embryo cells. Cell 16: 683–689

Kay M A, Rothenberg S, Landen C N et al 1993 In vivo gene therapy for haemophilia B. Sustained partial correction in factor IX deficient dogs. Science 262: 117–119

Kay M A, Landen C N, Rothenberg S R et al 1994 In vivo hepatic gene therapy: complete albeit transient correction of factor IX deficiency in haemophilia B dogs. Proc Natl Acad Sci USA 91: 2353–2357

Kotin R M 1994 Prospect for the use of adeno-associated virus as a vector for human gene therapy. Human Gene Ther 5: 793–801

Liu H-W, Ofosu F A, Chang P L 1993 Expression of human factor IX by microencapsulated recombinant fibroblasts. Human Gene Ther 4: 291–301

Lu D R, Zhou J M, Zheng B et al 1993 Stage 1 clinical trial of gene therapy for haemophilia B. Sci China [B] 36: 1342–1351

Lynch C M, Israel D I, Miller A D 1990 Toward gene therapy using endothelial cells. J Cell Biochem 14E (suppl): 222

Lynch C M, Israel D I, Kaufman R J et al 1993 Sequences in the coding region of clotting factor VIII act as dominant inhibitors of RNA accumulation and protein production. Human Gene Ther 4: 259–272

Markowitz D, Goff S, Bank A 1988 A safe packaging line for gene transfer: separating viral genes on two different plasmids. J Virol 62: 1120–1124

Miller A D 1990 Retrovirus packaging cells. Human Gene Ther 1: 5–14

Miller A D, Buttimore C 1986 Redesign of retrovirus packaging cell lines to avoid recombination leading to helper virus production. Mol Cell Biol 6: 2895–2902

Muenchau D D, Freeman S M, Cornetta K et al 1990 Analysis of retroviral packaging lines for generation of replication-competent virus. Virology 176: 262–265

Nilsson I M, Berntorp E, Loqvist T 1992 Twenty-five years experience of prophylactic treatment in severe haemophilia A and B. J Intern Med 232: 25–32

Palmer T D, Thompson A R, Miller A D 1989 Production of human factor IX in animals by genetically modified skin fibroblasts: potential therapy for haemophilia B. Blood 73: 438–445

Palmer T D, Rosman G J, Osborne W R A et al 1991 Genetically modified skin fibroblasts persist long after transplantation but gradually inactivate introduced genes. Proc Natl Acad Sci USA 88: 1330–1334

Pavirani A, Meulien P, Harrer H et al 1987 Two independent domains of factor VIII coexpressed using recombinant vaccinia viruses. Biochem Biophys Res Commun 145: 234–240

Perales J C, Fekol T, Beegen H et al 1994 Gene transfer in vivo: sustained expression and regulation of genes introduced into the liver by receptor-targeted uptake. Proc Natl Acad Sci USA 91: 4086–4090

Pittman D D, Kaufman R J 1989 Structure function relationships of factor VIII elucidated through recombinant DNA technology. Thromb Haemost 61: 161–165

Ponder K P, Gupta S, Leland F et al 1991 Mouse hepatocytes migrate to liver parenchyma and function indefinitely after intrasplenic transplantation. Proc Natl Acad Sci USA 88: 1217–1221

Scharfmann R, Axelrod J H, Verma I M 1991 Long term in vivo expression of retrovirus mediated gene transfer in mouse fibroblast implants. Proc Natl Acad Sci USA 88: 4626–4630

Smith T A G, Mehaffey M G, Kayda D B et al 1993 Adenovirus mediated expression of therapeutic plasma levels of human factor IX in mice. Nature Genet 5: 397–402

Stratford-Perricaudet L D, Makeh I, Perricaudet M et al 1992 Widespread long term gene transfer to mouse skeletal muscles and heart. J Clin Invest 90: 626–630

Thomason D B, Booth F W 1990 Stable incorporation of a bacterial gene into adult rat skeletal muscle in vivo. Am J Physiol 258: C578–C581

Toole J J, Pittman D D, Orr E C et al 1986 A large region (~95kDa) of human factor VIII is dispensable for in vitro procoagulant activity. Proc Natl Acad Sci USA 83: 5939–5942

Tuddenham E G D, Schwaab R, Seehafer J et al 1994 Haemophilia A: database of nucleotide substitutions, deletions, insertions and rearrangements of the factor VIII gene, second edition. Nucleic Acids Res 22: 4851–4868

Wells D J, Goldspink G 1992 Age and sex influence expression of plasmid DNA directly injected into mouse skeletal muscle. FEBS Lett 306: 203–205

Wion K L, Kelly D, Summerfield J A et al 1985 Distribution of factor VIII mRNA and antigen in human liver and other tissues. Nature 317: 726–729

Wolff J A, Malone R W, Williams P et al 1990 Direct gene transfer into mouse muscle in vivo. Science 247: 1465–1468

Wu G Y, Wilson J M, Shalaby F et al 1991 Receptor mediated gene delivery in vivo. Partial correction of genetic analbuminemia in Nagase rats. J Biol Chem 266: 14338–14342

Yao S-N, Kurachi K 1992 Expression of human factor IX in mice after injection of genetically modified myoblasts. Proc Natl Acad Sci USA 89: 3357–3361

Yao S-N, Kurachi K 1993 Implanted myoblasts not only fuse with myofibers but also survive as muscle precursor cells. J Cell Sci 105: 957–963

Yao S-N, Smith K J, Kurachi K 1994 Primary myoblast-mediated gene transfer: persistent expression of human factor IX in mice. Gene Ther 1: 99–107

Zabner J, Couture L A, Gregory R J et al 1993 Adenovirus-mediated gene transfer transiently corrects the chloride transport defect in nasal epithelia of patients with cystic fibrosis. Cell 75: 207–216

Zatloukal K, Caten M, Berger M et al 1994 In vivo production of human factor VIII in mice after intrasplenic implantation of primary fibroblasts transfected by receptor-mediated, adenovirus-augmented gene delivery. Proc Natl Acad Sci USA 91: 5148–5152

Zenke M, Steinlein P, Wagner E et al 1990 Receptor mediated endocytosis of transferrin–polycation conjugates: an efficient way to introduce DNA into haematopoietic cells. Proc Natl Acad Sci USA 87: 3655–3659

Index

Abetalipoproteinemia, hereditary, 11
ABO blood groups, 78, 210
Abortion, recurrent spontaneous (RSA),
    22, 23, 26
Activated partial thromboplastin time
    (APTT), 3, 103
Activated protein C (APC), 50
    antiphospholipid antibodies and, 25
    resistance, 24, 26, 49, 55–60
        investigations/treatment, 62–63
        key points, 63
        molecular mechanisms, 56–58
        population frequencies, 56–57
        and protein C deficiency, 51, 60–61
        and protein S deficiency, 52, 60–61
        test, 55, 57–58, 62
        venous thromboembolism risk, 49,
            55, 58–60, 73
        see also Factor V, Arg506Gln mutation
Activated prothrombin complex
    concentrate (FEIBA), 237, 243
Adeno-associated virus (AAV), 263, 265
Adenoviral vectors, 263, 264–265
    in haemophilia, 269, 271
Alcohol consumption, 168
α_2-antiplasmin, 163, 164
α_2-macroglobulin, 165
Aminocaproic acid, 227
Anaesthesia, fibrinolytic effects, 165–166
Ancrod, 75, 85
Angina
    thromboprophylaxis in, 150
    unstable
        antithrombins in, 42–43, 189–190
        aspirin/anticoagulant therapy,
            150, 151
        aspirin therapy, 39
        platelet activation, 38
Angiography, pulmonary, 100
Angiotensin converting enzyme (ACE)
    inhibitors, 165
Animal models, haemophilia, 267, 272
Anticardiolipin antibodies (ACA), 21–22,
    23

pathophysiology, 24–25
Anticoagulants
    in pregnancy, 103–106
    see also Heparin; Warfarin
'Anticonvertin', 5
Anti-factor VIII antibodies/inhibitors,
    237–238, 242–244
    concentrates for, 237–238
    management, 243–244
    tolerizing regimens, 243–244
Anti-factor IX antibodies, 244
Antifibrinolytic agents, in von Willebrand
    disease, 226–227
Antiphospholipid antibody (APA)
    syndrome, 19–27, 88
    primary, 22–23, 88
    alloimmune, 20
    antigenic targets, 19–22
    autoimmune, 20
    classification, 20
    clinical features, 22–23
    key points, 27
    pathophysiological mechanisms, 23–25
    treatment, 26
Antiplatelet agents, 74, 185–188
    in atherosclerosis/arterial thrombosis,
        39–42
    in von Willebrand disease, 224
    see also Aspirin
Antiplatelet Trialists Collaboration, 77–78
Antithrombin III, 5
    deficiency, 49, 62, 86–87
Antithrombins, 42–43, 187, 188–191
Antithrombotic agents, new, 183–195
APC, see Activated protein C
Apolipoprotein A-II, 134
Aprotinin, 167
Arterial bypass graft surgery, peripheral,
    73, 79, 150
Arterial disease, 73, 89
    peripheral, 73, 81, 171
Arterial thrombosis
    altered haemostasis and, 35–37
    anaesthesia and, 165–166

in antiphospholipid antibody (APA)
  syndrome, 22, 23
antiplatelet prophylaxis/therapy, 39–42
antithrombins in, 42–43
APC resistance and, 60, 88
fibrinolysis and, 174
haemostatic risk factors, 72–73, 77, 79,
  91
pathogenesis, 34–35
plasma fibrinogen and, 73, 74, 75, 76,
  80–84
platelets in, 37–39, 43, 184–185
warfarin in prevention, 142–151
see also Ischaemic heart disease; Stroke
Aspirin, 141, 185
antiplatelet effects, 39, 40–41, 43, 77
in atherosclerosis, 39–41, 43
in atrial fibrillation, 74, 143, 146, 147
combined with warfarin, 150–151
fibrinolysis and, 167
in myocardial ischaemia prevention,
  148–149, 150–151
in pregnancy, 26, 106, 167
in prosthetic heart valves, 148
Atheroma, 33
Atherosclerosis, 33–43
altered haemostasis in, 35–37
antiplatelet prophylaxis/therapy, 39–42
antithrombins in, 42–43
pathogenesis, 34–35
plasma D-dimer and, 36, 89
plasma fibrinogen in, 35–36, 84
platelet activation in, 37–39
types of lesions, 33–34
see also Ischaemic heart disease
Atrial fibrillation (AF), 89
antithrombotic prophylaxis, 74
warfarin therapy, 74, 142–148
  bleeding complications, 145–147
  recommendations, 147–148

β₂-glycoprotein I (β₂GPI), 21, 22
Bleeding
c7E3 monoclonal antibody-associated,
  186
hirudin-associated, 42, 189, 190, 191
LMW heparin-associated, 193
in von Willebrand disease, 206–207,
  224
warfarin-associated, 145–147, 150–151,
  153
Bleeding time
in treated vWD, 228–229
in von Willebrand disease, 208, 210,
  222, 223
Blood groups, 78, 211
Budd–Chiari syndrome, 59

C4b-binding protein (C4BP), 52–54

C7E3 monoclonal antibody, 41–42,
  185–186
Caerphilly and Speedwell Studies, 75, 77,
  78, 79
Calf-vein thrombosis
in pregnancy, 98
warfarin therapy, 153
Cancer, fibrinolysis in, 172–173
Cardiolipin, 20
Cardiopulmonary bypass, 167
Cardiovascular disease, fibrinolysis and,
  174
CD4 counts, in haemophilia, 251–252
Central venous catheters
in haemophilia, 240–241
thrombosis prevention, 142, 152
Chest radiography, plain, 100
Cholesterol, serum, 72, 125
Chylomicrons, 127
Claudication, intermittent, 73, 171
Clopidogrel, 187
Clot lysis times, 89–90, 161
Coagulation
cascade/waterfall hypothesis, 2–3, 14
classic theory, 1
contact system, 2, 130–131
extrinsic pathway, 2, 3
factor VIIa–TF pathway, 3, 4–5
intrinsic pathway, 2, 3
revised hypothesis, 12–14
Collagen, vWF binding, 203
Collagenases, 36–37
Contact system of coagulation, 2,
  130–131
Contraceptive pill, oral, 59–60, 73, 88,
  227
Coronary angioplasty, percutaneous
  transluminal, 186, 189
Coronary artery bypass surgery, 150
Coronary heart disease, see Ischaemic
  heart disease
Cryoprecipitate
in haemophilia, 242, 251
in von Willebrand disease, 227, 229

D-dimer, plasma
in atherosclerosis, 36, 89
predicting thrombosis risk, 74, 88–89
in pulmonary embolism (PE), 106
Deep vein thrombosis
antiphospholipid-protein antibodies
  and, 24
in APC resistance, 59
haematological risk factors, 73
low molecular weight heparin
  (LMWH), 192–193
in pregnancy, 97
  clinical suspicion, 98
  diagnosis, 98–100

pathophysiology, 97–98
warfarin therapy, 153–154
11-Dehydro-thromboxane B₂, 38, 39
Dermatan sulphate, 193–194
Desmopressin
  in haemophilia A, 225
  side-effects, 85–86, 226
  in von Willebrand disease, 224–226, 229,
    230
Diabetes mellitus
  insulin-dependent, fibrinolytic activity,
    171
  non-insulin-dependent (NIDDM)
    fibrinolytic activity, 171
    PAI-1 polymorphisms, 166, 171
Dicoumarol, 141
Diet
  coronary heart disease and, 125
  fibrinolysis and, 168–169
  plasma factor VIIa and, 119, 128–129,
    130, 131–133
2,3-Dinor-6-keto-prostaglandin F₁ₐ, 38
2,3-Dinor-thromboxane B₂, 38, 39
Direct mutation detection (DMD),
    213–215
Disseminated intravascular coagulation
    (DIC), 195
DNA
  direct injection, 263, 265–266
  ligand conjugates, 263, 265

Embolism
  pulmonary, see Pulmonary embolism
  systemic, prevention, 142–148
Endothelial cells
  in atherosclerosis, 34, 37
  factor VIII gene transfer, 266
  markers of thrombosis risk, 78–79
  platelets and, 40–41
  TFPI production, 10, 11
  vWF synthesis, 201, 204
Erythrocyte sedimentation rate (ESR),
    75
European Atrial Fibrillation Trial (EFAT)
    study, 143, 145, 146
Exercise
  fibrinolysis and, 164, 169
  platelet activation and, 40–41

Factor V, 50
  activated (Va), 50
    antibodies, 25
  Arg506Gln mutation (FVa:Q⁵⁰⁶; factor
    V Leiden), 49, 56–58, 87–88
    heterozygotes, 57, 58–60, 62
    homozygotes, 57, 58–59, 62
    with other genetic defects, 60–61
    PCR analysis, 62
    population frequencies, 56–57

see also Activated protein C (APC),
    resistance
Factor VII, 2, 4, 111–120
  activated, see Factor VIIa
  activation in absence of TF, 130–131
  amidolytic assay (VII:Am), 114–115
  antigen (VII:Ag), 114, 127
    dietary fat and, 128–129, 130,
      131–132
    plasma triglycerides and, 127, 128
  coagulant activity (VII:C), 111
    assays, 115
    clinical significance, 117, 118–119
    dietary fat and, 131–132
    ischaemic heart disease and, 85, 117,
      118, 126
    phospholipase C sensitivity, 114
    plasma triglycerides and, 127–128,
      129
  deficiency, 3
  dietary fat and, 119, 128–129, 130,
    131–133
  plasma, 126–127
    assay methods, 114–115, 126–127
    in atherosclerosis, 35
    forms in, 113–114
    significance, 117–118
    warfarin therapy and, 114
  zymogen, 4–5, 112, 113–114, 126
Factor VIIa, 4–5, 111–120
  plasma, 111, 112, 113–114, 126
    assay methods, 114–115, 126–127
    clinical perspectives, 118–119
    dietary fat and, 119, 128–129, 130,
      131–133
    half-life, 112
    key points, 119–120
    significance, 117–118
    sTF-based assay, 116–117, 119, 127
  recombinant (VIIa), 237–238
  standard concentrate, 116
Factor VIIa–tissue factor (TF) complex,
    3, 4–5, 111–113, 126–127, 183
  inhibition by TFPI, 7, 8, 9, 133–134
  in revised hypothesis of coagulation, 12,
    13, 14
  therapeutic inhibition, 194–195
  in von Willebrand disease, 223
Factor VIII, 2, 203
  antibodies/inhibitors, see Anti-factor
    VIII antibodies/inhibitors
  coagulant activity (VIII:C), 85–86
    arterial thrombosis and, 78, 79,
      85–86
    venous thrombosis and, 79, 86
  concentrates, see Factor VIII(–vWF)
    concentrates
  gene, 261–262
  gene transfer studies, 266, 267

plasma, in von Willebrand disease, 210,
    222, 224
post-translational modification, 266
recombinant (rVIII), 261
    in haemophilia A, 236–237
    in von Willebrand disease, 230
vWF binding activity, 209–210
Factor VIII(–vWF) concentrates
continuous infusion, 241
in haemophilia prophylaxis, 240–241
in haemophilia treatment, 235–236
high-purity, 227–228, 235–236
in HIV positive patients, 251–253
immunogenicity, 242–243
intermediate-purity, 227–228, 242
in patients with anti-factor VIII
    antibodies, 243
plasma-derived (pd), 235–236
porcine (Hyate C), 237, 241, 243
very-high-purity, 227
viral inactivation methods, 245, 248
viral safety, 244–248
viruses transmitted by, 249–253
in von Willebrand disease, 227–229,
    230, 236
Factor IX, 2, 3
antibodies, 244
concentrate
    continuous infusion, 241
    prophylactic use, 240–241
    therapeutic use, 239–240
    viral inactivation methods, 245, 248
    viral safety, 244–248
    viruses transmitted by, 249–253
gene, 261–262
gene transfer studies, 268–272
post-translational modification, 266
recombinant, 261
Factor X, 2
Factor Xa, 4–5
inhibition by TFPI, 5–6, 7–8, 9, 12
Factor XI, 2
deficiency, 3, 12–13
in revised hypothesis of coagulation,
    12–14
Factor XII, 2
contact activation, 2, 130–131
deficiency, 3, 86
Fat, dietary
coronary heart disease and, 125
fibrinolysis and, 168–169
plasma factor VII/VIIa and, 119,
    128–129, 130, 131–133
Fatty acids see Polyunsaturated fatty acids;
    Saturated fatty acids
Fatty streaks, 33, 34
FEIBA (activated prothrombin complex
    concentrate), 237, 243
Fibrates, 84

Fibre, dietary, 132, 169
Fibrin, 161–162
in atherosclerosis, 36
formation, 183
sealant (glue), 238
Fibrinogen, 161–162
Aα chain, 162
Bβ chain polymorphism, 83–84
plasma
    agents lowering, 84
    assays, 82–83
    in atherosclerosis, 35–36, 84
    predicting thrombosis risk, 73, 74,
        75, 76, 80–85
    serum lipids and, 134
    smoking and, 71–72, 81–82
receptor inhibitors, 41–42, 185–187
Fibrin(ogen) degradation products (FgDP
    & FbDP), 88–89, 161–162
urinary, 173
see also D-dimer, plasma
Fibrinolysis, 161–175
biological regulation, 167–169
in cancer, 172–173
cardiovascular disease and, 174
in diabetes mellitus, 170–171
exercise and, 164, 169
genetic aspects, 166
inflammation and, 170
insulin resistance and, 170–171
key points, 174–175
lifestyle factors and, 168–169
platelets and, 166–167
in renal disease, 173
in skin disease, 173–174
thrombosis risk and, 89–90
Fibrinopeptide A
plasma, 35, 36, 239
urinary, 173
Fibroatheroma, 33
Fibroblasts
factor VIII gene transfer, 266, 267
factor IX gene transfer, 268–269
Fish oils, 133, 134, 168–169
Foam cells, TF expression, 4, 33, 36
Framingham study, 81

Gene therapy
approach, 261–262
gene delivery systems, 262–266
in haemophilia, 261–272
    future directions, 272
    studies to date, 266, 267–272
    target tissues/choice of transfer
        strategy, 266–267
Glomerulonephritis, 173
Glycosaminoglycans, 191–194, 195
see also Heparin
Growth hormone deficiency, 171

Haematocrit, 75
Haematopoietic tissue, factor VIII gene
    transfer, 266, 267
Haemodialysis, chronic, 193
Haemodilution, 75
Haemolytic uraemic syndrome, 170
Haemophilia
  Haemophilia A
    anti-factor VIII antibodies, 237–238,
      242–244
    desmopressin therapy, 225
    gene therapy, 266, 267
    ischaemic heart disease risk, 85
    therapeutic products, 235–238
    vs. type 2N von Willebrand disease,
      210, 224
    animal models, 267, 272
  Haemophilia B
    anti-factor IX antibodies, 244
    gene therapy, 266–267, 268–272
    therapeutic products, 238–240
  gene therapy, 261–272
  hepatitis C infection, 249–250
  HIV infection in, 235, 249, 251–253
  mechanism of bleeding, 1, 12
  plasma factor VIIa, 116
  prophylactic therapy, 240–241
  treatment, 235–253
  viral safety of concentrates, 244–248
Haemostasis, 183–184
  vWF in, 203
  see also Coagulation
Haemostatic risk factors for thrombosis,
    see Risk factors for thrombosis,
    haemostatic
Heart valves, prosthetic, see Prosthetic
    heart valves
Heparan sulphate, 194
Heparin, 191–193
  arterial thrombosis prevention, 41, 42,
    150
  low-affinity (LAH), 194
  low-molecular-weight (LMWH),
    191–193
    in pregnancy, 105, 106–107
  in pregnancy, 26, 103, 104–106
  TFPI and, 8, 10–11
  unfractionated (UFH), 191–193
Hepatitis A virus (HAV), 245–246
Hepatitis B virus (HBV), 245, 246
Hepatitis C virus (HCV)
  in factor concentrates, 245, 246
  infection in haemophilia, 249–250, 252
Hepatitis D virus (HDV), 245, 246
Hepatitis G virus (HGV), 245
Hepatocellular carcinoma, 250
Hepatocytes, factor IX gene transfer, 269,
    271–272
High-density lipoprotein (HDL)

TF expression and, 134
TFPI binding, 5, 9
Hirudin, 187, 188–191
  in ischaemic heart disease (IHD), 42,
    189–190
  polyethylene glycol-conjugated (PEG-
    hirudin), 188
  recombinant, 188
Hirulog, 42–43, 188, 190, 191
Histidine-rich glycoprotein (HRG), 165
HIV
  infection, in haemophilia, 235, 249,
    251–253
  transmission in factor concentrates,
    245, 247
Hormone replacement therapy (HRT),
    84
Human immunodeficiency virus, see HIV
Hyate C (porcine factor VIII), 237, 241,
    243
Hypertension, 72
  in atrial fibrillation, 147
  primary pulmonary, 154–155

Immune abnormalities, in haemophilia,
    251–252
Immunoglobulin, intravenous, 230
Impedance plethysmography (IPG), 99,
    103, 105
Inferior vena cava filters, 104
Inflammation, and fibrinolysis, 170
Insulin resistance
  fibrinolysis and, 90, 170–171
  syndrome, 71, 170–171
Integrelin, 186, 187
Interferon-α, in haemophilia, 242, 250
International normalized ratio (INR),
    103, 142
Intracoronary stents, 150
Intracranial bleeding
  hirudin-associated, 190
  warfarin-associated, 145–146, 147
Ischaemic heart disease (IHD)
  altered haemostasis in, 35–36
  antiphospholipid-protein antibodies
    and, 24
  dietary fat and, 125
  haemostatic risk factors, 71–72, 75–85,
    87, 89–91
  hirudin in, 42, 189–190
  new antiplatelet therapies, 41–42, 186
  PAI-1 polymorphisms and, 166
  plasma factor VII/VIIa and, 85,
    117–118, 126
  platelet activation in, 38, 39
  primary prevention, 149, 151
  see also Angina; Myocardial infarction

Jejuno-ileal bypass surgery, 169

Kaposi's sarcoma, 251
Keratinocytes, factor IX gene transfer, 269, 270
6-Keto-prostaglandin $F_{1\alpha}$, 40
High molecular weight kininogen, 2

Left ventricular dysfunction, 148
Lifestyle, fibrinolysis and, 168–169
Linkage analysis, von Willebrand factor gene, 215
Lipids, serum, 125–135
  key points, 134–135
  plasma factor VIIa and, 117, 119, 128–131
  plasma fibrinogen and, 134
  TF expression and, 134
  see also Triglycerides, plasma
Lipofection, 263
Lipoprotein-lipase deficiency, familial, 129, 130–131
Lipoproteins
  factor VII:C association, 127, 129
  lipolysis, in factor VII activation, 131
  TF expression and, 134
  TFPI binding, 5, 6, 9
Liver
  disease, in haemophilia, 249–250
  TFPI production, 10
Low-density lipoprotein (LDL), TFPI binding, 5, 9
Low-density lipoprotein (LDL) receptor related protein (LRP), 11
Lupus anticoagulant (LA), 20, 21, 24–25, 88
Lupus erythematosus, systemic (SLE), 20, 22, 24–25
LY 53857, 187
Lymphoma, non-Hodgkin's, 251

MCI-9042, 187
Megakaryocytes, vWF synthesis, 201, 203, 204
Metastasis, tumour, 172
Mitral stenosis, rheumatic, 142, 148
MK-383, 186
Moloney murine leukaemia virus (MoMLV), 268
Monocytes, TF expression, 4, 36, 134
Murine leukaemia viruses (MLV), 263
Myoblasts
  factor VIII gene transfer, 266, 267
  factor IX gene transfer, 269, 270–271
Myocardial infarction, 126
  antithrombin therapy, 189, 190
  APC resistance and, 60
  embolism prevention after, 148
  evolving, 41
  non-Q-wave, 151
  PAI-1 polymorphisms and, 166

plasma factor VIIa and, 118
platelet activation and, 38, 39
primary prevention, 39, 40, 149, 151
secondary prevention, 39–40, 142, 149–150
Myocardial ischaemia, prevention, 148–151

N-3 fatty acid ethyl ester, 134
N-3 polyunsaturated fatty acids (fish oils), 133, 134, 168–169
Northwick Park Heart Study (NPHS), 77, 78, 85, 115, 117–118, 126

Obesity, 71, 169
Oestrogens
  plasma fibrinogen and, 84
  in von Willebrand disease, 227
  ω-3 (n-3) polyunsaturated fatty acids (fish oils), 133, 134, 168–169
Oral anticoagulants, 141
  in antiphospholipid antibody syndrome, 26
  plasma factor VIIa levels and, 116
  in protein C deficiency, 51
  see also Warfarin
Oral contraceptive pill, 59–60, 73, 88, 227
Org 10172, 193

Parvoviruses, 245, 247, 248
Pentasaccharide, synthetic antithrombin-binding, 194
Peripheral arterial disease, 73, 81, 171
Peripheral artery bypass graft surgery, 73, 79, 150
Phospholipids, 19, 20
  binding proteins, 20–22
Plasma
  fresh frozen, 227
  viscosity, 75, 76
Plasmin, 162
  in atherosclerosis, 36–37
  inhibitors, 165–166
Plasmin–antiplasmin (PAP) complexes, glomerular, 173
Plasminogen
  activators, 162–165
  in atherosclerosis, 36
Plasminogen activator inhibitor 1 (PAI-1)
  anaesthesia and, 165–166
  in atherosclerosis, 36, 37, 174
  in cardiovascular disease, 174
  in diabetes mellitus, 171
  gene polymorphisms, 166, 171
  in inflammation, 170
  in insulin resistance, 170–171
  in leg ulcer patients, 174
  lifestyle factors affecting, 168–169

mutations, 166
  in platelets, 167
  predicting thrombosis risk, 74, 90
  renin–angiotensin system and, 165
Plasminogen activator inhibitor 2 (PAI-2),
    in cancer, 172–173
Platelet factor 4, 38
Platelet glycoprotein Ib, 203
Platelet glycoprotein IIb/IIIa
  inhibitors, 185–187
  monoclonal antibodies (c7E3), 41–42,
    185–186
  vWF binding, 203
Platelets
  activity tests, 77
  antiphospholipid-protein antibodies
    and, 23
  in arterial thrombosis, 37–39, 43,
    184–185
  concentrates, 229
  counts, 77
  fibrinolysis and, 166–167
  in haemostasis, 183, 184
  inhibitors, see Antiplatelet agents
  mean volume (MPV), 77
  receptor antagonists, 41–42, 43
  TFPI content, 10
  thrombosis risk and, 77–78
  in von Willebrand disease, 207
  vWF in, 203, 204
Plethysmography, impedance (IPG), 99,
    103, 105
Polycythaemia, 75
Polymerase chain reaction (PCR), 62,
    213, 215
Polyoma virus, pseudocapsid, 272
Polyunsaturated fatty acids, 130, 132, 133
  n-3 (fish oils), 133, 134, 168–169
Pregnancy
  antiphospholipid antibody syndrome,
    23, 26
  APC resistance and, 59, 73
  aspirin in, 26, 106, 167
  plasma factor VIIa levels, 116
  in valvular heart disease, 105–106
  venous thromboembolism in, 97–107
    diagnosis, 98–103
    future prospects, 106–107
    key points, 107
    pathophysiology, 97–98
    treatment, 103–104
    women with previous history,
      104–105
  von Willebrand disease therapy, 229
Prekallikrein, 2, 167
Preoperative haemostatic tests, 73
Prospective Cardiovascular Münster
    (PROCAM) study, 81, 85,
    117–118

Prostacyclin, 185
  in atherosclerosis, 37, 38, 43
Prosthetic heart valves
  aspirin/warfarin therapy, 150–151
  pregnancy and, 105–106
  warfarin therapy, 142, 148
Protease inhibitors, Kunitz-type, 6–7
Protein C
  activated, see Activated protein C
  anticoagulant pathway, 50
  antiphospholipid antibodies and, 25
  deficiency, 51, 60–61, 86–87
    heterozygous, 51
    homozygous, 50, 51
    treatment, 62
    type I, 51
    type II, 51
Protein S, 50, 52
  C4BP interaction, 52–54
  deficiency, 51–54, 60–61, 86–87
    treatment, 62
    type I, 52, 53, 54
    type II, 52
    type III, 52, 53, 54
  gene mutations, 54
  plasma free, 52, 53, 54
  plasma total, 52, 53
Prothrombin
  complex concentrates
    activated (FEIBA), 237, 243
    thromboembolic complications,
      238–239
  fragment 1+2, 35, 36, 239
  lupus anticoagulant and, 21
Prothrombin time, 2–3
Pro-urokinase (scuPA), 163, 164
  platelets and, 167
  prophylactic use, 163
  therapeutic use, 163
P-selectin, 37
Pulmonary angiography, 100
Pulmonary embolism (PE)
  antiphospholipid-protein antibodies
    and, 24
  in APC resistance, 59
  aspirin prophylaxis, 40
  low molecular weight heparin, 192
  in pregnancy, 97
    clinical suspicion, 100
    diagnosis, 100–103, 106
    warfarin therapy, 153
Pulmonary hypertension, primary,
    154–155

Recurrent spontaneous abortion, 22, 23,
    26
Renal disease, fibrinolysis in, 173
Retroviral vectors, 262–264
  in haemophilia, 267, 268, 269, 270

RGDS motif, 202, 203
Rheological variables, 72, 75
Rheumatoid arthritis, 170
Ridogrel, 42, 187
Risk factors for thrombosis, 24
  genetic, 49, 86–88
  haemostatic, 69–91
    biological issues, 70, 71–72
    clinical utility, 70, 72–74
    key points, 91
    predictive value of individual, 75–90
    statistical issues, 69–70
  see also specific factors
Ristocetin cofactor activity (RiCoF), 208,
    210, 222, 223
Ristocetin-induced platelet agglutination
    (RIPA) assay, 208, 222, 223
Ro-44, 186

Saturated fatty acids
  dietary intake, 125
    plasma factor VII and, 130, 132–133
  factor XII activation, 130–131
SC-54684A, 186–187
Scottish Heart Health Study, 80
scuPA, see Pro-urokinase
Serotonin receptor antagonists, 187
Shea butter diet, 133
Skin disease, fibrinolysis in, 173–174
Smoking, cigarette, 71–72, 81–82, 171
Smooth muscle cells, in atherosclerosis,
    34
SR 46349, 187
Stearic acid, 130–131, 133
Stents, intracoronary, 150
Streptokinase, 39
Stroke
  fibrinolytic activity and, 90
  hirudin-associated, 42, 190
  plasma fibrinogen and, 80, 81, 82
  platelet activation in, 38
  prevention, 39–40, 143
  see also Intracranial bleeding
Stroke Prevention in Atrial Fibrillation
    (SPAF) studies, 143, 145, 146–147
Stromelysin, 37
Surgery
  preoperative haemostatic tests, 73
  venous thromboprophylaxis, 152
Syndrome X (insulin resistance syn-
    drome), 71, 170–171
Syphilis, serological tests for (STS),
    20–21
Systemic lupus erythematosus (SLE), 20,
    22, 24–25

tcuPA, see Urokinase
Testosterone, plasma, 171
Thrombin

in atherosclerosis, 37–38
  generation, 183–184
  inhibitors, see Antithrombins
  pro- and anticoagulant effects, 50
  receptor inhibitors, 187–188
Thrombin–antithrombin III, plasma, 35,
    36, 239
Thrombocytopenia
  in antiphospholipid antibody syndrome,
    23
  heparin-induced, 193
  in von Willebrand disease, 229
Thromboembolism,
  see Venous thrombosis/
    thromboembolism
β-Thromboglobulin, plasma, 38, 78
Thrombolysis
  therapeutic, 39, 163
  see also Fibrinolysis
Thrombomodulin, 50
  gene defects, 54–55
Thrombophilia, familial, 49–63
  investigation/treatment, 62–63
  multiple genetic defects in, 60–62
  pregnancy and, 104
  see also Activated protein C (APC),
    resistance
Thrombophlebitis, superficial, 59
Thrombosis
  in antiphospholipid antibody (APA)
    syndrome, 22, 23–25, 88
  in APC resistance, 58–60, 87–88
  mechanism of, 183–185
  risk factors, see Risk factors for
    thrombosis
  see also Arterial thrombosis; Venous
    thrombosis/thromboembolism
Thromboxane A_2, 38, 40, 43
Thromboxane B_2, 40
Ticlopidine, 84, 185
Tissue factor, 1, 4, 111–113,
    133–134
  in atherosclerosis, 4, 33, 34, 36
  cells expressing, 4, 112
  function, 113
  serum lipids and, 133–134
  soluble truncated (sTF), 113
    in factor VIIa assay, 116–117, 119,
      127
  see also Factor VIIa–tissue factor
    complex
Tissue factor pathway inhibitor (TFPI),
    3, 5–14, 133–134
  antibodies (anti-TFPI-IgG), 12
  history, 5–6
  inhibitory properties, 7–8
  physiology, 9–11
  plasma, 9, 10–11
  recombinant, 9–10, 11, 195

in revised hypothesis of coagulation,
12–14
structure, 6–7
Tissue plasminogen activator (tPA), 162,
163–164
alcohol consumption and, 168
in atherosclerosis, 36, 37
cholinergic-mediated release, 168
gene polymorphisms, 166
knock-out mice, 164–165
platelet activation, 39
predicting thrombosis risk, 90
in renal disease, 173
tPA, see Tissue plasminogen activator
Tranexamic acid, 227
Triglycerides, plasma
factor VII and, 127–128, 129
PAI-1 and, 171
Tumour necrosis factor-α (TNF-α), 170
Tumours, fibrinolysis in, 172–173

Ultrasonography
in deep vein thrombosis, 99, 103, 105
in thrombolysis, 162
Universal heteroduplex generator (UHG),
213–215
uPA, see Urokinase-type plasminogen
activator
Urokinase (tcuPA), 163, 164
in atherosclerosis, 36, 37
in cancer, 172
receptor (uPAR), in cancer, 172, 173
in renal disease, 173
Urokinase-type plasminogen activator
(uPA), 162–163
knock-out mice, 164
single-chain (scuPA), see Pro-urokinase
total plasma antigen (uPA:Ag), 163
two-chain (tcuPA), see Urokinase

Valvular heart disease
pregnancy and, 105–106
warfarin therapy, 142, 148
Vasodilatation, plasmin-induced, 162
Venereal Disease Research Laboratory
(VDRL) test, 20–21
Venography, in pregnancy, 98–99, 100
Venous thrombosis/thromboembolism
(VTE)
in antiphospholipid antibody (APA)
syndrome, 22, 23, 24
in antithrombin III deficiency, 86–87
antithrombin therapy/prophylaxis,
190–191
APC resistance and, 49, 55, 58–60, 73,
87–88
aspirin prophylaxis, 40
fibrinolysis and, 174
fibrinolytic activity and, 90

genetic risk factors, 49, 86–88
haemostatic risk factors, 72, 73, 75, 91
low molecular weight heparin, 192–193
plasma factor VIII activity and, 79, 86
plasma fibrinogen and, 85
plasma vWF and, 79
platelets and, 78
in pregnancy, see Pregnancy, venous
thromboembolism in
in protein C deficiency, 51, 86–87
in protein S deficiency, 52, 86–87
prothrombin complex concentrates and,
238–239
warfarin in, 151–154
see also Deep vein thrombosis;
Pulmonary embolism
Venous ulcers, fibrinolysis in, 173–174
Very-low-density lipoproteins (VLDL)
factor VII:C association, 127
TFPI binding, 5, 9
Viruses
in factor VIII/IX concentrates, 244–248
inactivation methods, 245, 248
Viscosity, plasma, 75, 76
von Willebrand disease (vWD), 201,
204–216, 221–231
clinical diagnosis, 206–207
diagnosis and classification, 221–224
genetic diagnosis, 213–215
genetics, 211–213
inheritance, 211
key points, 216
nomenclature, 205–206
phenotypic diagnosis, 207–211,
222–224
platelet-type, 206
pseudo-, 206
treatment, 224–231, 236
general principles, 224
key points, 230–231
non-transfusion therapies, 224–227
patients with vWF antibodies,
229–230
in pregnancy/delivery, 229
transfusion therapy, 227–229
type 1, 205, 223
diagnosis, 208, 209, 211, 222
gene defects, 212
inheritance, 207, 211
treatment, 225, 226, 229
type 2, 205, 211, 212, 223–224
type 2A, 205, 207, 223
diagnosis, 208, 209, 222
gene defects, 212
treatment, 225, 226
type 2B, 205, 207, 209, 223
diagnosis, 208, 222
gene defects, 212
treatment, 225, 226, 229

type 2M, 205, 223
  diagnosis, 208, 222
  treatment, 225
type 2N, 205, 207, 223–224
  diagnosis, 208, 209–210, 222
  gene defects, 212
  treatment, 225, 226
type 3, 205, 224
  diagnosis, 208, 209, 222
  gene defects, 212
  inheritance, 211
  treatment, 225, 226, 229–230
  with vWF antibodies, 224, 225,
    229–230
von Willebrand factor (vWF), 201–204,
    221
  alloantibodies, 224, 225, 229–230
  antigen (vWF:Ag), 210, 222
  in atherosclerosis, 37
  biological activity, 203–204
  concentrates, see Factor VIII–vWF
    concentrates
  gene, see VWF gene
  plasma multimer profile, 208, 209, 222
  platelet multimer profile, 208–209, 222
  predicting thrombosis risk, 73, 74, 78,
    79
  protein biochemistry, 201–203
  ristocetin cofactor activity (RiCoF),
    208, 210, 222, 223
  ristocetin sensitivity (RIPA assay), 208,
    222, 223

very-high-purity concentrate, 227
von Willebrand syndrome, acquired, 205,
    206, 228, 230
V/Q lung scan, 100, 102
vWF, see von Willebrand factor
VWF gene, 204
  direct mutation detection, 213–215
  linkage analysis, 215
  mutations causing disease, 212–213

Warfarin, 141–156
  in arterial thrombosis prevention,
    142–151
  in atrial fibrillation, 74, 142–148
  combined with aspirin, 150–151
  INR recommendations, 142
  key points, 155–156
  in myocardial ischaemia prevention,
    142, 148–151
  plasma factor VII and, 114
  postpartum use, 103, 104
  in pregnancy, 105
  in primary pulmonary hypertension,
    154–155
  in prosthetic heart valves, 142, 148
  teratogenicity, 104, 105
  in venous thromboembolism, 151–154
    prevention, 142, 152
    treatment, 142, 152–154
  very-low-dose, 152
Weibel–Palade bodies, 203
White cell count, 75, 76